An Overview of the Human Services

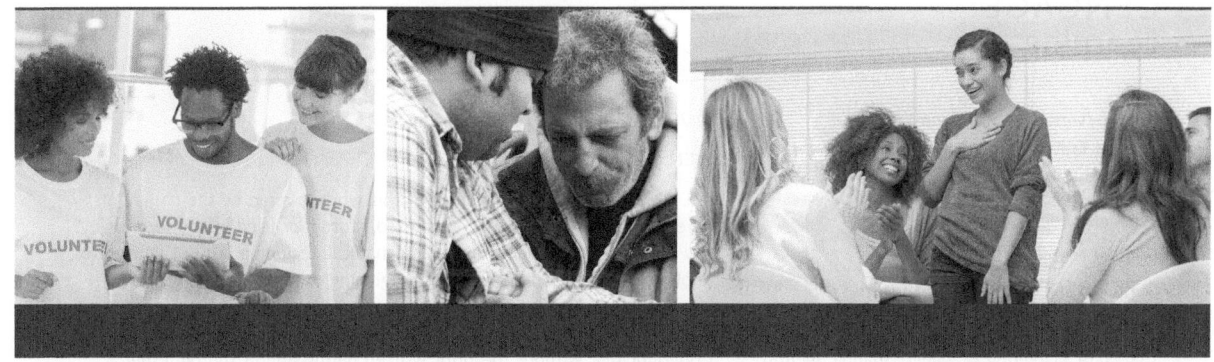

An Overview of the Human Services

SECOND EDITION

KRISTI KANEL
California State University, Fullerton

Contributing Author:
MELANIE HORN MALLERS,
California State University, Fullerton

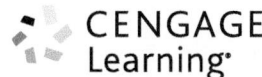

Australia • Brazil • Mexico • Singapore • United Kingdom • United States

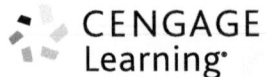

An Overview of the Human Services, Second Edition
Kristi Kanel and Melanie Horn Mallers

Product Director: Jon-David Hague

Product Manager: Julie Martinez

Content Developer: Wendy Langerud

Product Assistant: Kyra Kane

Associate Marketing Manager: Shanna Shelton

Art and Cover Direction, Production Management, and Composition: Lumina Datamatics, Inc.

Manufacturing Planner: Judy Inouye

Cover Image(s): Smiling patient standing and telling her problems: © wavebreakmedia/Shutterstock; Cheerful volunteers looking at a tablet pc: © wavebreakmedia/Shutterstock; Homeless Male Crying: © Kevin Russ/E+/Getty Images; Volunteers painting wall: © Hill Street Studios/ Eric Raptosh/Blend Images/Getty Images

© 2016, 2008 Cengage Learning

WCN: 01-100-101

ALL RIGHTS RESERVED. No part of this work covered by the copyright herein may be reproduced, transmitted, stored, or used in any form or by any means graphic, electronic, or mechanical, including but not limited to photocopying, recording, scanning, digitizing, taping, Web distribution, information networks, or information storage and retrieval systems, except as permitted under Section 107 or 108 of the 1976 United States Copyright Act, without the prior written permission of the publisher.

> For product information and technology assistance, contact us at
> **Cengage Learning Customer & Sales Support, 1-800-354-9706.**
> For permission to use material from this text or product,
> submit all requests online at **www.cengage.com/permissions**.
> Further permissions questions can be e-mailed to
> **permissionrequest@cengage.com**.

Library of Congress Control Number: 2014938124

ISBN: 978-1-285-46510-4

Cengage Learning
20 Channel Center Street
Boston, MA 02210
USA

Cengage Learning is a leading provider of customized learning solutions with office locations around the globe, including Singapore, the United Kingdom, Australia, Mexico, Brazil, and Japan. Locate your local office at **www.cengage.com/global**.

Cengage Learning products are represented in Canada by Nelson Education, Ltd.

To learn more about Cengage Learning Solutions, visit **www.cengage.com**.

Purchase any of our products at your local college store or at our preferred online store **www.cengagebrain.com**.

Printed in the United States of America
Print Number: 02   Print Year: 2019

This is dedicated to my mother, Joyce

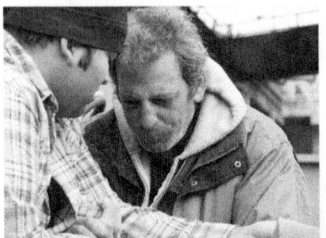
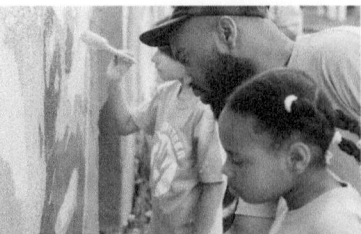
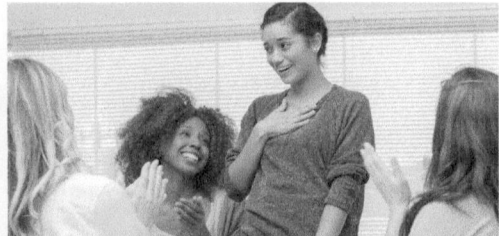

Preface

GENERAL OVERVIEW OF THE BOOK

Human Services has evolved tremendously as a distinct discipline over the past 40 years. It was first studied in colleges and universities in response to societal changes in the 1960s and 1970s (changes that had already been evolving over the previous century) regarding the value of helping the disadvantaged, and it succeeded in creating an increased willingness on the part of both individuals and the government to become involved in providing services for those in need.

This book has been written for students who are just beginning to study the field of human services. It is intended to be an easy-to-read, practical guide to the field; it provides students with a nuts-and-bolts overview of the myriad facets that make up the field; and it offers students a glimpse of what they can expect to experience as they continue their education and begin working in the field.

Because the field of human services encompasses so many career opportunities, skills, client populations, and job duties, this book was written not only to introduce students to the field but also to help them find their place in the field by guiding them toward a specific area of human services that might interest them. By the end of the book, students should have a clearer idea what they want to do, whom they want to help, and where they want to work.

Having taught introduction to human services for over 25 years and having consistently heard student complaints about not feeling connected to the often dry and impersonal textbooks used, Dr. Kanel felt compelled to write a textbook that would inspire a sense of involvement with the subject matter. When Dr. Horn Mallers joined the Human Services Department and began teaching Introduction to Human Services, she was inspired to make revisions and additions to the first edition of this textbook. She also brings a vital background in issues related to gerontology and family studies. *An Overview of the Human Services*, second edition, avoids pure lecture by providing numerous opportunities for students to engage in role-plays and other in-class activities. We believe that students who are genuinely interested in the course and are actively engaged with the material will gain more from the course than they would if they feel distanced from the text, teacher, and other students. This textbook challenges students to become active learners via self-reflection, case studies, real-world scenarios, applied activities, and inventories. All of these applied and experiential activities bring theoretical concepts to life for students and help prepare them to serve in agency settings as beginning interns and volunteers.

CHAPTER-BY-CHAPTER WALK THROUGH

Organized into 13 chapters, *An Overview of the Human Services* proceeds in a cumulative manner from basic concepts and history to specific aspects of the human services field and finally to in-practice considerations such as delivery to clients, stress management, and program evaluation and development. Although students interact with and internalize the material throughout the book, the "Human Services Career Inventory" Appendix asks students to give themselves a final self-assessment of their aptitude toward and interests within the field.

Chapter 1: Human Services: Foundational Concepts and Historical Background

This chapter provides a succinct definition of the term *human services*, offers an overview of the different types of human services workers, defines the key terms used in the field, outlines the various places human services workers are employed, and explores the reasons why people should or should not choose a career in the human services. In addition, the chapter provides several case examples to help students begin to understand the practical nature of the book. In order to show students the evolution of human services to its present-day incarnation, this historical overview section discusses how early societies dealt with behaviors that were seen as deviant and how eventually human compassion came to take the place of punishment. The historical overview begins as far back as early humans and traces the evolution of human services through ancient civilizations, the early Christian era, the Dark Ages, the Age of Reason, the 19th century, the 20th century, and finally the 21st century. Throughout the chapter, students are shown how the values of the time greatly influence who receives help and how mental health services, social welfare, correctional services, and educational services have evolved over time.

Chapter 2: Modern-Day Human Services: Policies and Programs, Interventions, and Demographic Considerations

This chapter discusses modern-day human services with expansive information on 21st-century programs, services, and policies related to mental health, social welfare, correctional, and educational systems. This includes an overview of the role of nonprofits within these systems. Also discussed are current interventions used in the field, including those in the primary, secondary, and tertiary levels. The roles of current demographic trends and sociocultural influences on multiethnic human services delivery are discussed.

Chapter 3: Ethical and Multicultural Issues in the Human Services

Because ethics are crucial in the field of human services, this chapter not only defines ethics but also presents a number of ethical dilemmas for students to navigate. The chapter begins with a general definition of ethics and a discussion of the importance of ethics in the human services field. It then presents specific ethical issues such as confidentiality, dual relationships, countertransference, and values clarification, which are illustrated with many examples of appropriate and inappropriate ethical behaviors. A discussion about continuing education emphasizes the importance of ongoing training to maintain ethical standards throughout one's human services career. Multicultural issues are discussed in the context of ethical practice.

Chapter 4: Human Services Workers

Expanding upon a list first proposed by the Southern Regional Education Board, this chapter begins with definitions and examples of typical functions and roles that human services workers play and then outlines the educational levels of human services workers and the four types of human services agencies. Finally, the chapter ties together these sections by listing career options within each type of agency based on educational level. Questions in the Critical Thinking/Self-Reflection box and a table of actual job postings help students to begin the process of deciding in what capacity they might want to work and what education level they will need to achieve their goals.

Chapter 5: Basic Counseling Skills, Personal Characteristics of Human Services Workers, and Theoretical Approaches in Counseling

The purpose of this chapter is to introduce students to basic helping skills, what personal qualities can often lead to successful helping, and how to achieve assertive communication skills. The chapter begins with an outline of the general goals of effective communication, then defines and provides examples of specific effective communication skills, and finally presents examples of personal characteristics that human services workers should have. A table summarizing the various effective communication skills and personal characteristics is provided along with numerous real-world scenarios. The Critical Thinking/Self-Reflection boxes help students to internalize the material.

The second part of this chapter focuses on psychological models, outlining the psychological theories of psychoanalysis, existential-humanist therapies, behaviorism, and cognitive therapies and explains the implications of each theory in terms of human services delivery. A table summarizing the key elements of all the psychological models of causality is provided, and students are asked to reflect upon and internalize the material throughout the chapter. Evidence-based practice is introduced as well.

Chapter 6: Crisis Intervention, Suicide Prevention, PTSD, Community Disasters and Trauma Response, and Military Trauma

This chapter introduces the reader to the function and process of crisis intervention, including a detailed discussion on how to conduct a suicide assessment and offer suicide prevention. Trauma response as related to community disasters and PTSD is also explored. Finally, the reader will be introduced to various issues facing veterans, especially in relation to PTSD and military trauma.

Chapter 7: Humans Services Populations

This chapter discusses the needs and issues of client populations that utilize human services, specifically children, adolescents, and the aged, including updated information on prevalence, causality models, and approaches to delivery.

Chapter 8: Mental Illness, Poverty, Disabilities, Crime/Violence, and Substance Abuse

This chapter provides a broad overview of mental illness, poverty, disabilities, crime/violence, and substance abuse, including prevalence rates, needs and issues, causal and risk factors, as well as human services delivery and prevention approaches.

Chapter 9: Interpersonal Partner Abuse, Sexual Assault, HIV/AIDS, and LGBT Issues

This chapter provides detailed information about the populations affected by interpersonal partner abuse, sexual assault, HIV/AIDS, and LGBT issues. The specific issues, needs, and interventions for these populations are discussed.

Chapter 10: Stress Management

Because stress is a major part of the human services field, this chapter focuses on this important topic. The chapter begins with brief definitions of stress and burnout. Thereafter, the chapter focuses on the symptoms and impacts of stress and burnout and how to reduce and manage stress and burnout by using cognitive reframing, maintaining a healthy lifestyle, improving interpersonal communication, learning how to be assertive, and maintaining a sense of humor. Numerous examples throughout the chapter illustrate these methods of stress management.

Chapter 11: Case Management

This chapter defines case management duties and the philosophy behind it. The reader will be introduced to the duties of case managers, such as assessment, case notes, progress notes, and reports.

Chapter 12: Macro-Level Practice

This chapter discuses macro-level human services practice, with emphasis on conducting needs assessments and evaluations, writing grants and proposals, and involving in efforts critical to success in the field of human services, including social action, advocacy, and lobbying.

Chapter 13: Leadership and Organizational Structure

This chapter focuses on different types of leadership styles found in nonprofit human services agencies and in public human services agencies. Additionally, the structures and norms for each type of agency are explored.

SPECIAL FEATURES

As mentioned earlier, the primary goal of this book is to inspire in students a sense of personal involvement with the subject of human services. To that end, this edition contains a number of pedagogical features to help students personalize the chapter material via self-reflection (e.g., Critical Thinking/Self Reflection Corner and Suggested Applied Activities) and to actualize the material by seeing abstract concepts played out in a real-world context (e.g., True Stories From Human Services Workers and Case Presentation and Exit Quiz). Other special features, such as Chapter Review Questions and a chapter Glossary of Terms, are provided to review and reinforce concepts presented in the chapters.

- **Critical Thinking/Self Reflection Corner:** Developing self-awareness is an important challenge for those entering the helping professions. As a result, each chapter contains Critical Thinking/Self-Reflection Corner boxes with questions aimed to catalyze students to explore their own values as well as emotional and cognitive reactions to the topics discussed in the chapters. These boxes appear throughout each chapter, in close proximity to the topics to which they relate, and they can be answered outside of class as students read the chapters, can be opened up to small-group discussions in class, or both.

- **True Stories From Human Services Workers:** These boxed items feature real-life experiences of human services workers in the field. Placed in close proximity to the topics to which they relate, the boxes are intended to help students visualize the topics under consideration in a real-world context.

- **Suggested Applied Activities:** Following each chapter's summary, these activities bring chapter concepts to life and help students to personalize what they have read by asking them to reflect on their own lives, role play with other students, make observations outside of class, interview people, visit human services agencies, and so on.

- **Chapter Review Questions:** At the end of each chapter, students are presented with several open-ended, short essay questions related to key points from the chapter. These questions may be used as course exam questions or by students to help clarify which chapter points they understand and which they may need to revisit.
- **Glossary of Terms:** These are key terms that have been boldfaced within each chapter and are listed in alphabetical order at the end of corresponding chapters, along with succinct definitions. Students should review these pivotal terms prior to moving on to subsequent chapters in which knowledge of these terms will be assumed. The terms may also be included on multiple-choice quizzes.
- **Case Presentation and Exit Quiz:** At the end of each chapter, a case presentation related to concepts covered in that particular chapter provides students with further opportunities to see chapter concepts played out in a real-world context. The 5 to 12 multiple-choice questions at the end of each case presentation relate directly to the case and reinforce chapter topics.
- **Appendix:** Human Services Career Inventory—this inventory consists of 15 questions designed to aid students in formulating their career goals. The questions help students narrow their career focus in terms of what types of agency they would like to work in, what types of clients they would like to deal with, what duties they want to perform, and what educational level they want to complete.

MAJOR REVISIONS

Chapter 1

Chapters 1 and 2 from the first edition are combined and made into one chapter. The chapter has been renamed as "Human Services: Foundational Concepts and Historical Background."

Chapter 2

This chapter is renamed as "Modern Day Human Services: Policies and Programs, Interventions, and Demographic Considerations." Information on government policies, harm reduction models, and demographic and cultural shifts on human services population (including aging, immigration, and ethnic/racial status) has been added. More current, relevant examples of delivery, as well as a discussion on the current health care system, are provided. Suggested Applied Activities emphasize personal reflection of biases toward others and competencies to work with diverse populations.

Chapter 3

This is now the chapter on ethics, which was Chapter 11 of the previous edition. Multicultural issues are discussed into this chapter as a component of ethical practice. The standards and ethical practices outlined by NOSE are emphasized.

Chapter 4

This chapter on human services workers is Chapter 3 of the previous edition. Salary ranges are updated to reflect current economic trends.

Chapter 5

This chapter now combines Chapter 4 with the second half of Chapter 5 of the previous edition. The discussion on the biological and medical model and Gestalt therapy have been removed from the textbook altogether. Evidence-based practice is explored in this chapter.

Chapter 6

This is newly named "Crisis Intervention, Suicide Prevention, PTSD, Community Disasters and Trauma Response, and Military Trauma" and includes new information on crisis intervention, suicide prevention, PTSD, military issues, and community disaster and trauma response.

Chapters 7 through 9 of this edition include a discussion of a variety of client populations. The intervention strategies at all levels are embedded in the chapter related to the topic.

Chapter 7

This chapter includes current, updated prevalence data; added information in the section on children about blended and bi-nuclear families and the impact of divorce and custody on children; and more adolescent-related issues, such as gang membership and self-mutilation. Heavier focus is given to aging-related issues, including health conditions, functional ability, elder abuse, alcohol abuse, poverty, and Alzheimer's disease.

Chapter 8

This chapter includes updated prevalence data and examples of current, innovative interventions. A more comprehensive overview of risk factors and causal models, particularly for addiction, has been added.

Chapter 9

The current, updated prevalence data in this chapter includes a discussion on military sexual trauma alongside sexual assault. LGBT issues are discussed here rather than in a chapter on cultural diversity.

Chapter 10

A section on harm reduction is included here.

Chapter 11

This chapter has been renamed "Case Management." It explores the definition of case management and the forms, intakes, notes, and reports from Chapter 8 of the previous edition are now included in this chapter.

Chapter 12

More emphasis on the development of government policy, funding announcements, reasons for developing grant writing skills, and types of evaluations have been included in this chapter. An additional section on advocacy and policy practice has been added, and examples of current legislation have been included.

Chapter 13

This is a new chapter titled "Leadership and Organizational Structure" includes material from Chapter 12 of the first edition about agency leadership styles and norms of agencies. It discusses nonprofit and public-type agency practices.

INSTRUCTOR'S RESOURCES

The Instructor's Resources for *An Overview of the Human Services*, 2nd edition, provides teaching suggestions, numerous multiple choice and true/false exam questions and answers, suggested answers to the student text's chapter review questions, and a sample course outline.

ONLINE TEST BANK

The Online Test Bank is provided for assessment support, and the updated test bank includes true/false, multiple choice, matching, short answer, and essay questions for each chapter.

ONLINE INSTRUCTOR'S MANUAL

The instructor's manual contains a variety of resources to aid instructors in preparing and presenting text material in a manner that meets their personal preferences and course needs. It presents chapter-by-chapter suggestions and resources to enhance and facilitate learning.

ONLINE POWERPOINT®

These vibrant Microsoft® PowerPoint® lecture slides for each chapter assist instructors in lecturing by providing concept coverage using images, figures, and tables directly from the textbook.

COURSEMATE

Available with the textbook is Cengage Learning's CourseMate, which brings course concepts to life with interactive learning, study, and exam preparation tools that support the printed textbook. CourseMate includes an integrated ebook, glossaries, flashcards, quizzes, downloadable forms, and end-of-chapter activities. CourseMate also includes Engagement Tracker, a first-of-its-kind tool that monitors student engagement in the course.

HELPING PROFESSIONS LEARNING CENTER

Helping Professions Learning Center is designed to help students bridge the gap between coursework and practice. The Helping Professions Learning Center offers centralized familiarity with the principles that govern the life of the helping professional. The interactive site consists of six learning components: video activities organized by curriculum area and accompanied by critical thinking questions; ethics, diversity, and theory-based case studies; flashcards; practice quizzes; a professional development center; and a research and writing center.

ACKNOWLEDGMENTS

I would like to give my sincerest appreciation to my mother, Joyce Kanel, who spent much time and energy reading the rough draft of this text. She is proficient at expository English and helped ensure that the writing made sense.

I would also like to thank Ray Estrella, a former student of mine, who researched some of the material for the chapters. I also thank my human services students, who have given me feedback about what they would like to see in an introductory text.

Also, I thank Glennda Gilmour, a human services instructor, who has taught this course for many years. She gave me valuable ideas about what to include, especially the idea of creating exit quizzes.

Many, many thanks to the following manuscript reviewers who carefully assessed drafts of this book and provided detailed and thoughtful comments to help keep the book on track and in focus:

> Lisa Boone, Community College of Baltimore County
> Nancy Calleja, University of Detroit Mercy
> Ray Feroz, Clarion University
> Gigi Franyo, Stevenson University
> Charles Hennon, Miami University Oxford
> MaryJo Jakab, University of Maine at Augusta
> Donna Oropall, University of Bridgeport
> Victoria Schultz, Wharton County Junior College
> Valerie Wise, South Suburban College

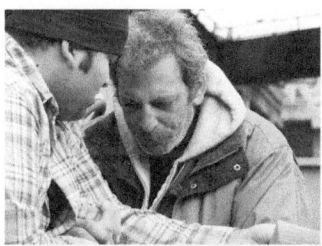
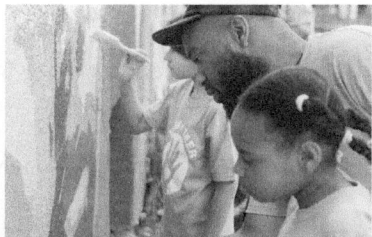
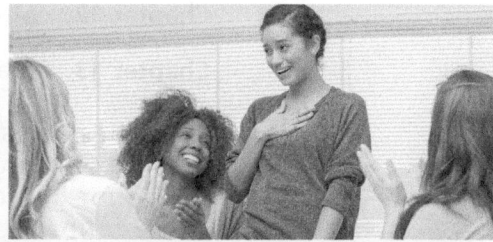

Brief Contents

Chapter 1 Human Services: Foundational Concepts and Historical Background 1

Chapter 2 Modern-Day Human Services: Policies and Programs, Interventions, and Demographic Considerations 31

Chapter 3 Ethical and Multicultural Issues in the Human Services 54

Chapter 4 Human Services Workers 81

Chapter 5 Basic Counseling Skills, Personal Characteristics of Human Services Workers, and Theoretical Approaches in Counseling 108

Chapter 6 Crisis Intervention, Suicide Prevention, PTSD, Community Disasters and Trauma Response, and Military Trauma 144

Chapter 7 Humans Services Populations 162

Chapter 8 Mental Illness, Poverty, Disabilities, Crime/Violence, and Substance Abuse 190

Chapter 9 Interpersonal Partner Abuse, Sexual Assault, HIV/AIDS, and LGBT Issues 224

Chapter 10 Stress Management 246

Chapter 11 Case Management 270

Chapter 12   Macro-Level Practice   294

Chapter 13   Leadership and Organizational Structure   311

REFERENCES   325
APPENDIX: HUMAN SERVICES CAREER INVENTORY   337
NAME INDEX   340
SUBJECT INDEX   343

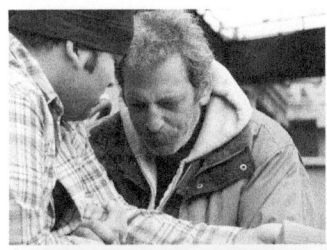
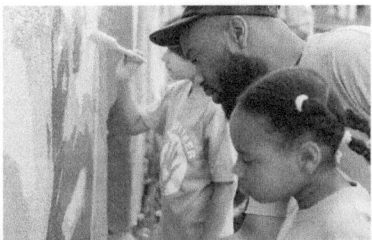
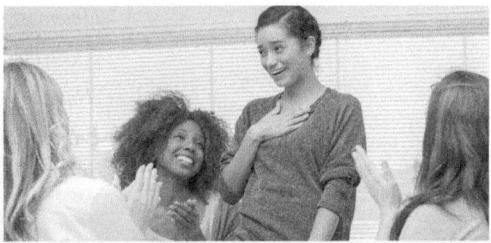

Contents

PREFACE vi

Chapter 1 Human Services: Foundational Concepts and Historical Background 1

Introduction 1
Defining Human Services 2
Human Services Workers 2
   Professional, Paraprofessional/Nonprofessional 2
   Volunteers and Interns 3
   Where Do Human Services Workers Perform Their Duties? 4
Key Terms Used in the Human Services 5
   Clients 5
   Clients with Multiple Needs 5
   Model 5
   Multidisciplinary Team Approach 6
   Bias 6
   Disparity 6
   Prejudice 7
   Discrimination 7
   Stereotypes 7
   Sexism 7
   Racism 7
   Ageism 7

Heterosexism 8

Classism 8

Ableism 8

Ethnocentrism 8

The Generalist Model 8

Biopsychosocial Model 8

Why Choose a Career in Human Services? 9

Reasons Not to Choose a Career in Human Services 9

CRITICAL THINKING/SELF-REFLECTION CORNER 9

A Brief History of the Human Services: From Prehistoric People to the 20th Century 10

Prehistoric Humans 10

Ancient Civilizations: Scientific Inquiry Evolves 11

Early Christianity and the Middle Ages 12

The Age of Reason: Scientific Discovery and Rational Politics Are Revitalized During This Renaissance 14

The 19th Century: Laying a Foundation for Modern Human Services 16

The 20th Century: Science Flourishes and Government Funds Human Services 18

TRUE STORIES FROM HUMAN SERVICE WORKERS: Grassroots Movement Agencies 21

Chapter Summary 22

Suggested Applied Activities 23

Chapter Review Questions 23

Glossary of Terms 25

1. *Case Presentation and Exit Quiz* 27

2. *Case Presentation and Exit Quiz* 29

Chapter 2 Modern-Day Human Services: Policies and Programs, Interventions, and Demographic Considerations 31

Introduction to the 21st Century 31

The 21st Century: Mapping Change for New Approaches 32

Modern-Day Mental Health Agencies and Programs 32

Modern Social Welfare Programs 34

Modern Correctional System 35

Modern Educational System 36

More on Nonprofits 37

CRITICAL THINKING/SELF-REFLECTION CORNER 39

Interventions 39
    Primary, Secondary, and Tertiary Interventions 39
    Harm Reduction Models 40
CRITICAL THINKING/SELF-REFLECTION CORNER 41
Demographic Shifts and Considerations 41
    The Graying of America 41
    Immigration 42
    Ethnic/Racial Considerations 42
    Multicultural Programs and Policies 43
    Sociological Considerations 44
CRITICAL THINKING/SELF-REFLECTION CORNER 45
Chapter Summary 46
Suggested Applied Activities 46
Chapter Review Questions 50
Glossary of Terms 51
Case Presentation and Exit Quiz 52

Chapter 3 Ethical and Multicultural Issues in the Human Services 54

Introduction 54
What Are Ethics? 54
Why Are Ethics Necessary? 55
    The National Association of Human Services 56
Confidentiality 60
    Exceptions to confidentiality 61
Dual Relationships 62
    Definition of Dual Relationships 62
    Why Should Dual Relationships Be Avoided? 63
    Examples of Dual Relationships 63
Values and the Need to Monitor Them 65
    Examples of Self-Monitoring of One's Values 66
    The Benefits of Self-Awareness 67
CRITICAL THINKING/SELF-REFLECTION CORNER 67
Ensuring Ethical Competence with Continuing Education 68
Multicultural Competence 69
    Culture Defined 69
    Gender 70

CRITICAL THINKING/SELF-REFLECTION CORNER   70
    Sexual Orientation   71
    Ethnicity   71
    Religious Issues   74
Chapter Summary   75
Suggested Applied Activities   75
Chapter Review Questions   76
Glossary of Terms   76
Case Presentation and Exit Quiz   77

Chapter 4   Human Services Workers   81

Introduction   81
Job Functions of Human Services Workers   82
    Administrators and Assistants   82
    Advocates   82
TRUE STORIES FROM HUMAN SERVICE WORKERS: Administration in Human Services Agencies   83
    Behavior Changer   83
TRUE STORIES FROM HUMAN SERVICE WORKERS: Advocates' Responsibilities   84
TRUE STORIES FROM HUMAN SERVICE WORKERS: Focus on Changing Behaviors   84
    Brokers   85
    Caregivers   85
    Caseworkers   85
    Consultants   85
    Crisis Workers   86
    Evaluators   86
    Educators   87
    Fundraisers   87
    Grant Writers   87
    Outreach Workers   87
    Therapists   88
CRITICAL THINKING/SELF-REFLECTION CORNER   88
Educational Requirements for Human Services Workers   88
    High-School Diploma   88
    Associate's Degree   89

TRUE STORIES FROM HUMAN SERVICE WORKERS:
A Human Services Worker Shares Her Experiences Working
in Human Services After Obtaining a Two-year Degree   89

    Bachelor's Degree   90

TRUE STORIES FROM HUMAN SERVICE WORKERS:
Job Description for Human Services Worker   91

    Master's Degree   92

    Doctoral Degree   93

    Medical Degree   93

CRITICAL THINKING/SELF-REFLECTION CORNER   94

Human Service Agencies and Jobs Based on Educational Attainment   94

    Social Welfare Agencies   94

    Mental Health Agencies   96

TRUE STORIES FROM HUMAN SERVICE WORKERS:
Career Opportunities for Workers with Bachelor's Degrees   98

TRUE STORIES FROM HUMAN SERVICE WORKERS:
Master of Science in Counseling Leads to More Challenges, Pay,
and Status in Mental Health   99

    Correctional Facilities   100

    Specialized Education Programs   100

Chapter Summary   101

Suggested Applied Activities   102

Brief Career-Decision Inventory   102

Chapter Review Questions   103

Glossary of Terms   103

Case Presentation and Exit Quiz   104

Chapter 5 Basic Counseling Skills, Personal Characteristics of Human Services Workers, and Theoretical Approaches in Counseling   108

Introduction   108

Part I: Effective Communication Skills of Human Services Workers   109

    General Goals of Effective Communication   109

TRUE STORIES FROM HUMAN SERVICE WORKERS:
Building Trust in the Real World   111

    Specific Effective Communication Skills   111

CRITICAL THINKING/SELF-REFLECTION CORNER   112

    Other Things to Consider   115

CRITICAL THINKING/SELF-REFLECTION CORNER   121

Part II: Theoretical Approaches to Counseling   121
   Evidence-Based Practice   *121*
   Psychoanalysis   *123*
CRITICAL THINKING/SELF-REFLECTION CORNER   125
   Object-Relations Theory   *126*
CRITICAL THINKING/SELF-REFLECTION CORNER   127
   The Neo-Freudians   *127*
   Existential/Humanistic Approaches   *128*
   Behavioral Approaches   *130*
   Cognitive Approaches   *132*
   Family Therapy   *133*
Chapter Summary   134
Suggested Applied Activities   *136*
Chapter Review Questions   *137*
Glossary of Terms   *138*
Case Presentation and Exit Quiz   *140*

Chapter 6 Crisis Intervention, Suicide Prevention, PTSD, Community Disasters and Trauma Response, and Military Trauma   144

Crisis Intervention   144
   The ABC Model of Crisis Intervention   *145*
Suicide Prevention   146
   Stages Used in Suicide Assessments   *146*
CRITICAL THINKING/SELF-REFLECTION CORNER   149
Posttraumatic Stress Disorder (PTSD)   150
   Other Interventions for PTSD   *151*
Response to Traumatic Community Disasters   152
TRUE STORIES FROM HUMAN SERVICE WORKERS: Critical Incident Debriefing after a Bank Robbery   152
   Manmade Disasters   *153*
Military Trauma   154
   PTSD and Military Service   *155*
   A 2008/2009 Research Study of Veterans and PTSD   *156*
   Traumatic Brain Injury (TBI)   *157*
   Other Interventions for Veterans   *157*
Chapter Summary   158
Suggested Applied Activities   *158*

Chapter Review Questions 158
Glossary of Terms 159
Case Presentation and Exit Quiz 160

Chapter 7   Humans Services Populations   162

Introduction 162
Children 162
- *Child Maltreatment* 162
- *Prevalence* 163
- *Causality Models* 163
- *Human Services Delivery in Child Abuse Situations* 164
- *Other Childhood Considerations* 167

CRITICAL THINKING/SELF-REFLECTION CORNER 168

Adolescence 169
- *Prevalence: At-Risk Behaviors* 169
- *Causality Models* 171
- *Human Services Delivery to At-Risk Adolescents* 172
- *Other Adolescent Considerations* 175

CRITICAL THINKING/SELF-REFLECTION CORNER 176

Aging Adults 176
- *Prevalence* 177
- *Elder Mistreatment* 177
- *Alcohol Abuse* 178
- *Poverty* 178
- *Frail Elderly* 179
- *Alzheimer's Disease* 179
- *Causality Models* 179
- *Human Services Delivery to Aging Adults* 180
- *Other Aging-Related Considerations* 182

CRITICAL THINKING/SELF-REFLECTION CORNER 183

Chapter Summary 183
Suggested Applied Activities 183
Chapter Review Questions 184
Glossary of Terms 186
Case Presentation and Exit Quiz 187

Chapter 8 Mental Illness, Poverty, Disabilities, Crime/Violence, and Substance Abuse 190

Mental Illness 190
- *Historical Background* 190
- *Definition of Mental Disorders* 191
- *Prevalence* 191
- *Causality Models* 191
- *Needs and Issues* 193
- *Human Services Delivery for Mental Illness* 193

CRITICAL THINKING/SELF-REFLECTION CORNER 195

Poverty 195
- *Historical Background* 195
- *Definition of Poor/Poverty* 195
- *Prevalence* 196
- *Causality Models/Needs and Issues* 197

TRUE STORIES FROM HUMAN SERVICE WORKERS:
The Needs of Those Living in Homeless Shelters 199
- *Human Services Delivery for Those Living in Poverty* 199

CRITICAL THINKING/SELF-REFLECTION CORNER 201

Disabilities 201
- *Historical Background* 201
- *Definition of Disabilities* 201
- *Prevalence* 202
- *Causality Models/Needs and Issues* 202
- *Human Services Delivery to Persons with Disabilities* 202

CRITICAL THINKING/SELF-REFLECTION CORNER 205

Crime/Violence Perpetrators 206
- *Historical Background* 206
- *Definition of Crime or Violence Perpetrator* 206
- *Prevalence* 206
- *Causality Models* 207
- *Needs and Issues* 207
- *Human Services Delivery for Crime and Violence Perpetrators* 208

CRITICAL THINKING/SELF-REFLECTION CORNER 210

Substance Abuse 211
- *Historical Background* 211
- *Definition of Substance Abuse* 211

Causality Models   213

Needs and Issues   214

Human Service Delivery for Substance Abuse   214

CRITICAL THINKING/SELF-REFLECTION CORNER   218

Chapter Summary   218

Suggested Applied Activities   218

Chapter Review Questions   219

Glossary of Terms   220

Case Presentation and Exit Quiz   222

Chapter 9   Interpersonal Partner Abuse, Sexual Assault, HIV/AIDS, and LGBT Issues   224

Interpersonal Partner Abuse   224

Women and Domestic Violence   224

Prevalence   225

Battered Women's Syndrome   225

Feminist View of Domestic Violence   226

Human Services Delivery in Domestic Violence Situations   226

TRUE STORIES FROM HUMAN SERVICE WORKERS: Working with Battered Women at a Shelter   227

Sexual Assault   229

Prevalence   229

Military Sexual Assault   231

Human Services Delivery in Sexual Assault Situations   232

TRUE STORIES FROM HUMAN SERVICE WORKERS: Crisis Intervention with Sexual Assault Survivors   233

HIV/AIDS Issues   234

Historical Background   234

Definitions of HIV and AIDS   235

Prevalence   235

Causality Models   236

Needs and Issues   236

Human Services for AIDS and HIV Clients   237

Issues Facing the Lesbian, Gay, Bisexual, and Transgender (LGBT) Community   239

Some Basic Definitions   240

Issues Facing the LGBT Community 241

Intervention with LGBT Persons 242

Chapter Summary 242

Suggested Applied Activities 243

Chapter Review Questions 243

Glossary of Terms 243

Case Presentation and Exit Quiz 244

Chapter 10 Stress Management 246

Introduction 246

CRITICAL THINKING/SELF-REFLECTION CORNER 246

Stress and Burnout 247

What Is Stress? 247

What Is Burnout? 248

The Impact of Stress and Burnout 249

Physical Symptoms 250

Cognitive and Emotional Symptoms 250

Social Deterioration 250

Behavioral Deterioration 250

Impairments in Work Performance 251

CRITICAL THINKING/SELF-REFLECTION CORNER 252

Managing Stress and Burnout 252

A Four-Pronged Approach to Managing Stress 253

Recognize Your Own Problem Areas 254

CRITICAL THINKING/SELF-REFLECTION CORNER 255

Work on Your Own Problem Areas 256

Improving Interpersonal Communication 259

Maintaining a Sense of Humor 263

Chapter Summary 264

Suggested Applied Activities 264

Chapter Review Questions 265

Glossary of Terms 266

Case Presentation and Exit Quiz 266

Chapter 11 Case Management 270

Introduction 270

What Is Case Management? 270

Types of Treatment Frequently Suggested for Recipients of
Human Services   271
    Micro Level   *271*
    Mezzo Level   *272*
    Macro Level   *275*
    Specific Types of Treatment   *275*
CRITICAL THINKING/SELF-REFLECTION CORNER   278
Specific Tasks of Case Managers   278
    The Intake Process   *278*
    Treatment Planning   *282*
    Progress Notes   *283*
    Report Writing   *286*
CRITICAL THINKING/SELF-REFLECTION CORNER   288
Chapter Summary   288
Suggested Applied Activities   *288*
Chapter Review Questions   *288*
Glossary of Terms   *289*
Case Presentation and Exit Quiz   *290*

Chapter 12   Macro-Level Practice   294

Introduction   294
Developing Programs and Policies   295
Evaluating Programs and Policies   301
CRITICAL THINKING/SELF-REFLECTION CORNER   303
Advocacy and Policy   303
CRITICAL THINKING/SELF-REFLECTION CORNER   306
Chapter Summary   306
Suggested Applied Activities   *307*
Chapter Review Questions   *307*
Glossary of Terms   *308*
Case Presentation and Exit Quiz   *309*

Chapter 13   Leadership and Organizational Structure   311

Introduction   311
General Characteristics of Human Services Agencies   312
    Norms   *312*
    Shadow Organization   *313*

Leadership Styles 313
Number Numbness 314
Types of Human Services Agencies 314
Public Agencies 314
Nonprofit Agencies 315
TRUE STORIES FROM HUMAN SERVICE WORKERS: Bureaucracy in a Public Mental Health Agency 316
TRUE STORIES FROM HUMAN SERVICE WORKERS: Working at a Nonprofit Agency 318
CRITICAL THINKING/SELF-REFLECTION CORNER 319
Chapter Summary 319
Suggested Applied Activities 320
Chapter Review Questions 321
Glossary of Terms 321
Case Presentation and Exit Quiz 322

REFERENCES 325
APPENDIX: HUMAN SERVICES CAREER INVENTORY 337
NAME INDEX 340
SUBJECT INDEX 343

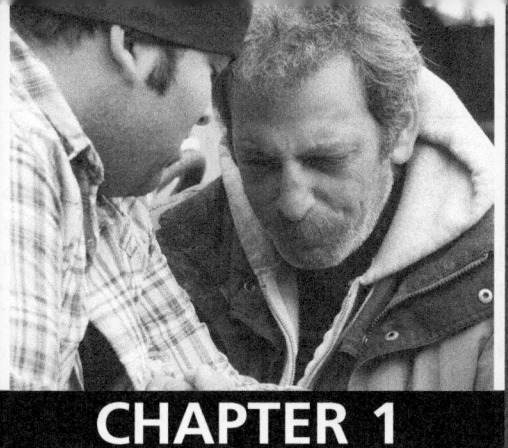

CHAPTER 1

Human Services: Foundational Concepts and Historical Background

INTRODUCTION

When someone hears the words **human services** for the first time, he or she might wonder, "Is this a college major or a department in the federal government?" The answer is "yes" to both questions. Or one might ask, "If it is a viable college major, why doesn't it end in "ology" like psychology, sociology, anthropology, biology, criminology, and other traditional majors?" The study of human services involves studying certain aspects of all those "ologies" and more. Human services uses a **multidisciplinary** (when several different human services workers trained in different areas of expertise work together for one consumer of service), **holistic** (viewing a person and his or her needs from many different perspectives such as physical, psychological, spiritual, and cultural), and **eclectic** (intervening with a person in need using a variety of theories and strategies based on those theories) approach to helping people with various needs.

President Franklin Roosevelt (FDR) established the Department of Human Services within the federal government in the 1930s, during the Great Depression, to assist people who were down on their luck. The Department of Human Services grew stronger throughout the 1960s and 1970s as U.S. residents began to assert their rights to be treated fairly and to have their basic needs met. Human needs and rights became a part of the federal government's focus.

Some might believe that those who study or work in human services are "jacks of all trades but masters of none." This text, however, supports the view that the **generalist human services model** enables those who work in the human services to become "masters of all trades." In other words, successful human services workers must know a variety of psychological, biological, and sociological theories so they can understand the causes of human behavior and use a variety of intervention strategies that take into consideration all models available. Putting the knowledge of these many and varied approaches to use can help human services workers successfully help their **clients** deal with their various problems.

DEFINING HUMAN SERVICES

Generally, "human services" is a broad term that includes services and programs provided to meet the needs of a person, a family, or an entire community. These services and programs are varied and ever changing as the needs and demands of society change. Maslow (1968) developed his hierarchy of needs that human services workers often focus on when providing services. Based on Maslow's model, one might suggest that activities that aim to meet the physiological needs, safety needs, social needs, self-esteem needs, and the need for self-actualization are human services. Alle-Corliss and Alle-Corliss (1998) present a simple definition of human services as "encompassing professional services provided to those in need."

HUMAN SERVICES WORKERS

A **human services worker** can be anyone, from psychologists and social workers to data managers. Neukrug (1994) describes a human services worker as "a person who has an associate's or bachelor's degree in human services or a closely related field." Others use "helper" and "human services professional" interchangeably to refer to a wide range of practitioners, including social workers, clinical and counseling psychologists, marriage and family therapists, pastoral counselors, community mental health workers, and rehabilitation counselors" (Corey & Corey, 1993).

Teachers, coaches, the clergy, guidance counselors, probation officers, gang-prevention specialists, outreach workers, and advocates may also be considered human services workers.

Professional, Paraprofessional/Nonprofessional

Many believe that human services workers attain **professional** standing when they have earned at least a master's degree or a state license. **Paraprofessional** usually refers to community workers who have not completed a bachelor's degree but have completed some training or education at a community college, university, or human services agency (for example, at many clinics, rape counselors must undergo 60 hours of training to be considered paraprofessionals). Both professionals and paraprofessionals in human services usually receive a salary rather than work as volunteers. Many agencies could not provide the services needed without hiring paraprofessionals, who often receive a lower salary than their professional counterparts. Paraprofessionals can be as competent and effective as professionals, although their responsibilities may be different.

Volunteers and Interns

Anyone who works at an agency without pay is considered a volunteer. **Volunteers** often donate their time for altruistic reasons. They do not receive credit from a school and are not considered **interns**. Volunteers are integral to the operation of most nonprofit agencies. Professionals who have been working in the field for years may choose to volunteer to work alongside those with little or no experience in the human services. Services provided by agency volunteers aren't less effective or of poorer quality than paid workers. Volunteers often bring an enthusiasm to a situation that longtime employees may lose. Volunteers should be treated with the same respect as employees no matter what their education and abilities. The fact that they are helping clients and the agency because they truly care gives them a special place in an agency.

Volunteers may provide medical services at free clinics, serve food at homeless shelters, nurture babies at homes for abused children, and answer phone calls at crisis center hotlines.

Interns are usually enrolled in a college and work at an agency for course credit. Interns' experiences at agencies may be discussed in class or with an advisor and are essential to a student's overall education. Some internships are paid, whereas others are not. The purpose of an internship is to use the theories learned in class with actual on-the-job experience. Interns are often encouraged to reflect on their personal reactions to working at the agency as well. Interns are also expected to gain awareness of how their agency experience fits into their career goals. For example, an intern might discover that after working with elderly people at a senior center, she definitely does not want to work with that population during her experience as a case manager. She may, however, find that she is much more effective and therefore prefers working with children after interning at a home for abused and neglected children. An internship experience should match an intern's level of training. Students may be encouraged to begin their first internship by shadowing (following and observing) an agency employee with considerable experience. As interns gain confidence in their ability to work effectively with clients, they may seek out more direct client contact. Instead of merely observing a support group, they may choose to interact with clients and offer educational presentations. At some point, students feel confident enough to work with clients as if they were employees of the agency.

Participating in an internship is an invaluable opportunity. Not only does it provide experience, skills, and confidence, it may also increase the chances of finding full-time work in the future. Interns must adhere to the same ethical standards and work ethic as the employees who work in the agency. Interns are often required to meet an agency's highest expectations, despite the behavior of the full-time staff. For example, some employees may show up late to work. An intern would not be given the same latitude but be expected to display a strong work ethic. Internships may take place at daycare centers, at homes for abused children, at outreach programs that work with teenagers, at after-school programs, at centers for senior citizens, at shelters for battered women, and at state and local social service departments.

Where Do Human Services Workers Perform Their Duties?

Many different types of agencies and organizations employ human services workers. These range from community organizations, large and small nonprofits, and **public** and **private agencies**. Many operate using volunteers, interns, and salaried staff, all of whom have different backgrounds and levels of education.

Nonprofit Agencies According to Kramer (1981), a **nonprofit agency** is a bureaucratic organization that is governed by an elected, volunteer board of directors employing professional, paraprofessional, and volunteer staff to provide ongoing services to its clients. Funding for nonprofit agencies may come from private donations, fundraisers, and both private and government grants. There are two types of nonprofit agencies. The first type provides face-to-face service to various client populations. It is usually staffed primarily by volunteers and interns, with a few administrative paid workers and serves victims of domestic violence, child abuse, and rape; seriously ill people with limited income; and people who are battling alcoholism and other addictions. The second type of nonprofit is more of an administrative organization whose main function is fundraising for a specific cause, such as the United Way, Easter Seals, and the American Heart Association. They provide community education and distribute money to direct-service organizations.

Public Agencies These are agencies funded by government taxes at the city, county, state, or federal level. Sometimes consumers pay to receive services. Some public agencies don't provide direct services but are administrative or provide community education. Such city-level agencies include senior centers, park and recreation centers, and gang units in police departments. At the county level, human services agencies include the departments of social services and welfare, the department of mental and behavioral health, and the department of corrections. State- and federal-level human services agencies include the department of rehabilitation, state regional centers for developmentally disabled persons, and the department of social security.

Private Agencies These agencies are funded by consumer fees and usually operate on a for-profit model, such as some hospitals or convalescent homes. Clinicians who engage in private practice as mental health counselors also fit into this category. Perhaps the most widely used types of private agencies are health maintenance organizations (HMOs). HMOs began to replace private medical and mental health insurance usage in 1980s. HMOs also provide educational information and treatment for substance abuse. HMOs tend to utilize more professional-level workers. Some may use volunteers, but their role is less vital to the daily operation of an HMO than to nonprofits and public agencies. Funding for HMOs comes partially from client co-payments and partially from insurance carriers, primarily acquired from clients' place of employment, and some may also receive third-party payments from Medicare and Medicaid.

Agencies, organizations, and institutions that focus on mental and behavioral health, social welfare, education, and correctional needs are usually the places in which human services workers are employed. These facilities may be nonprofit, public, or private. The specifics of these agencies will be discussed in Chapters 2 and 13.

KEY TERMS USED IN THE HUMAN SERVICES

Clients

A client, or recipient, is any individual, family, group, or organization that seeks assistance from a human services worker. Some people refer to clients as consumers.

Patients in psychiatric hospitals, people on probation (probationers), abusive parents, students, children who have survived abuse, survivors of rape or domestic violence, the elderly attending a senior center, and people struggling with addiction who are attending 12-step programs are all considered clients.

Clients with Multiple Needs

While a client may only have one need and therefore require service from one human services worker (e.g., seeing a guidance counselor who recommends a class to take), other clients may come in with many different concerns and would then need the assistance of a variety of workers. Some refer to clients who have many needs as **multineeds clients**.

For example, it is not rare for a client to have emotional issues, such as depression; to need housing and food stamps; to be involved in child custody disputes; and to struggle with substance abuse. Each issue requires the collaboration of different human services workers to meet this client's needs. While one human services worker may sometimes be designated as the case manager (this is true in cases where a child has been removed from the client or if the client is on probation), all the workers servicing the client must work together cooperatively for the benefit of a client. Difficulties that may arise include trying to separate out which need came first. Was the client depressed first and then abuse her child? Did the client lose her job, become poor, lose her home, and then become depressed? These questions become irrelevant at some point. The main goal is to assess all the needs of the client and then set up plans that can address them all.

Model

A **model** is a theory or approach that is used to understand a situation or to help work through a problem. It usually includes related terms that attempt to explain something.

Examples of models include the psychoanalytical model, the generalist model, the humanistic model, and the behavioral model, all of which offer strategies to use to help clients and understand their needs. Additional models are presented in Chapter 5.

Multidisciplinary Team Approach

The reason that a **multidisciplinary team approach** is needed is because many individuals and families have multiple problems and needs. In human services agencies, it is typical for several workers to provide services for one client, each with a different duty, all working collaboratively.

For example, a case manager might assess a family's financial eligibility for welfare, a psychiatrist might prescribe antidepressant medication for the mother's depression, a social worker might investigate a report of child abuse made on the father, and a probation officer might monitor compliance with terms of probation on the teenager in the family who sold drugs. Although each team member would focus on the family member who they are best qualified to assist, they all would communicate and coordinate care with one another.

Another typical example often occurs in a group home for abused and neglected children. A child will usually have an individual counselor (possibly a master's degree–level therapist) who provides ongoing counseling to deal with long-standing emotional and behavioral issues related to prior abuse and neglect and issues related to being separated from parents. Additionally, if a child demonstrates serious psychiatric symptoms or unmanageable behaviors, a psychiatrist may be called in to prescribe medication. On a daily basis, this child will interact with paraprofessional case workers and child-care workers who may lead groups and provide continuity of care and ongoing support and who may step in for crisis management situations. A child may also have an assigned social worker from the state department of social services who oversees the entire treatment plan and consults with all service providers. At times, the child may see a psychologist for more intense therapy or psychological testing.

The following foundational terms deal with the sociopolitical aspects of our society. Human services workers are strongly encouraged to understand these ideas and how they may affect clients and their own attitudes toward recipients of human services.

Bias

Bias is a preconceived point of view about a person, a group of people, or an issue. Biases may stem from beliefs of your own cultural background, your family's, or even your neighborhood's. Bias occurs when judgment about a situation or a group is based on generalities and personal opinion rather than on an objective, dispassionate point of view.

Disparity

Disparity refers to an imbalance, usually when people are treated unequally. The result of disparity is that certain groups do not receive the same appropriate and effective services as others simply because of the cultural group to which they belong.

Prejudice

Prejudice is the emotional and attitudinal component of group antagonism. It can refer to a negative attitude about an entire category of people and often leads to rejection of people who belong to a certain group. Prejudice usually involves a one-sided opinion based on generalities, such as disliking someone merely because of that person's affiliation with a certain group (Sears, Peplau, & Taylor, 1991; Schaefer, 1988).

Discrimination

Discrimination is the "behavioral component of group antagonism. People discriminate against the disliked group by refusing its members access to desired jobs, educational opportunities, country clubs, restaurants, places of entertainment, and so on" (Sears et al., 1991, p. 550). Discrimination is illegal and politically incorrect, but it is experienced all too often, especially by people of highly vulnerable groups who are reluctant to assert their rights (such as illegal immigrants). Discrimination puts prejudicial beliefs into action and denies members of a group access to certain rights that are available to others. Not all discriminatory behaviors coincide with prejudice. One can be prejudiced but not discriminate (Schaefer, 1988).

Stereotypes

Stereotypes are generalized beliefs about the characteristics of a group's members. A stereotype may be positive or negative and can lead to prejudice, discrimination, and bias. Some stereotypes may include some objective truth, but basing human services practice on them is considered culturally insensitive. Instead, human services workers are encouraged to understand certain group patterns and values but always keep in mind that not every member of a certain cultural group is alike in every way.

Sexism

Sexism is negative attitudes and behaviors toward a person because of his or her gender identity. Sexism is prejudice and discrimination against someone based only on that person's gender.

Racism

Racism is prejudice and discrimination against someone based only on that person's ethnic or racial identity.

Ageism

Ageism is age-specific prejudice and discrimination. In our society, elderly people tend to be victims of ageism. They are often rejected socially, receive inferior treatment by medical workers, and are asked to leave their jobs or are not hired at all because of their age.

Heterosexism

Heterosexism is having negative attitudes and behaviors based solely on a person's sexual orientation. Heterosexism is the belief that heterosexuality is superior to homosexuality.

Classism

Classism is holding negative attitudes and behaviors toward a person because of the economic class to which he or she belongs. Typically, classism is most likely to be experienced by the poor and often results in a disparity of services.

Ableism

Ableism considers people with developmental, emotional, physical, or psychiatric disabilities to be inferior (of less worth) than those who are supposedly able-bodied and -minded (*Free Online Dictionary, Thesaurus and Encyclopedia*, 2/14/2012).

Ethnocentrism

Ethnocentrism is the belief that one's own culture and way of life are superior to all others. Ethnocentrism judges all other cultures in the context of one's own cultural group and often views other cultures as being inferior (Schaefer, 1988), believing that members of these other cultures would be better off living according to the standards of one's own culture.

The Generalist Model

A **generalist model** takes a flexible, all-inclusive approach to helping clients deal with their problems. Rather than using one theoretical model or one duty or function, a generalist considers which theories and interventions are most appropriate to meet a client's needs. Rosenthal (2003) sees human services workers as functioning as "generalists, like general practitioners, who are the primary contact." Rosenthal also suggests that most human services workers view themselves as generalists with a multitude of skills who can work with a vast range of difficulties and perform a variety of functions.

Biopsychosocial Model

The generalist human services worker uses a holistic approach that looks at the biological, psychological, and social aspects of a client. Zastrow (1995) stresses the importance of considering all systems within the social environment and the interactions between a person and his or her physical and social environments when trying to understand a client. For example, when working with someone diagnosed with depression, one would not solely focus on the biomedical aspects of the disease but also take into account the person's social support system, personality, and lifestyle.

WHY CHOOSE A CAREER IN HUMAN SERVICES?

There are many reasons to seek a degree in human services and help others in need. This is an exciting field with much opportunity for professional enrichment, job promotion, and personal fulfillment and lifelong meaning. It is a chance to encounter people who are both different and the same as you. Human services workers can gain a sense of pride for contributing to the well-being of others. Human services jobs allow for autonomy and varied job duties. While some human services jobs conduct business during the traditional hours of 9 a.m. to 5 p.m., many offer flexible scheduling. There is constant growth—both personal and professional—for those who work in human services. Challenges abound, and this can be an intellectually rewarding occupation as well.

REASONS NOT TO CHOOSE A CAREER IN HUMAN SERVICES

If your goal is to make a million dollars and retire by age 55, human services may not be for you. Other motivations such as a need to save others and take care of others or a need to be depended on or to control others, may not be appropriate reasons to enter the helping field either. Sometimes a well-meaning helper may inadvertently use clients to meet his or her own personal emotional needs rather than focusing on the client's needs. If a person's motivation to enter the helping field is to feel good because someone else needs him or her or if the helper feels powerful when someone depends on him or her, the prospective human services worker should discuss these feelings with a counselor or an instructor. It isn't fair to clients to use them to meet our own emotional needs.

While one can make a decent living in this field, money is usually not the primary goal of those in human services. The field can be personally taxing, and dedication to helping others live better lives is key. Also, this is not just an easy degree that anyone can obtain. Many of the classes are both academically and emotionally difficult. Working on a daily basis with people who suffer from emotional and physical problems can be difficult. A person who works in human services must be committed to ongoing self-development and self-examination. These processes are part of the training for human services workers. For those who find these challenges appealing, human services may be a good career choice.

Critical Thinking/Self-Reflection Corner
- What is your motivation to enter the helping profession?
- What are your strengths and weaknesses?
- How committed do you feel to this field?
- What do you think it would be like to work with people suffering, people engaging in deviant behaviors, and people with many challenges?

A BRIEF HISTORY OF THE HUMAN SERVICES: FROM PREHISTORIC PEOPLE TO THE 20TH CENTURY

While the term "human services" is rather new, services provided to people in need by governments, religious organizations, and communities have been around since recorded time. There has always been a need to take care of people in the community, whether it be the disabled members of tribes of prehistoric days, the lepers from biblical times, the sick during the leech-sucking days of Aristotle, or the "possessed witches" of the Middle Ages. Taking care of those around us was most likely a way to ensure survival of the species, which is an intrinsic drive in all species. It wasn't until Queen Elizabeth of England created the **Elizabethan Poor Laws** in 1547 that the government stepped in and officially declared its part in assisting those in need. Since then, programs have become more sophisticated and complex, but the type of individuals who receive assistance seem to stay the same. Let's go on a brief journey into the past to better understand the state of affairs in the 21st century.

Prehistoric Humans

Picture yourself walking through jungles, deserts, and icy tundras with heavy loads of food and other survival gear such as hides for ensuring warmth and weapons. What would you do with a member of your tribe who was physically disabled? How would you manage that cousin who suffered from mental retardation? Who would assist the elderly that were often too frail to travel? On the other hand, what should the tribe do if someone steals food or items from another? Worse, how would a murderer be handled? Would that oddly behaving uncle be given charity, or would he be punished? The members of the tribe had to decide whether to punish, take care of, or abandon these individuals. Although much change has occurred throughout time regarding how to manage deviance and assist those in need, modern-day human services still operate under the same perspective of ancient man for the most part. Those in the human services field still approach those in need with charity and take care of them, or if deemed to be purposefully bad, punish them; sadly, sometimes those in need are abandoned, neglected, and excluded. Just as it was probably confusing back then as to who was deserving of charity and who deserved punishment, it is still sometimes confusing today who is entitled to services and who is not. Much of this confusion is due to the way in which human services workers attribute the causes of the problems.

One of the causal theories that anthropologists believe was adhered to by prehistoric civilizations is **animism**, in which spirits were believed to inhabit inanimate objects (Clodd, 1997). At times, evil spirits were thought to inhabit a person's brain and cause deviant behaviors, similar to what we now call psychotic delusions and hallucinations. A technique used to rid a person of evil spirits was called **trepanning** (see Figure 1.1), in which a hole was drilled into the skull of

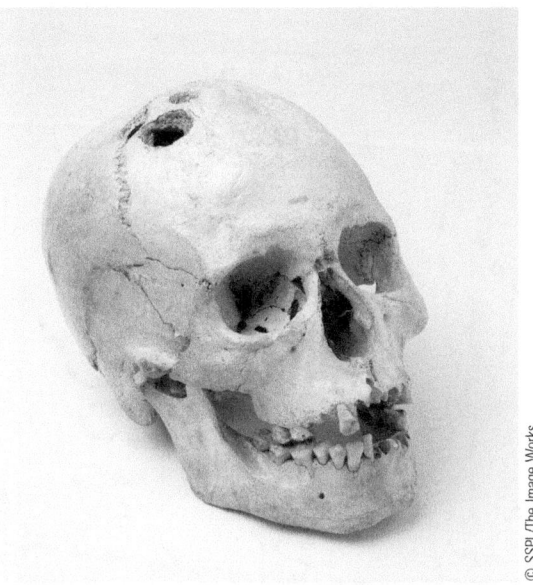

FIGURE 1.1 Trepanning, the procedure of boring a hole in the skull, is the earliest known medical operation. Some anthropologists believe that trepanning was performed on people with mental illnesses to drive out evil spirits from their heads. This skull dates from the Bronze Age, 2200–2000 B.C.

the affected person to release evil spirits. This may have been one of the first attempts to treat mental illness, and it was certainly one of the first surgical procedures practiced. Trepanning, sometimes referred to as trephining, might still be performed today on certain individuals. Sophisticated tools are used to relieve pressure from the brain caused by skull fracture or cerebral abscess.

While this sounds barbaric, when one compares it to a frontal-lobe **lobotomy** practiced in the 1930s and 1940s, it is not so unthinkable. Lobotomies were performed by using an ice pick through a slot above the eye into the brain to excise the frontal lobe—the part of the brain theorized to control aggressive and violent behaviors. The theory of causes may be different from our earliest ancestors, but the practice of trepanning may have been effective in the same way lobotomies were effective in managing psychotic behaviors. While modern-day psychiatry does not perform lobotomies with ice picks anymore (this was deemed too barbaric), some individuals suffering from severe mental disorders still undergo **psychosurgery**, in which parts of the brain are excised. History does repeat itself! But with the introduction of antipsychotic medications, the once widespread use of lobotomy in America was all but extinguished (El-Hai, 2004).

Ancient Civilizations: Scientific Inquiry Evolves

Enlightened Greeks, circa 600 B.C., such as **Hippocrates** (see Figure 1.2), Aristotle, Socrates, and Plato, began exploring humans physically, mentally, and politically as

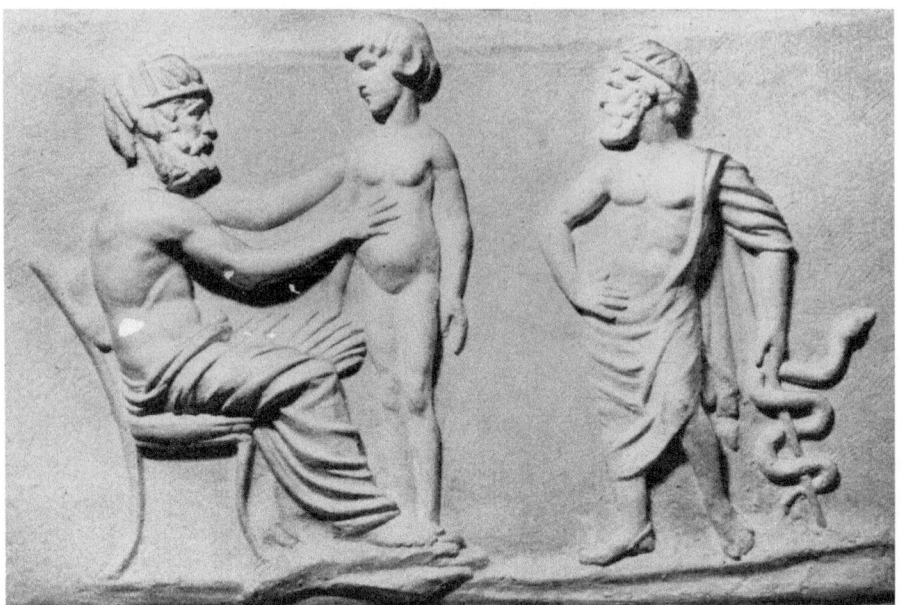

FIGURE 1.2 Hippocrates, who is seen in this Greek bas-relief watching as a doctor treats a young patient, believed that most diseases were chiefly organic in origin. For example, Hippocrates believed that the brain was the center of intelligence, and mental disorders, therefore, were due specifically to the malfunctioning of the brain.

their civilizations grew and became strong. Unlike their primitive predecessors, they proposed a scientific explanation for illness. Hippocrates, for whom the physicians' Hippocratic Oath was named (Miles, 2003), believed that human diseases, including deviant behaviors, resulted from an imbalance in four bodily fluids referred to as **humours**. This theory led to such practices as blood-letting and leeching, used to rid the body of excess fluids, thereby restoring the balance. An interesting point to consider is that many people in modern times use these methods on themselves when depressed (e.g., cutting oneself with razor blades to see blood and inducing vomiting to be thin and feel purified). Use of leeches to extract disease is still used by modern physicians as well. Also, although modern-day psychiatrists and physicians might not believe that illness is due to imbalance in blood, phlegm, and stomach acids, beginning in the 1950s when psychiatrists began to prescribe antipsychotic medications to mentally ill patients, the idea of biochemical imbalances as the cause of deviance has become strong and the predominant causal theory for 20th- and 21st-century practice. The perception by psychiatrists that biochemical imbalances cause many mental health disorders dictates intervention by many psychiatrists and physicians working in public and private agencies. Instead of having patients induce vomiting or release blood, modern-day human services workers prescribe medications to balance biochemistry.

Early Christianity and the Middle Ages

Dealing with deviance, poverty, and human needs looks decidedly different from the perspective of the societies in which religious leaders ruled. Prior to

Christianity, most deviant behavior was punished by putting the offender in stocks and gallows and having the public stone him or her for his or her misbehaviors.

The basis of criminal law in early civilizations was most likely based on the Semitic law of "an eye for an eye" and the earliest legal code, known as the **Code of Hammurabi** (see Figure 1.3), in which equal retaliation was the basis for criminal justice (Harper, 2002).

In John 8:7, Jesus challenges a crowd, saying, "Let he who is without sin, cast the first stone" (Tyndale, 1611). Such renowned quotations may have reflected the changing attitudes of the time from punishment to compassion. Jesus's stance toward the unfortunate may have led to a trend toward forgiveness and empathy rather than the punitive stance that viewed people with struggles as being morally deficient.

As the Roman Empire lost its stronghold on the world by about 500 A.D., the era usually referred to as the Middle Ages began and continued until about 1500 A.D. The first 300 years of the Middle Ages are often referred to as the Dark Ages because there was a lack of cultural achievements in contrast to the literary and scientific achievements during the classical period of the Roman Empire (Mommsen, 1942). The Dark Ages most likely occurred due to the growing strength of Christianity and focus on faith rather than on science as was seen in the classical era of the Greeks and Romans. The clergy was growing strong in terms of its influence on societal laws and norms. Lack of faith became the primary societal focus to explain deviance during these Dark Ages, and faith

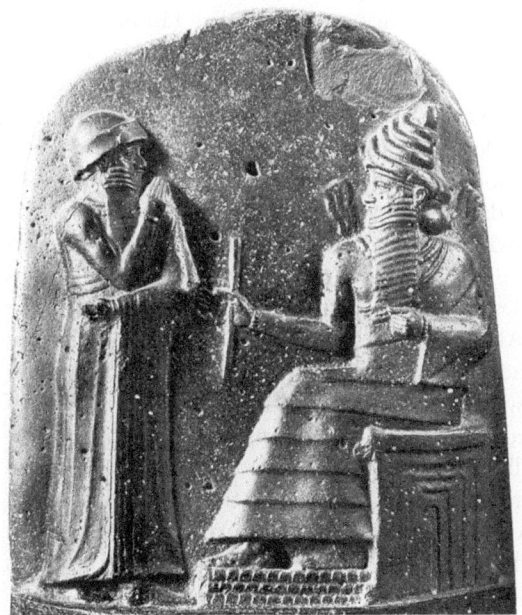

F I G U R E   1.3 The Code of Hammurabi is engraved on the black basalt of this stele, which is 2.25 meters (7 feet, 5 inches) high and was made in the first half of the 18th century B.C.

continued to be the primary explanatory model throughout the rest of the Middle Ages.

At times, prayer and faith healing were used to help those in need, along with compassion and charity. Later in the Middle Ages (during the time of the Spanish Inquisition between 1100 and 1300), the church dealt with perceived deviance by more punitive measures. Those who studied science or were associated with unexplained phenomena were considered heretics and in league with the Devil, and the church often ordered them to be burned at the stake or to undergo exorcisms in which demons were ordered to leave the body of the person. Many women during this time were ordered to enter deep water after those in power filled their clothes with stones. If they drowned, it was proof they weren't heretics, and they would go to heaven. If they survived, they were witches and would be executed. The *Malleus Maleficarum* (a book written by clergy during the second half of the Middle Ages) was written to prove the existence of witches and warlocks and to instruct witch hunters in how to identify them and how to treat or help them (Summers, 1969). The sick, the poor, and the needy were considered sinners and were left to die without any care. Only the very wealthy and most powerful were allowed to be educated.

The Age of Reason: Scientific Discovery and Rational Politics Are Revitalized During This Renaissance

Fortunately, society made it through the Middle Ages, and science and rational politics returned, and at a more advanced level than those of the ancient Greeks, Romans, and Egyptians. Monarchies ruled most countries, and the royals in power established civil governments that studied science systematically. Human services were developing during this Renaissance in a very systematic way as well. Although average citizens had no access to education and those accused of crimes were at the mercy of those in power, humanitarian philosophies influenced services established to aid poor, disabled, and infirmed people. In 1601, Queen Elizabeth of England created the Elizabethan Poor Laws that authorized the British government to provide for the needs of people who were unable to care for themselves, such as children, the disabled, and the poor (Dean, 1996). Shelters and workhouses provided for these populations. Modern-day social welfare is largely based on these same principles. Children and the disabled have priority in receiving governmental assistance. Although the shelters and services available in those days didn't focus on truly ameliorating the problems (they may have been a way to hide them), they do show that changes were being made in regard to these populations. At least they were being noticed by the governing class.

During that time, the mentally ill, mentally retarded, and criminals also received more humanitarian treatment than was given in the Middle Ages. In 1247, Bethlem Royal Hospital, popularly known as **Bedlam**, the first asylum for the insane, was built in London to care for those with psychiatric illnesses (Hollingshead, 2004).

In France, institutions had been established to deal with members of its society who were insane and who broke the law by locking them in chains until they died. By the late 1700s, however, such institutions were being reformed, influenced largely by the work of **Philippe Pinel** (see Figure 1.4). Pinel was a physician who promoted the moral treatment of those who were institutionalized, not only by removing their chains but also by offering them food, shelter, and clothing (Weiner, 1979).

In colonial America, civil government was developing, and the country was governed administratively rather than by theocracy or monarchy during the 1700s. As the government became strong and independent, it developed public health and human services for children, the sick, and the poor largely because it was important to keep the streets clean from those afflicted with the plague and other public health nuisances. Although some people during this time period held punitive stances toward those exhibiting deviant behaviors (many people were called witches and burned at the stakes, such as during the Salem witch trials), it's possible that the Christian base of the growing nation allowed for humanitarian treatment of those in need. Also, the foundation of this new country was based on individual rights and the pursuit of happiness. The government may have been compelled to take care of its citizenry in order to fulfill the dream of happiness and opportunity that was the foundation of the constitution.

Education in the United States was also undergoing major improvements. **Horace Mann**, known as the "great equalizer" (Compayri & Frost, 2002), worked with Thomas Jefferson to create mandatory education for everyone.

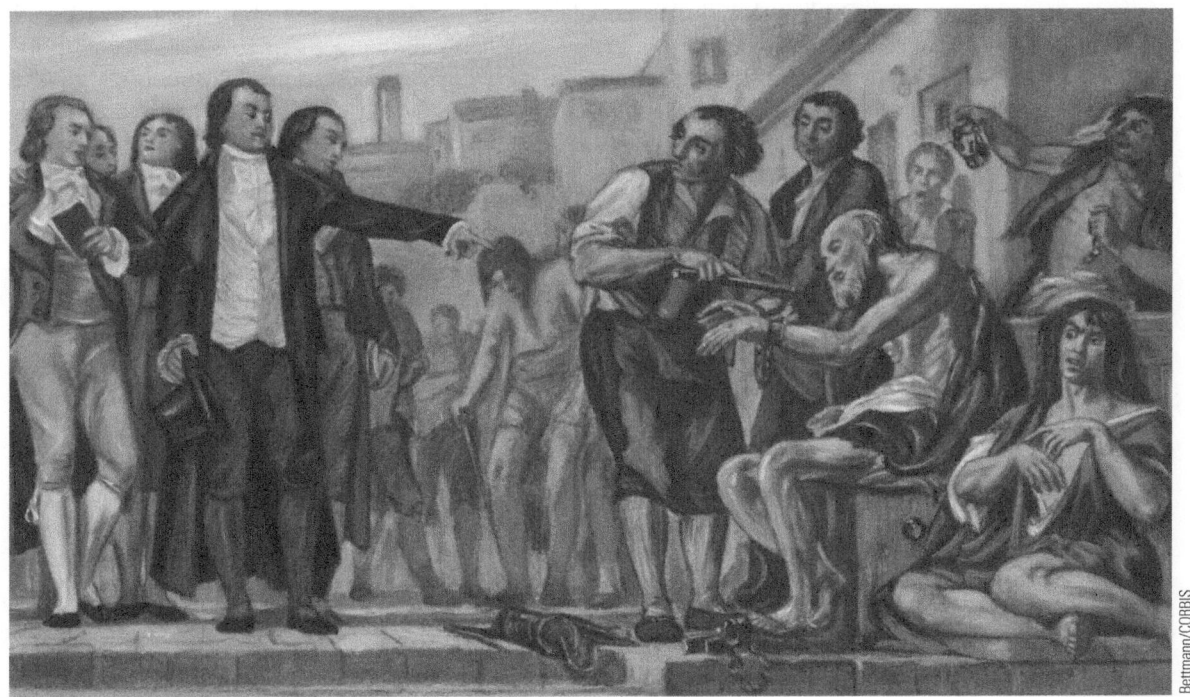

FIGURE 1.4 French physician Philippe Pinel supervises the unchaining of mentally ill patients in this painting by Charles Muller.

Prior to that, only the wealthy and the powerful had access to education. Mann's reforms marked the beginning of government-funded school systems that would be regulated and would provide all U.S. residents access to literature and the fundamentals of learning that were the foundations of a prosperous standard of living.

The 19th Century: Laying a Foundation for Modern Human Services

Scientific interest in the causes of deviant behavior increased during the 1800s and led to different schools of thought about the causes of such problems as crime, mental illness, and poverty. **Cesare Lombroso** began the systematic study of criminals, and scientists separated them from individuals thought to be mentally ill (Lombroso & Ferrero, 2004). **Emil Kraepelin**'s practice of dividing mental illnesses into different categories set the stage for modern-day diagnoses. He is particularly well known for establishing the clinical pictures to diagnose schizophrenia and manic depression (Columbia University Press, 2006).

Sigmund Freud developed his **psychoanalytic theory**, which not only proposed a model for understanding abnormal and normal human behaviors but also introduced a systematic method for treating patients. His approach was novel in that he was the first physician to propose that mental health problems served a psychological function for the individual. He likened people to machines and suggested that failure in brain machinery may lead to mental illness. Rather than judge people or subject them to punishment or pity, Freud proposed that people could be helped by allowing them to speak freely about their problems and their thoughts to a doctor who would then interpret for the patients why they are suffering. His introduction of "talk" therapy was monumental in the field of mental health. Although many modern-day mental health workers use other approaches in their counseling practices, Freud must be credited with introducing the idea that a patient-therapist relationship can help people overcome emotional problems. For this, Freud probably deserves being considered the father of modern mental health.

Social welfare was also developing systematically during the 1800s. **Dorothea Dix** (see Figure 1.5) was well known for crusading on behalf of the insane, poor, and criminals (Grob, 1994). She championed the causes of prison inmates, the mentally ill, and the destitute. Her work began when she began to volunteer to teach Sunday class for women inmates at the East Cambridge Jail. She noticed horrific experiences for the inmates, which included crowded, unheated, unfurnished, and despicable-smelling quarters. Many of the inmates, aside from being criminals, were mentally ill, and when she asked why the jail was in its current state of conditions, she was told the insane do not feel heat or cold. This ignited Dorothea to take action; she visited jails and almshouses (where the mentally ill where typically housed) throughout Massachusetts and eventually submitted a document to the Massachusetts legislature about the nature of the care provided to the mentally ill. Eventually, due to Dorothea's conviction and passion, the legislature agreed to provide support and set aside funds for the expansion of a state hospital. She took her crusade to other states,

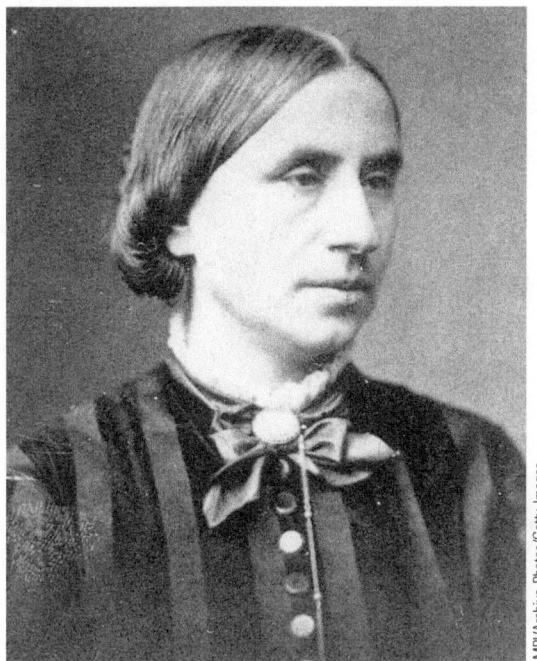

FIGURE 1.5 American reformer Dorothea Dix championed the causes of prison inmates, the mentally ill, and the destitute.

persuading other state governments to take better care of and responsibility for their mentally ill citizens. In this way, she became the "voice for the mad." As a result of her work, by 1843 there were 13 mental hospitals in the country; by 1880, there were 123. Dix's work changed the thinking of the time. While most people during this time believed that the mentally ill could not be treated, Dorothea understood that people could get better if their environmental conditions got better. In 1843, the New York Association for Improving Conditions of the Poor was created. Social workers of the time attributed poverty to "moral deficiency" and divided poor people into two categories: either unworthy or worthy. Sadly, many people today still adhere to this theory about the poor.

During the Industrial Revolution of the late 1800s, hundreds of thousands of people immigrated to the United States seeking a better quality of life. Another person interested in meeting the social welfare needs of people, **Jane Addams** (see Figure 1.6), founded **Hull House** as a settlement house to assist these immigrants in adjusting to their new homeland. Other similar houses were created in an initial attempt to provide housing assistance to the poor (Davis, 1990). Addams also founded the National Consumers League (NCL), America's oldest national consumer organization that focused on improving federal labor laws, as well as national health insurance, food and drug safety laws, social security legislation especially for the elderly or disabled, and unemployment insurance.

Headway was being made in the criminal justice system during this century as well. Based on results of scientific studies, criminals who demonstrated signs of

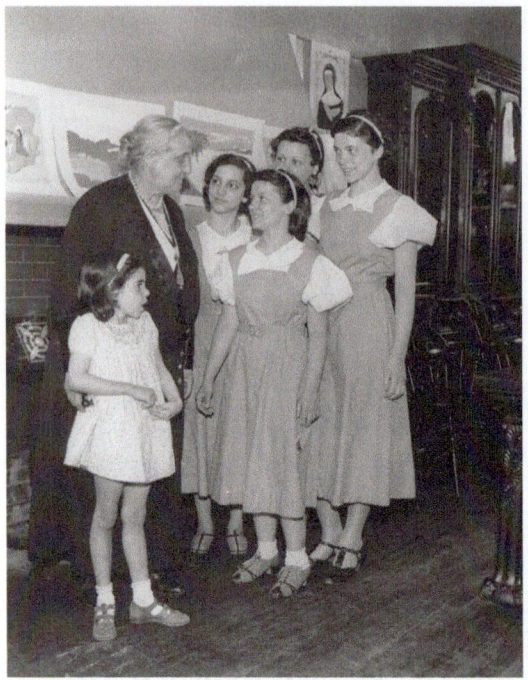

FIGURE 1.6 In 1889, Jane Addams, seen here greeting girls at Hull House, founded Hull House, a center for welfare work in Chicago. Fueled by Addams's exuberant personality, Hull House championed the causes of labor reform, public education, and immigrants' rights. Addams's book, *Twenty Years at Hull House*, details her service and social justice work in Chicago.

rehabilitation were being released from prison before the terms of their sentence were up. The **Elmira Reformatory** in Pennsylvania was the first U.S. prison to use the practice of "time off for good behavior." Past attempts at prisoner rehabilitation had failed, but prisoners given the chance of early release were more likely to reform their ways.

The 20th Century: Science Flourishes and Government Funds Human Services

Developments in Mental Health Freud certainly set the stage for modern-day counseling with his psychoanalytic approach to treating emotionally troubled people. The idea that a practitioner would sit with a patient and talk about problems was unique. Of course now, we take this practice for granted, and various types of therapists and counselors abound in modern times. Psychoanalysis as a mental health theory and treatment model predominated until the 1940s when humanistic models such as Carl Rogers's nondirective approach (currently referred to as person-centered therapy, which is a form of humanistic counseling) became popular. Also, behavioral approaches (the use of rewards and restrictive methods to change behaviors) to treat certain problems were being used in schools, prisons, and mental hospitals.

In the early 1940s, **Gerald Caplan** and **Eric Lindemann** developed crisis intervention counseling through their work at the Wellesley Project in Boston (an institute involving research to learn about the reactions of survivors who had experienced serious trauma and grief). It also served as a training ground for people interested in providing crisis intervention. Their work was precipitated by the Coconut Grove Nightclub fire, in which almost 500 people died and many more were injured (Lindemann, 1944). Using concepts and intervention strategies based on the psychoanalytic, humanistic, and behavioral models, Caplan and Lindemann developed ways in which individuals could benefit from short-term intervention. Caplan's preventive psychiatry, as it was first called, would ensure that individuals suffering from a life crisis wouldn't deteriorate and develop serious psychiatric illnesses. It promoted psychological and emotional growth and led to an acceptance of mental health consultation among the general public (Slaikeu, 1990). The practice of crisis intervention flourished over the next 50 years, and today's HMOs and many public and private agencies encourage its use. Besides being economically efficient, short-term therapy is effective in helping people return to a normal state of functioning and in preventing suicide and other dangerous behaviors.

In the 1950s, psychiatrists began studying family therapy models. In the 1960s, other approaches to counseling were developed, such as gestalt therapy (which involves creating balance within an individual) and reality therapy (in which individuals are encouraged to take responsibility for their behaviors and to engage in more socially acceptable behaviors). Cognitive therapy (which focuses on how a person's perception of a situation can lead to emotional problems) became popular in the 1970s and 1980s.

In the 1980s and 1990s, when health insurance companies began using **managed care** (which requires that treatment plans be preapproved before a person can receive care), **crisis intervention** (which focuses on coming to terms with a specific event that is keeping a person from functioning at a normal level) predominated, and it still does in the 21st century.

In 1955, there were over 500,000 patients in mental hospitals, which was the highest number in U.S. history. With the introduction and widespread use of psychiatric medications such as thorazine and lithium in the 1950s, patients who suffered from chronic mental illness could be managed in the community, which led to the **deinstitutionalization of the mentally ill** over the ensuing two decades, in which that same population was down to about 200,000 (Cutler, Bevilacqua, & McFarland, 2003). In 1955, Congress established the Joint Commission on Mental Illness and Health and found that three out of every four individuals treated for mental illness were in public mental hospitals, and by 1960, the Joint Commission recommended that the mentally ill be cared for in the community and that federal financial assistance would be provided to the states to accomplish this (Library of Congress, retrieved 12/20/2012). President Kennedy was very interested in community mental health as there was someone in his own family with a mental disability, and in 1963 he proposed a new National Mental Health Program.

Community Mental Health Centers Act of 1963 The **Community Mental Health Centers Act of 1963** is federal legislation that provided funding to communities to create mental health centers. The goal of this act was that by 1980 there would be one community mental health center per 1,000 individuals, or 2,000 such centers nationwide. In 1967 Congress reaffirmed the goal of having 2000 community mental health centers built, but by 1980 there were only 768 centers, which may have been the cause of the high homeless population among the mentally ill. Kennedy also emphasized the need to provide services to children, families, and adults suffering from the effect of stress and programs were to be comprehensive and available to anyone (Cutler et al., 2003). In 1963, Kennedy addressed Congress and suggested poverty was a cause of mental illness. As a result, he called for community prevention specifically directed toward low-income people and formed an interagency taskforce on mental health.

In subsequent years, states have developed their own laws and ethical standards to implement community mental health and not without controversy in some areas.

During the antiestablishment era of the 1960s and 1970s, **grassroots** movements (programs and services that community activists started without government financing or a professional staff) established nonprofit agencies where people could go and talk about problems, often in support-group style. These were run by paraprofessionals and depended heavily on volunteers. These centers still exist today as viable alternatives for mental health treatment.

Social Welfare Development In the 20th century, social welfare has undergone many changes since the days of orphanages, settlement houses, and charity wards in hospitals. During the Great Depression of the late 1920s and 1930s, Franklin Delano Roosevelt's **New Deal** provided people in need with food, clothing, and other basic necessities of life and also created work programs so that people could earn a living wage (Davis, 1990). Under the leadership of President Roosevelt, government became strong in its focus on social problems, and the notion of disparity (inequality and differences) among socioeconomic classes (social class based on income per year; usually divided into upper, middle, and lower classes) was studied by social scientists. This disparity, especially between minorities and mainstream society, eventually led to the civil unrest of the 1960s in which minorities insisted on equality and reform.

In the 1960s, President Lyndon Johnson waged a **War on Poverty**, resulting in the passage of the 1964 Economic Opportunity Act, which created such programs as affirmative action, welfare, food stamps, low-cost housing, and federally funded medical insurance (Howard, 1972). While the welfare system has changed since the 1960s, the basic premise of government aid to those in need still exists. The implementation of these welfare programs required the employment of thousands of social workers across the country. This catalyzed the formal study of social welfare in colleges, the increased usage of social workers in various agencies, and the sociopolitical premise that certain people are entitled to government charity.

Prison Reform The 20th century also brought reform to U.S. prison systems. In response to substantiated proof that there is a direct relationship among poverty, violence, and criminal behavior, the prison system has begun to focus on more humanistic approaches to rehabilitation. The proven connection between crime and poverty has made crime more of a social problem. Probation and parole programs were set up to allow probationers and parolees to live in society under the supervision of human services workers who monitored their behaviors. Allowing certain individuals these freedoms seemed more economically efficient than sending all violators to prison. Many law enforcement and correctional agency workers began to receive training in social and psychological theories so that they could better understand criminal behaviors. Even recent television dramas often have a character whose job is to analyze the criminal mind.

True Stories from Human Service Workers

Grassroots Movement Agencies

A Free Clinic for Women

The Anaheim Free Clinic, a community agency in California, was created in 1973 by two women interested in offering community residents concerned about issues of confidentiality an alternative to visiting a family doctor or a government-funded clinic. This clinic is a classic example of a grassroots agency. It was established during the time when women in America were beginning to assert their right to equal treatment. In particular, women wanted to be able to make decisions about their bodies. *Roe vs. Wade*, which gave women the constitutional right to terminate a pregnancy, had just been decided by the U.S. Supreme Court. The Free Clinic was developed to provide birth-control counseling, as well as birth control itself, and pregnancy testing and counseling. Participants didn't even have to give their real names or show identification.

I (the author) began interning at the Free Clinic in 1978, when I was a junior in college working toward my degree in human services. I chose that agency because I was interested in women's rights and in creating a safe place for women to learn and make choices about their bodies that could affect them for the rest of their lives. At the Free Clinic, I worked with physicians who volunteered because they also believed women needed to receive accurate information and testing so they could make informed decisions that would benefit them both physically and mentally.

In my role as an intern, I ran support groups, information groups, and pregnancy tests and counseled the woman about their options. Most of the clients were women and teenage girls who thought they might be pregnant or have a sexually transmitted disease or who wanted some form of birth control. Because sexuality was the primary issue at the clinic, it was vital to create a strong feeling of trust and confidentiality with the clients. All services were free. We did ask for donations from clients when possible. We held fundraisers in the community and sought donations from many companies to keep the clinic operating. I believe this clinic epitomizes a grassroots organization. Although I worked there more than 25 years ago, I still remember vividly my experiences there. It was a political as well as a healing agency.

A Safe Place for Battered Women

Battered women's shelters, another outgrowth of the women's rights movement of the 1970s, are also examples of grassroots agencies. The first such shelter was created in the mid-1970s to provide a safe haven for woman who were victims of

(Continued)

domestic violence. At the same time that women were asserting their sexual rights, they were also realizing that putting up with physical and emotional abuse from a partner was unacceptable. This was and continues to be a political issue to this day as various legislations dealing with domestic violence gets passed.

At first, these shelters were very small, involving women helping women. Over the years, they have become more elaborate agencies, with services ranging from employment counseling and legal advocacy to mental health treatment and child care. I also worked at a battered woman's shelter, and the following is a description of my experience there.

I remember immediately noticing the difference between this agency and the county mental health department, where I was a mental health worker for four years. At the shelter, clients were treated with more respect. The workers were motivated to make a difference in each of their clients' life. Everyone talked about women's rights issues. Paperwork, while it existed, was not as extensive as it was at the county agency. The shelter focused on helping women feel empowered. Many of the advocates and counselors at the agency had survived abusive relationships themselves. The atmosphere was supportive, educational, and political. While furniture was somewhat old and dingy, it felt more homey than the county facility. Money was always a concern, but the autonomy gained from not having to abide by government regulations was worth the frantic, ongoing search for funding.

Educational Reform Education also progressed during the 20th century. Although mandatory education had been around for a while, the quality of education was in no way the same for every child living in the United States. In the 1950s and 1960s, **Martin Luther King Jr.**, and other civil rights leaders, campaigned for an equal quality of education for minorities. Until the 1950s, and even into the 1960s and 1970s in some places, blacks and whites in the South were not allowed to attend the same schools. The **civil rights movement** of the 1960s focused national attention on the inequalities and abuses brought about by segregation and racism. Public schools throughout the country slowly became integrated.

Eventually, state governments began passing legislation that funded special programs in the public schools so that learning-disabled and developmentally delayed children, as well as children with physical limitations, could be provided with the same educational opportunities as their peers. These growing programs required public school systems to hire human services workers to evaluate students' needs and to provide counseling to them and their families.

CHAPTER SUMMARY

The field of human services includes a wide range of activities that focus on helping people meet a variety of needs. Human services workers perform many functions and are skilled to perform many duties. This generalist approach is one of the hallmarks in the field of human services and allows for an interdisciplinary approach to working with clients. Human services workers may use a variety of theories and interventions, may be volunteers or paid employees, and may be highly educated or have minimal formal education. The history of human services can be traced back to prehistoric man, and it seems there has always been a need to provide societal interventions for a variety of problems. Human services workers provide service in mental health systems, social welfare agencies, correctional facilities, and educational institutions. They work in nonprofit agencies, public agencies, and the private sector.

Suggested Applied Activities

1. Interview someone who works in human services in a nonprofit agency, a public agency, and a private agency. Ask this person to describe the types of other workers he or she deals with regularly. Inquire about the multiple needs of the clients who come into the agency. See if you can determine whether this person uses a generalist approach.

2. Create a chart that compares the human services models used today to the societal interventions of previous eras. Include the predominant theoretical perspective of that era that attempted to explain deviant behavior and sickness.

Chapter Review Questions

1. What is meant by a generalist approach?

   _____

   _____

2. Why is an eclectic approach considered necessary for being an effective human services practitioner?

   _____

   _____

3. What are the differences and similarities between an intern, a volunteer, and an employee?

   _____

   _____

4. Name two appropriate reasons to work in human services.

   _____

   _____

5. Name two inappropriate reasons to work in human services.

6. What is trephining, and why was it used?

7. How does trephining relate to modern-day mental health treatment?

8. How did the ancient Greeks view physical and mental health problems, and how did they treat them?

9. How did the clergy tend to view deviance, and how did they provide help to those in need?

10. When did modernized human services first begin?

11. Which populations tend to be considered deserving of human services?

12. What was the War on Poverty?

13. How did modern-day psychotherapy practice begin?

14. What was an important outcome of Caplan's and Lindemann's Wellesley project?

15. Name five people who created reforms in social welfare and corrections.

Glossary of Terms

Addams, Jane was a 19th-century social worker who founded Hull House.

Animism was a belief held by early civilizations that spirits inhabited inanimate objects and sometimes a person's brain.

Bedlam was an institution in London built in the 13th century that provided humanitarian care to the mentally ill and others who demonstrated deviant behavior.

Biopsychosocial model is a theoretical model for understanding what causes deviance that includes physiological, psychological, and sociological theories.

Caplan, Gerald was considered the "father of crisis intervention" because he developed preventive psychiatry, a new approach to counseling that he used to treat victims of the Coconut Grove Nightclub fire in 1942.

Civil rights movement began in the 1950s and 1960s. Many Americans worked to end racism and the inequities endured by the majority of black people in the United States. Many people engaged in protests and marches in support of these causes.

Client is a person who receives human services.

Code of Hammurabi is the earliest criminal justice code, which stated that equality of retaliation should be used when someone breaks the law.

Community Mental Health Centers Act of 1963 is federal legislation that provided government funding for treating severely mentally ill patients throughout the country.

Crisis intervention is a short-term approach focused on returning clients to a functioning level after they experience a traumatic event.

Deinstitutionalization of the mentally ill refers to the release of thousands of mentally ill patients who were hospitalized in government-funded mental hospitals during the 1950s and 1960s, after development of the antipsychotic medication thorazine, which enabled many psychotic patients to live outside the confines of a hospital.

Disparity is when things are not equal.

Dix, Dorothea was a 19th-century crusader for the rights of criminals, the mentally ill, and the poor.

Eclectic approach uses a variety of theoretical models and interventions to deal effectively with clients.

Elizabethan Poor Laws were laws set up by Queen Elizabeth as a system of assistance for the worthy poor in England during the 16th century.

Elmira Reformatory was an 18th-century prison in Pennsylvania known for its reforms that included giving prisoners time off for good behavior.

Freud, Sigmund was a 19th-century physician who developed the psychoanalytic approach to understanding and treating individuals with mental disorders.

Generalist human services model uses a variety of theoretical models and interventions to assist clients.

Grassroots movements started in the 1960s during times of civil unrest and lack of faith in the government to take care of the public's needs.

Hippocrates was an ancient Greek physician who proposed a biological basis for human illness and set ethical standards for doctors.

Holistic is an approach that considers the clients in their entirety, including their biological, psychological, and social needs.

Hull House was a settlement house founded by Jane Addams in 1889.

Human services are services provided to help people with various needs live better lives.

Human services worker is any person employed by or volunteering in a human services agency.

Humours refers to Hippocrates's proposition that an imbalance of four bodily fluids could cause mental and physical disturbances. This theory led to the practice of bloodletting and the use of leeches.

Intern is a person who works in the field of human services as part of formal education.

King, Martin Luther Jr. was an African American minister who was a prominent civil rights leader during the 1950s and 1960s and used passive resistance to protest racial segregation and inequalities. He was assassinated in 1968.

Kraepelin, Emil was a social scientist of the late 1800s who categorized human deviance into separate illnesses such as schizophrenia and manic-depressive psychosis.

Lindemann, Eric was one of the pioneers in the development of crisis intervention who worked extensively with Caplan on the Wellesley project. Lindemann worked extensively with many forms of loss including working with women grieving over the loss of infants through miscarriages and stillborn births.

Lobotomy is the practice of removing brain tissue in the frontal lobe to rid the patient of aggressive tendencies. It first began in the 1930s with the use of ice picks in the eyeball sockets.

Lombroso, Cesare was a social scientist of the late 1800s who began to understand the psychology and social needs of criminals.

Mann, Horace was the great equalizer who worked with Thomas Jefferson to create mandatory education in the United States.

Managed care was created in the 1980s as a way for medical insurance companies to monitor treatment and offer more affordable care to families.

Model is an approach that usually has a theoretical basis that helps workers understand clients and help them out with their problems.

Multidisciplinary team approach is an approach that requires collaboration and open communication among various workers to best meet the needs of clients with multiple problems.

Multineeds clients are individuals or families with a variety of needs who seek assistance from human services. Such clients require workers to be knowledgeable and resourceful.

New Deal was a program created by Franklin Roosevelt in the 1930s during the Great Depression that provided some basic needs and set up work programs to help destitute people.

Nonprofit agencies are community organizations funded by donations, fundraisers, and charity whose focus is providing service and effective programs rather than focusing on making a profit.

Paraprofessionals are human services workers who do not have a professional degree or license.

Pinel, Philippe was a physician who humanized institutions not only by removing chains but also by offering food, shelter, and clothing to inmates.

Private agencies are organizations that are not funded by municipal, state, or federal government programs.

Professional is a human services worker with a college degree or license.

Psychoanalytic theory/psychoanalysis was developed by Sigmund Freud in the late 1800s and focused on talk therapy and uncovering unconscious forces.

Psychosurgery is a surgical procedure used in the latter half of the 20th century to excise brain material from mentally ill patients.

Public agencies are agencies that are government run or funded.

Trepanning/trephining is a procedure whereby a hole is drilled into the skull to release spirits or pressure and is theorized to have been used by prehistoric man.

Volunteers are people who serve at a human services agency without pay and not for educational credit.

War on Poverty was President Lyndon Johnson's program to help minorities and other citizens living in poverty to increase their standard of living.

1. Case Presentation and Exit Quiz

General Description and Demographics

Jenny is an unmarried 27-year-old woman with three children, all of whom have different fathers. She has never been married and is currently four months pregnant with a child from yet another man. Jenny has never worked nor graduated from high school. She survives through financial assistance from Aid to Families with Dependent Children (AFDC) but has recently been told that she must find a job or enroll in a vocational-training program. Jenny and her children live in a two-bedroom apartment in federally subsidized housing, receive monthly checks from AFDC, and are enrolled in state-funded medical programs. Two of her children go to public school where they get free breakfast and lunch. Jenny stays at home during the day to care for her two-year-old. She has yet to seek prenatal care for her current pregnancy.

Jenny was raised by her mother, had very little contact with her father, and has one brother, three years her senior, who is in jail. Her mother works, lives close by, and often baby-sits for Jenny. Despite this help, Jenny and her mother are not close, but Jenny's children feel very close to their grandmother.

Problems That Need Assistance

Both of Jenny's school-aged children often show up at school improperly dressed and unwashed. But recently, Jenny's eight-year-old daughter, Rebecca, came to school with bruises on the backs of her legs. The teacher reported this to the child protective agency within the state department of social services.

Jenny has had drug problems for the past 10 years. She uses crystal methamphetamine between three and five times a week, even when the children are home, and hangs out regularly with other crystal meth users. Despite this, she prepares dinner for her children every night and never leaves them alone.

First Human Services Worker Involved in the Case

When the report of child abuse came in to the department, the case was assigned to an emergency investigative social worker. He met with Rebecca at her school and spoke with Jenny at her home; he then referred the case to another social worker who began to develop a case plan.

Based on the details of this case, respond to the following questions. The concepts in this quiz have been discussed in this chapter.

Exit Quiz

1. Jenny is an example of
    a. a client with a very specialized need
    b. a multineed client
    c. a client who is undeserving of service because of her drug use
    d. none of the above

2. The most effective way for the social worker to deal with this case would be to
    a. conduct one-on-one counseling with Jenny
    b. focus on the children and let Jenny find her own case worker
    c. collaborate with several other human services workers to help the entire family
    d. all of the above

3. If the social worker sets up a case plan that requires Jenny to participate in her own therapy and drug treatment, undergo an assessment for depression, and seek prenatal care, it would require
    a. a multidisciplinary team approach
    b. that each worker specialize in a specific task and let the others do their jobs as specialists
    c. that only the professionals be allowed to treat Jenny
    d. none of the above

4. If the social worker in this case understands Jenny and her children's various needs and is capable of coordinating all the necessary services, the social worker is considered
    a. a jack of all trades but a master of none
    b. a generalist worker
    c. ambivalent
    d. all of the above

5. The most effective way to understand Jenny's problems would be from a
    a. psychoanalytic view
    b. purely biological view
    c. biopsychosocial view
    d. none of the above

Exit Quiz Answers

1. b
2. c
3. a
4. b
5. c

2. Case Presentation and Exit Quiz

General Description and Demographics

Ann is a 39-year-old woman who has a four-year-old child and a seven-year-old child. She was divorced from her children's father a year ago and awarded primary custody. She receives $400 monthly for child support. Ann works full time for the phone company and makes $35,000 a year. Her seven-year-old attends public school, and her four-year-old goes to daycare while Ann works. The seven-year-old gets a ride to the daycare center after school by the daycare workers until Ann arrives at 6 p.m. to pick up both her children. She and the children live in a two-bedroom apartment, with the daughter sleeping in the same room as Ann. The apartment rent is $1,400 a month. Ann has $100 per month disposable income after all bills are paid. After the divorce, she was ordered to pay half of the liabilities incurred during the marriage even though her ex-husband earns twice what she earns. Ann couldn't afford a lawyer, so she was not represented during the divorce.

Although Ann has benefits from her company for mental health services, the HMO provided by her employer pays for only 20 visits a year, for which she must pay a $20 co-payment for each session as well.

While married, Ann was able to afford $70 a month for ongoing therapy with a private therapist. Now that she is divorced, she cannot afford a private therapist.

Problems That Need Assistance

Ann has been depressed on and off for more than 20 years. She has attempted suicide twice, was hospitalized once, and has seen five different therapists in the past 20 years. Her depression has been managed through antidepressant medications and therapy. Her family doctor has always prescribed the antidepressants, but he is retiring this year.

Ann must change therapists for financial reasons. When she doesn't see a therapist, her anxiety increases so much that she often feels unable to go to work. She must keep her job and wants to work. When she called her HMO to get a referral for a new therapist, she was told that there was a three-week waiting list. She then called a few county-funded mental health services, but they told her that she makes too much money to be eligible for services. Ann also called a nonprofit agency and was told that because of her income level, she would have to make a $35 co-payment for services.

Ann is getting more and more depressed and anxious. Based on this case, respond to the following questions. The concepts in this quiz have been presented earlier in this chapter.

Exit Quiz

1. Why might the nonprofit agency need to charge this middle-class client a $35 co-pay?
   a. The workers at the agency are usually highly trained professionals.
   b. They have many paid staff that must be paid.
   c. Many nonprofits have been receiving less funding from government grants.
   d. The client can easily afford the co-pay and must take responsibility for her problems.

2. What treatment would a doctor in ancient Greece, circa 600 B.C., use to treat Ann?
   a. lobotomy
   b. blood letting
   c. psychoanalysis
   d. prayer

3. What treatment would a doctor during the 1940s have used to treat Ann?
   a. leeches
   b. exorcism
   c. lobotomy
   d. public humiliation

4. What treatment would Ann receive in the Middle Ages?
   a. lobotomy
   b. blood letting
   c. exorcism
   d. person-centered therapy

5. Ann's HMO benefits her in all but one of the following ways:
   a. it permits her to receive the exact type of treatment she and her therapist think is best
   b. it permits her to receive medical benefits at a reduced rate
   c. it allows her to pay less per treatment session
   d. none of the above

Exit Quiz Answers

1. c   3. c   5. a
2. b   4. c

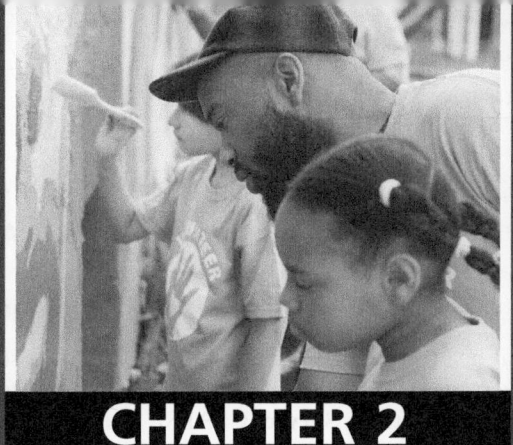

CHAPTER 2

Modern-Day Human Services: Policies and Programs, Interventions, and Demographic Considerations

INTRODUCTION TO THE 21ST CENTURY

As discussed in Chapter 1, human services has a rich history that has led to several important changes that affect us today. While our world has dramatically shifted, modern services, policies, and approaches are still in place to continue our rich history of advocating for and supporting individual independence, strong and healthy families and communities, and sustained well-being and general welfare of citizens. These shifts, in part due to demographic and cultural shifts (discussed in more detail later in this chapter), have made modern-day programs and services more complex and necessary than ever, requiring greater emphasis to be placed on creating equitable, sustainable, cost-efficient, and multicultural solutions in the delivery of human services.

THE 21ST CENTURY: MAPPING CHANGE FOR NEW APPROACHES

Modern-Day Mental Health Agencies and Programs

Mental health agencies include nonprofits (discussed later in this chapter) as well as government-funded programs such as **Child Protective Services** (CPS) and **Adult Protective Services** (APS). As discussed in Chapter 1, community mental health centers were first established following the **Community Mental Health Centers Act of 1963** and were primarily funded through the federal Short-Doyle Act. They were created to provide services for people with severe mental disorders, such as schizophrenia, and for people who were at risk of committing suicide. Each state was required to set up centers where clients could receive medication and crisis management. Many of the larger states funneled the money to the county systems, and county mental health facilities became the staple of mental health services for many years. Currently, the name of these centers has changed in many areas to "county behavioral health services." Because in the past mental health facilities had been used by clients who weren't severely impaired, administrators have instituted stricter guidelines for who may receive services. Typically, only those who demonstrate impairment in behavioral functioning are allowed to receive public mental health services, hence the name change to "behavioral health." "Mental health" may have been a bit too general and could have included many types of emotional problems that just weren't severe enough to warrant Short-Doyle funding. Because of these changes, many nonprofit agencies have been created to treat the higher functioning clients who previously used county mental health services.

In 1979, the National Alliance for the Mentally Ill (NAMI) was founded to provide support, education, and advocacy for people with mental illness, a growing population. Today, NAMI is the largest grassroots mental health organization in the United States. In 1997, President Clinton signed into law the Mental Health Parity Act of 1996. This landmark law, which received complete bipartisan support, began the process of requiring employers who offer mental health benefits to include similar insurance coverage for their employees who have mental illnesses or brain disorders, as compared to equally serious physical disorders. This was a promising step in decreasing negative stigmatization that often exists around mental illness in the workplace, although there were still limitations to its provisions. In 2008, Congress passed the Paul Wellstone and Pete Domenici Mental Health Parity and Addiction Equity Act, which closed many of the loopholes that existed and required that health insurance cover both mental health, including substance abuse, and physical health issues equally.

More recent mental health efforts include some states using lottery monies and cigarette and gasoline taxes to increase state-funded services, such as community mental health centers, which are designed to provide primary care for all patients irrespective of age, income, or income level on a sliding-scale fee basis. The New Freedom Commission on Mental Health, a key piece of the New Freedom Initiative (launched by President Bush in 2001), advocates for "fundamental transformation" of the mental health care delivery system. The goal is to give more power to consumers and families and revamp traditional bureaucratic and financial incentives especially as they pertain to the recovery process of adults and children with serious mental illnesses. Some of its strategies are to develop a more culturally competent workforce and to send the message that mental illness is treatable or manageable. Interestingly, the World Health Organization (WHO) has among its goals to also improve mental health care. One of its recommendations is that countries limit the number of mental hospitals and instead focus on self- and community care by building more community mental health services and integrating mental health services into primary health care settings.

Other examples of how government supports persons with mental health disturbances is through the U.S. Department of Health and Human Services (DHHS), which oversees several administrations (e.g., Centers for Disease Control and Prevention, National Institutes of Health, and Indian Health Services), designed to provide education, support, service coordination, and funding for individuals and groups who need mental health–related assistance. One agency, within the DHHS, is the Substance Abuse and Mental Health Services Administration (SAMHSA), whose mission "is to reduce the impact of substance abuse and mental illness on American's communities." This was established by Congress in 1992, and since then it has served as a leader in the advocacy and promotion of services, information, and research related to prevention, treatment, and recovery from mental health and substance use disorders. This is critical given that nearly 20 million people in 2012 did not receive the services they needed (www.SAMHSA.gov). The government also houses programs that protect one's mental health, due to abuse or neglect, including the Administration for Children and Families (also under the DHHS). The Child Abuse and Prevention Treatment Act was reauthorized in 2003 to continue to support the prevention, assessment, investigation, prosecution, and treatment of children who have been abused or neglected. States and localities are also principally responsible for protecting seniors and vulnerable adults from abuse and providing victims with protective services and treatment.

In the private arena, **health maintenance organizations** (HMOs) (discussed in greater detail in Chapter 11) provide or arrange managed care for health insurance. In most HMO plans, you must see health providers who are "in-network" for your plan or hospital. Often, HMOs provide a wide range of mental health care and services that are low cost to clients but that do not permit clinicians to provide long-term treatment for the most part. Also, HMOs have lowered the rates that clinicians receive for their services. For example, in 1984, the first author was able to collect 90 percent of her fee from most private indemnity insurance companies for psychotherapy services. Twenty years later in 2004, most clinicians received a set rate made by the HMOs for their services, which is often half of what they would charge if they billed indemnity insurance or half of what they would charge a cash-paying client. Additionally, it has been noted that primary care physicians in HMOs may be less likely than fee-for-service physicians to detect or feel confident in treating depression in their patients. On the other hand, many argue that HMOs' health care quality will be monitored, and the cost will be reduced for the taxpayer.

With the election of President Barak Obama and a majority Congress in 2009, the conversation of universal health care has gained importance. In 2010, President Obama signed a comprehensive health reform, the **Patient Protection and Affordable Care Act** (ACA), into law. The overall goal of the ACA is to ensure that all Americans have access to quality, affordable health care. The American Medical Association estimates the act will "expand health insurance coverage to 32 million more Americans" including those with mental health issues. Among the initial provisions are eliminating insurance restrictions with preexisting conditions, providing tax credits and no increases in premiums, and assisting young adults and retirees who are in need of insurance. It has been argued though that many negative unintentional consequences will result from the passage of the ACA, including lower quality care. Only time can tell how this new act will unfold.

Modern Social Welfare Programs

Today, international relief bodies, including the Red Cross, WHO, and United Nations Children's Fund (UNICEF), provide social welfare services throughout the world, especially during times of distress and disaster. In the United States, there are several forms of social welfare, including social insurance (e.g., social security, unemployment insurance, and general assistance); health services (e.g., **Medicare** and **Medicaid**); and food and shelter programs (e.g., food stamps and Section 8 housing). Overall, public assistance has become increasingly governed by state and federal control; for example, government funding is fairly strong for child protection services and services that protect the elderly and the disabled. Many programs offered through the federal government rely on public, private non-profit, and private for-profit organizations to cooperate in the provision of these programs, such as school lunch programs and housing for low-income individuals and families. Of course the nature of these welfare programs have changed over the past 40 years, but the states are still responsible for providing medical attention, food, shelter, child care, and utilities to needy children, disabled adults, and the elderly. Many other programs are government funded but delivered by private organizations. Thousands of workers are employed in social welfare agencies, and they are typical of bureaucratic organizations.

In 1996, President Clinton signed the Personal Responsibility and Work Opportunity Reconciliation Act (PRWORA), which is considered a major shift in the method and goal of providing assistance to the poor. The bill added a workforce development criterion encouraging employment among persons who are poor. President Clinton's goal was to "end welfare as we have come to know it" and discourage dependency on the system. This act, though, has received much bipartisan criticism, including Democrats arguing that many welfare recipients cannot easily get out of the cycle of poverty. Today, individual states can apply for a waiver for the work requirements and provide assistance even if their citizens cannot find employment.

In general, if a person is not an abused or needy child, a vulnerable or needy elder, or diagnosed with a disability, most government-run agencies will not provide social welfare. Nonprofit agencies, however, do provide resources for the nondisabled adults and other needy people. In fact, nonprofits today "have become a primary avenue for the provision of a wide array of employment-related, child care, emergency assistance, and counseling services" and serve as "street-level providers of public-funded programs" (Allard, 2008, p. 1). Smith (2002) notes that nonprofits are part of the modern safety net for the poor and even "have a more central role in society's response to social problems than ever before" (p. 50). Reliance on both secular and faith-based organizations is critical in providing for those who are in need, such as homeless shelters for families and adults.

Interestingly, as our country currently watches the unfolding of the ACA, nonprofit and grassroots partners will play an even greater role in assisting their clients and communities to engage in more self-governance regarding health and social welfare issues. In particular, they will continue to assist in improving communities; empowering residents, particularly those in high-poverty neighborhoods; and engaging in policy, advocacy, and public education activities. These services are increasingly necessary as demand for services will likely increase.

Modern Correctional System

Crime is a major problem in the United States, and unfortunately, the correctional system is overwhelmed by inmates. Correctional facilities exist at the city, county, state, and federal levels. These programs are usually part of a jail or prison system. Because these correctional facilities are often overcrowded, most communities have organized a Department of Probation, funded by state and county government agencies. The Department of Probation allows people convicted of crimes to live in the community while being monitored by probation officers. This system employs thousands of probation and deputy probation officers, juvenile hall counselors, and other human services workers.

Historically, emphasis had been placed on containing and or/punishing criminals. More recently, a human services model within prisons became more salient, with the goals of imprisonment to include opportunities for probation, counseling, and rehabilitation. For example, Congress passed America's Law Enforcement and Mental Health Project in 2000 to begin assisting states and communities to put into action approaches to divert offenders into treatment programs, particularly those with mental illness charged with nonviolent crimes. These programs include life skills training, vocational training, health care, and relapse prevention. The worker in the field of corrections oftentimes focuses on prevention, such as through work with at-risk youth, active gang members, and current juvenile offenders. A friend of the second author is a parole officer and explains that those who work in probation or parole oftentimes are like "street social workers," working to eradicate poverty, provide counseling, and assist with job placement. The Department of Justice (DOJ) oversees the Office of Juvenile Justice and Delinquency Prevention (OJJDP), which supports states' and communities' efforts to develop programs for the needs of juvenile offenders and their families. There also exists a restorative justice program, a community program that brings together offenders, victims, and families together for conflict resolution. Such programs are designed to reintegrate criminals safely back into society so that they may become productive, contributing members of society. Of course, when criminals pose a threat to the safety and well-being of citizens, they are still locked up and sometimes put to death.

Due to the overwhelming numbers of criminals in society, private organizations and people have taken it upon themselves to intervene in some cases. For example, Oprah Winfrey, a national host of a talk show, has given large sums of money to people whose identification of child abusers leads to their arrest. Another television show, *America's Most Wanted*, hosted by a man whose young son was abducted and murdered, presents case stories of criminals who are at large so that the American public might be able to identify these perpetrators. Such examples of enlisting the help of private citizens indicate the trend in the human services field of asking all members of society to intervene in dealing with those who engage in deviant behavior. The motivation behind private intervention is sometimes profit; often individuals receive rewards for their intervention.

A current trend is the privatization of rehabilitation services for the criminal population. It might be more cost effective for the government to pay private organizations to provide the necessary counseling and job-training services for this population than to house them in prisons, especially if they are assessed to be nonviolent and amenable to rehabilitation. Nonprofit agencies that rely on volunteers wouldn't have the overhead and other expenses that typical correctional facilities have. Unfortunately, whether government or private, most prison employees have little human services training, and as we see an explosion of prison, jail, parole, and probation populations, it is likely that a movement back toward containment and punishment will occur. This is further likely given that, according to the 2011 Pew Center on the States report on recidivism rates, more than four in ten offenders return to state prisons within three years of being released, despite a massive increase in spending on prisons.

Modern Educational System

All communities fund public schools for children in grades kindergarten through 12. Most communities also fund community college programs and even state-funded universities. Within these schools, special programs exist beyond classroom teaching. The educational system is a clear example of publicly funded human services that operate under a bureaucratic organizational structure.

Efforts throughout history to improve education are notable and continue today. In 1975, Congress enacted the Education for All Handicapped Children Act to support states in protecting the rights and meeting the needs of infants, toddlers, children, and youth with disabilities and their families. Prior to this, many states actually had laws that excluded children, such as those who were deaf, blind, or emotionally disturbed. Today, the majority of such children are oftentimes educated in neighborhood schools in typical classrooms with their non-disabled classmates. Another modern support system is the McKinney-Vento

Education for the Homeless Children and Youth Program, which aids children in managing their academic challenges due to being homeless. The act ensures, for example, the inclusion of homeless children into mainstream classrooms, provision of transportation, and designation of a liaison to identify and support homeless children. During the Bush administration (2000–2008), the No Child Left Behind program was proposed. The program was intended to expose all children to the same level of education and therefore increase literacy in our country. The current Obama administration has worked to reform some of the negative unintended consequences of this program, including too much emphasis on absolute scores versus growth and progress. Unfortunately, much work is still left to be done. For example, while it is true that public educational institutions have been studying the effects of racism and discrimination on academic achievement for many years, an efficient change in the educational system has not been markedly demonstrated.

Over the past 20 years, dissatisfaction with public schools has spurred interest in privatizing education. Many Americans (especially those in the middle and upper economic classes) enroll their children in private, for-profit schools because they do not believe their children will receive a rigorous and safe educational experience in the public school system. Because these schools operate on a for-profit basis and often offer more luxurious work environments, they may be enticing teachers and other human services workers away from public educational institutions. The effect of this might be a return, at some level, to segregation. Private schools may also attract the most qualified and experienced teachers and counselors, leaving the public schools with a staff of inexperienced teachers and administrators. Interestingly, many entrepreneur-minded individuals have taken advantage of out-of-pocket educational programs, opening private tutoring businesses. Wealthy citizens who can afford private schools and tutoring might then receive better education while the more poor (and often minority) students would receive inferior instruction and services.

Of course, this may only be an ominous hypothetical scenario, but it is a serious possibility nonetheless. Human services workers in the future must focus on understanding low achievement scores and how they relate to poverty and racial discrimination. Interventions should be aimed at motivating students to achieve higher standards. Human services workers, such as school counselors and counselors and social workers, could run educational groups for families and students and explain how success in school is related to adult success and economic opportunity. Unless these types of services are encouraged, the public educational system might remain deficient.

More on Nonprofits

According to the National Center for Charitable Statistics (2013), there are nearly 1.5 million nonprofits registered currently in the United States. Today, many are more dependent on various government grants for funding. They rely on volunteers and interns, and the pay for employees is often not comparable to those working for private agencies or public agencies. Unlike private or public agencies, nonprofit agencies maintain more autonomy from government regulations than other agencies and still operate from a strongly political perspective than other types of agencies. Additionally, nonprofits, oftentimes founded on grassroots efforts, increase community support and offer innovative and high quality services for those in need. For example, battered women's shelters now not only provide physical safety but also offer mental health support to their communities. The National Adult Protective Services Association is a national nonprofit that provides APS with solutions for improving the quality of services for victims of elder abuse and mistreatment and preventing such abuse, including its mental health consequences, when possible.

Nonprofit Social Welfare Agencies   Some communities have created nonprofit agencies that provide services for homeless people and others who may need food, child care, and clothing. These services may be provided through homeless shelters, church programs, or other agencies such as daycare centers. The focus is providing for basic needs until people can get back on their own feet and provide for themselves. These agencies have become vital in recent decades as governmental funding for financial assistance has been reduced.

Other nonprofit agencies have been developed to assist the child protective welfare system. Various group homes have been created that work collaboratively with county social workers to provide housing for abused children. Also, various nonprofit agencies have been created to provide parenting education for abusive parents who may have lost their children to county child protective services.

Nonprofit Mental Health Agencies   Many U.S. agencies provide mental health counseling for a low fee to their clients. They can offer lower fee services because the programs are funded by grants, donations, and fundraisers. These agencies use more paraprofessionals, volunteers, and interns than public agencies. They are the ideal setting for interns to learn and gain experience and for people to receive the help they need at a low cost.

Nonprofit Agencies That Deal with Correctional Issues   Some facilities contract with governmental agencies to provide monitoring, education, and counseling for people who have violated the law. Some are residential, such as halfway houses (places where convicts may live for up to one year after release from prison), while others are diversion programs at community centers for first-time offenders, such as a teenager caught with drugs. Other facilities offer drug testing and adjunct services, such as counseling, drug education, or anger management groups, for those on probation. These nonprofit programs usually work closely with government officials to ensure that proper services are provided and used by the client, who is often mandated by a judge to use the services.

Nonprofit Educational Programs   There may be some agencies that provide tutoring services for children and adults. One example might be a local library that provides remedial reading courses for adults. These services are usually provided by volunteers. There may not be many opportunities for paid employment in tutoring programs. However, one may tutor privately at any level for pay.

> **Critical Thinking/Self-Reflection Corner**
> - Do you think modern programs are better than those of the past? Why or why not?
> - Do you think current programs are effective? Why or why not?
> - What are some of the unintended, negative consequences of programs offered today to vulnerable populations?
> - What values and ethics do you think drive current programs and policies?
> - What sort of programs do you anticipate for the near future?

INTERVENTIONS

While many of the policies, programs, and approaches to human services delivery discussed here have assisted populations in making changes at a structural level, most of the problems that bring people to see human services workers today must be addressed at the individual or community level. Often, there are specific levels of intervention that are utilized: **micro-**level interventions focus on working with an individual; **mezzo-**level interventions involve working with families and small groups; **macro-**level interventions involve working with organizations and communities (Alle-Corliss & Alle-Corliss, 1999). These are discussed in greater detail in Chapters 11 and 12. Chapter 11 discusses case management, and Chapter 12 continues the discussion on modern-day programs and policies and makes a closer examination of macro-level interventions, including advocacy, lobbying, and program development.

Primary, Secondary, and Tertiary Interventions

Understanding the needs of people who seek services is necessary then to apply the appropriate solution(s) that can range from preventative to life maintenance. These different levels of solutions include primary, secondary, and tertiary interventions. The general notion of prevention evolved by Gerald Caplan (1964), who was introduced in Chapter 1, argued that emotional illness could be prevented through proactive, capacity-building skills. Today, we can apply this approach to all issues, not just psychiatric problems.

Primary Interventions **Primary intervention** usually includes efforts to prevent the occurrence of a disorder or a problem by counteracting circumstances or risk factors that could contribute to or cause the disorder or problem. These efforts are typically used with people who appear to be either functioning normally or at-risk but have not yet demonstrated a need for human services. Broadly speaking, this type of prevention includes social policy development aimed at reducing environmental stress and enhancing life opportunities and educational programs that offer adaptive skills and alternatives to at-risk populations (Price, Cowen, Lorion, & Ramos-McKay, 1988). Some well-known examples include the D.A.R.E. (Drug Awareness Resistance Education) program offered to elementary school children, Scared Straight (a program in which at-risk teens visit prisons and speak with convicts), Project Head Start (a program for low-income, disadvantaged preschoolers), and parenting classes for adolescents in high school. Other examples include child or elder abuse prevention, violence, school safety, disaster or crisis, and divorce.

Secondary Interventions **Secondary interventions** include efforts to assist people who have already demonstrated early signs of dysfunction or problematic behaviors or to reduce the duration of the problem. Such interventions should be immediate, and if provided early enough, the problem's prognosis is good. **Crisis intervention** is one of the best examples of secondary intervention. The goal is to prevent people from developing **chronic** problems and to maintain functioning in as many areas as possible. Many of the problems that are suited for this level of intervention result from situational stress. Some are emergency situations and may have a life-threatening component, such as an attempt at suicide or the onset of psychotic behavior. Others may not necessarily be considered emergencies but should still be dealt with quickly. The crises may arise from normal transitional and developmental situations, such as the birth of a baby, marriage, or adolescent rebellion. Crises may also result from unexpected traumatic events, such as rape, divorce, unemployment, death, diagnosis of an illness, or extreme natural or human-caused disasters, as in the terrorist attacks of September 11, 2001, and Hurricane Katrina's destruction in New Orleans in 2005.

Tertiary Interventions **Tertiary interventions** are typically used with people who suffer from chronic problems and have difficulties caring for themselves. The goal often is to reorient individuals and return them to a more productive capacity. Many of these people are in a state of chronic distress and need ongoing rehabilitation and possibly even long-term institutionalization. Examples of tertiary care include long-term stays at psychiatric hospitals, ongoing psychotherapy or attendance at Alcoholics Anonymous meetings, incarceration, and indefinite periods in residential facilities.

Unfortunately, secondary and tertiary programs receive the largest portion of government funds (Newton, 1988). It might be more useful to fund programs that prevent problems from occurring rather than waiting for problems to materialize before fixing them.

Harm Reduction Models

Although controversial, many human services workers and practitioners support **harm reduction models**, an approach to looking at and responding to self-destructive problems, such as drug abuse, that does not require complete abstinence. It is based on the stages of change model, which suggests that people go through stages in the process of changing themselves and their behaviors. The focus of this approach shifts from the drug use to the harm associated with it. This approach may be useful for clients who are not willing to stop using drugs but who still need assistance. Treatment providers work to meet the clients where they are and not where they wish they would be in terms of usage. Many argue that this provides a more nonjudgmental, noncoercive approach to providing services and increasing one's motivation for achieving a healthier life overall.

> **Critical Thinking/Self-Reflection Corner**
> - If you were a human services worker in prevention, which level of prevention would you be most interested to engage in? Why?
> - What skills are required of human services workers to effectively work at the primary, secondary, and tertiary levels of prevention? Do you think these skills differ or vary depending on the level of prevention?
> - What are your thoughts on harm reduction models? Do you think this approach is more useful for certain problems or populations than others? Explain.

DEMOGRAPHIC SHIFTS AND CONSIDERATIONS

Modern-day human services policies, approaches, and programs are highly influenced by the needs of the population. As mentioned at the beginning of this chapter, population shifts and demographic changes have made approaches to human services more complex than ever and require that human services workers consider the unique cultural needs of people more critically than ever before, especially when designing and implementing policies, programs, and services. **Culture** can be thought of as operating both within and outside of us. At the individual level, it refers to a person's values, beliefs, explanatory systems, and behaviors that are learned in the family and within social groups (Hogan-Garcia, 1999). A consideration of culture often includes age, gender, race and ethnicity, socioeconomic status or social class, sexual orientation, religion, and disability or functional level, some of which are discussed in the sections that follow.

The Graying of America

One of the greatest changes in our society is attributed to the increasingly aging population, oftentimes referred to as the graying of America. According to the National Institutes on Aging, today people age 50 and over comprise 24 percent of the U.S. population, with 17 million Americans between 75 and 85 years old. By 2060, the population age 65 and older is projected to reach 90 million, with 23 percent of the population being 85 and older by 2050 (Himes, 2002). These changes are in part due to the decreases in mortality and concurrent increases in life expectancy such as due to better nutrition, safety, and advanced technology, as well as the fact that **baby boomers** (those born between 1946 and 1964, the post–World War II baby boom), nearly 76 million of them, are entering older adulthood. Overall, between 2000 and 2020, the U.S. population will add

19 million older adults with the number of older adults in this country, growing by 138 percent in the next 50 years. By the year 2050, one in five Americans will be age 65 or older.

Within this population, there exists significant cultural variation due to gender, race and ethnicity, and economic status—major factors when addressing aging clients in the field of human services. For example, a growing percentage of older adults will be racially and ethnically diverse, particularly due to the increase in Asian and Hispanic older adults; this requires that our health care workforce be more multilingual and culturally competent than in previous years. Additionally, the projected demand for human services from older adults likely outweighs what is currently available, or unfortunately, the demand is being met by professionals with limited training on supporting older adults. The increasing need for competent professionals and paraprofessionals to serve older adults will also be affected by health insurance policies, emerging technologies, new models of care, and changes in health care delivery practices (Center for Health Workforce Studies, 2006).

Immigration

Another major source of demographic change is due to increased immigration. Over the last 20 years or so, immigration has expanded tremendously; 2010 census data indicates that the U.S. immigrant population was about 40 million or 13 percent of the total population. The number of unauthorized immigrants living in the United States also grew from 8.4 million in 2000 to 11.1 million in 2011 (Passel & Cohn, 2011). Interestingly, of this group, many have lived in the United States for over a decade. While public opinion varies across political groups, there is no denying that human services workers will need to address the needs of immigrants. Understanding cultural and ethnic differences among all those living in the United States is necessary for strong human services delivery. Unfortunately, this is often easier said than done. According to the Assistant Secretary for Planning and Evaluation (ASPE) through the U.S. DHHS (2011), "Immigrant eligibility for health and human service benefits is complicated by a confusing patchwork quilt of federal statutory provisions, state and local benefit program choices and decisions, the mixed citizenship/immigration status of members in many immigrant families (e.g., immigrant parents who may be ineligible, with citizen children who are eligible), and the varying immigration enforcement efforts and initiatives not only at the federal level, but more recently at the state and local levels as well. Recent enactment of health care reform provisions may further complicate the policy environment and result in additional challenges and opportunities affecting immigrant families' access to health and human services and the wellbeing of these families."

Ethnic/Racial Considerations

Additionally, human services delivery also varies widely by **ethnoracial** status. For example, health-seeking behaviors, adherence to medical regimens, self-care practices, and utilization of health care all are influenced by one's cultural heritage (Kar, Kramer, Skinner, & Zambrana, 1995). Unfortunately, many human services workers are lacking the necessary multicultural awareness training to appropriately develop and implement related programs and services. For example, many who are part of the Latino culture embrace *marianisma*, a value placed on women who are self-sacrificing and who place the needs of everyone else's above their own. Sometimes, such women will experience *ataque de nervios*, which can manifest itself in a combination of symptoms of depression, panic disorder, and generalized anxiety disorder (Kanel, 2005; Koss-Chioino, 1999; Liebowitz et al., 1994; Oquendo, 1995; Schechter et al., 2000). However, many sufferers may not seek traditional support but rather alternative health care providers, such as curanderos, spiritual and curing leaders who are popular among those who practice Mexican folk healing.

A second example of the importance of being aware of culture can be seen in the research by Kim, Liang, and Li (2003) and Uba (1994) with findings that Asian American communication styles, compared to other ethnic groups, tend to be less expressive and more reticent and restrained in nonverbal behavioral expression. In general, traditional Asian cultures value control over emotional expressiveness even among family members and consider such control a sign of strength (Hsu, Tseng, Ashton, McDermott, & Char, 1985). This behavior is vastly different from mainstream American culture that expects people to openly and directly express affection and other strong emotions with family and friends alike. These and other studies of Asian culture should help human services workers keep in mind the effect free emotional expression can have on their Asian clients and be conscious of not pushing them into doing so. Instead, workers should allow their clients to communicate in ways that are comfortable to them so that they can work through their problems and get their needs met, even if it means taking a more indirect approach than usual.

Overall, whether working with older adults, immigrants, various racial/ethnic groups, as well as religious groups (such as Protestants, Catholics, Jews, Muslims, or Buddhists), the disabled, lesbian, gay, bisexual, transgender, queer, and intersexed (LGBTQI) communities, or those from different social classes than your own, it is imperative that each person's or group's needs, strengths, and experiences are taken into account. Strong awareness of the prejudice, stereotypes, bias, and discrimination (defined in Chapter 1) these groups have likely experienced is critical. Thus, moving away from mainstream interventions and developing and implementing more culturally sensitive and appropriate services and policies are necessary.

Multicultural Programs and Policies

The U.S. DHHS houses the Office of Minority Health. It was created in 1986 and is dedicated to improving the health of racial and ethnic minority populations through policies and programs. In addition, many state-wide departments of mental health have offices offering multicultural services. These are charged with developing services that are multicultural and linguistically appropriate as

> ### The Impact of Culture on Humans
>
> Everybody has culture, even though some folks think they don't. Culture is ever present. It greets you when you and the sun first wake up in the morning and it rests with you when you get comfortable enough to fall asleep and say the day is over. Culture is how you love and who you choose to love. It's whether you eat cornbread or pumpernickel. It's how you respond to the dilemmas life offers and how you celebrate living. It shows itself without you knowing and it tells who you are without you speaking. Culture includes all your family, even those who are dead and gone because they are the ones who set the cultural patterns you follow ....
>
> —From *The Color of Culture* (1993) by Mona Lake Jones

well as ensuring that practitioners are trained to deliver appropriate health and social services for diverse communities. Whether providing services to the aged, disabled, AIDS/HIV community, or a specific ethnicity, it is critical that programs take into account the individual or community members' experiences, as well as feelings of power, safety, and needs. Culturally competent programs (Chin, 2000) must also ensure that (1) providers are well trained (e.g., can translate and interpret, know how to ask about and discuss cultural issues), (2) cultural and linguistic barriers to accessing care have been removed (e.g., lack of translated materials can make it hard to make appointments or understand necessary terminology), (3) processes ensuring service utilization are in place (e.g., many low-income immigrants and refugees from ethnic minority groups often delay entry into care and then overutilize high-cost emergency rooms because of cultural barriers), and (4) high-quality care is provided (e.g., many human services providers need more training to become aware of their own biases and assumptions about how they work with and treat their clients).

Sociological Considerations

While it is beyond the scope of this book to elaborate the true extent of the role of culture as it relates to modern-day human services, we urge readers to take it upon themselves to read about sociological theories of maladaptive behaviors, especially among vulnerable or at-risk populations. Briefly, **sociological theories** explain how societal phenomenon are caused by external (not internal to a person, such as biology and genetics) and environmental conditions that shape **social values** and **politics** (power and influence) and can lead to prejudice, stereotypes, and discrimination. These factors are salient considerations when developing and/or implementing multicultural programs. Sociological theories also explain how maladaptive behaviors, such as substance abuse, criminality, and violence, are shaped by social norms and by those who have influence.

Violence as an Example According to Levin and Rabrenovic (2007), there are a few overarching sociological theories that help to explain violence, each of which seeks to explain violence as a function of social structures and systems. These theories include strain theory (social structures and relationships cause frustration leading some to react with violence), social disorganization theory (physical factors in the neighborhood environment such as chaos and poverty create social conditions that leads to violence), and benefit theory (violence occurs when the social costs are low but the benefits are high, like affiliation with a gang that provides support and camaraderie for needy youth). These perspectives point to the social, community (a form of culture) influences of violence and not individual causes. Taking such viewpoints into account provides human services professionals more accurate, comprehensive, holistic, and, of course, multicultural approaches to preventing and solving problems prevalent in our society.

Violence against women has long been thought to be in part due to the lack of a zero tolerance of violence toward women in our society. Many women across many cultures have been socialized to accept that men have bad tempers and that women must stay with a man in order to have worth in society. This often leads to women enduring violence in relationships and to many men believing their violence is justified, especially if society offers no severe consequences for it.

A Multicultural Violence Prevention Program In 2007, MALDEF, the Latino Legal Voice for Civil Rights in America, together with the Asian Pacific American League Center (APALC) and the Los Angeles, California, Urban League, has created the Los Angeles Domestic Violence Prevention Collaborative—a cooperative to raise multicultural awareness of domestic violence. One of their goals is to provide community outreach, educational materials, and low-cost or free services. Many of these services are in both English and Spanish, with culturally and linguistically appropriate ads including such phrases as "Stand up for Respect!/Lucha por el Respeto!"

Critical Thinking/Self-Reflection Corner

- What culture(s) are you part of? How does this shape the way you work or will work with others?
- What stereotypes do you hold of others? Have you ever experienced prejudice? How did it feel? What did you do?
- What cultures are you not comfortable working with? Why?
- What are three things you can do to become more knowledgeable about other cultures and to become more comfortable working with them?
- If you understand that dysfunction is in part caused by environmental conditions, such as violence, poverty, or discrimination, how would you best provide services to your clients? What sort of programs would best address the related problems?

CHAPTER SUMMARY

Modern human services program, policies, and interventions reflect the rights that Americans have to life, liberty, and the pursuit of happiness. Compared to decades ago, Americans today thankfully have more rights to advocate for themselves and to improve the society. For example, there is a growing commitment to destigmatizing or deinstitutionalizing mental illness. While we continue asking some basic questions, such as "Who deserves help?" "Who has power or is given power?" and "To what extent are we responsible to help others?" We also now ask other relevant questions, including "How can we meet the needs of an ever-changing, multicultural society?" "What types of programs can we/should we develop to improve the well-being of Americans, especially of those in need?" and "What ethics and social values should continue to guide us in the field of human services?" In the future, human services professionals will face new challenges, and innovative ideas will be required. Whether working at the individual, family, community, or government level, efforts and commitment to improving accessibility, accountability, and coordination of service delivery to increase the quality of life of people remains a top priority.

Suggested Applied Activities

1. Working independently or in groups, develop ideas for primary, secondary, and tertiary programs or related activities for a topic or population of your choice, such as teen pregnancy, AIDS/HIV, child abuse, and dating violence.

2. Given the changing nature of society, make a list and describe at least five competencies human services workers must develop or enhance to be effective.

3. Complete the personal bias inventory. After you complete the inventory, review your responses and discuss them with classmates or another group of students. Compare and contrast your responses and explore where and why you responded as you did.

Personal Bias Inventory

Circle either true (T) or false (F) in response to each item.

T F 1. Men are smarter than women in math and science.
T F 2. Women can cook better than men can.
T F 3. Men do not have feelings such as sadness and loneliness.
T F 4. Women are less capable than men of controlling their emotions.
T F 5. More women than men are neurotic.
T F 6. Men don't need professional help as much as women do.
T F 7. Women are worse than men at driving.
T F 8. Women are better than men at parenting.
T F 9. Men are better than women at managing money.
T F 10. Women are more dependent on men than men are dependent on women.
T F 11. Gay men are promiscuous.
T F 12. Lesbians want to look like men.
T F 13. Homosexuals dress better than straight men do.

T F 14. Homosexuality is a sin against nature.
T F 15. Being gay is a symptom of deep psychological issues.
T F 16. Bisexuals just have identity issues.
T F 17. Someone who has a sex-change operation is deeply disturbed emotionally.
T F 18. Gay men are flamboyant.
T F 19. Most lesbians were raped or molested as children.
T F 20. Gay people try to turn straight people gay.
T F 21. Old people are stupid and only talk about boring things.
T F 22. Old people shouldn't be allowed to work because they are too slow.
T F 23. New college graduates are more energetic and deserve to be hired over middle-aged people.
T F 24. Teenagers are wild and cannot be trusted.
T F 25. Teenagers take drugs and drink alcohol and shouldn't be allowed to drive.
T F 26. Children should be seen and not heard.
T F 27. Poor people are lazy and enjoy handouts.
T F 28. Wealthy people are ruthless and arrogant.
T F 29. Blue-collar workers have average intelligence.
T F 30. Muslims cannot be trusted because any one of them could be a terrorist.
T F 31. Muslims are stupid because they dress in old-fashioned clothing.
T F 32. Buddhists will never go to heaven because they don't believe in God.
T F 33. Atheists are immoral people.
T F 34. Christians are the only people who will go to heaven.
T F 35. Catholics are ignorant because they don't use birth control.
T F 36. Protestants try to convert everyone to their religion.
T F 37. Jewish people are greedy and stingy.
T F 38. God will not let Jews into heaven because they don't worship Jesus.
T F 39. Latinos are all uneducated and ignorant.
T F 40. Most Mexicans who live in the United States are here illegally.
T F 41. African Americans are better athletes than those of other races.
T F 42. African Americans aren't smart enough to get into college unless they have an athletic scholarship
T F 43. Asians are smarter than other races.

T	F	44. Arabs are sneaky and shouldn't be allowed to live in the United States.
T	F	45. Latino men are male chauvinist pigs.
T	F	46. Asians are obedient.
T	F	47. Arab women have low self-esteem.
T	F	48. Mentally retarded people are of no use to society.
T	F	49. Caucasians think they are better than all other races.
T	F	50. All Native Americans are alcoholics.

4. Complete the Fourteen Personal Competencies Self-Test (Hogan, 2013) by rating yourself on a scale of 1 (low) to 5 (high) in each of the competencies. These competencies are important for developing competency in cultural diversity. After you complete the inventory, review your responses and discuss them with classmates or another group of students. Compare and contrast your responses and explore where and why you responded as you did. Reflect on your answers and your commitment to becoming more culturally aware.

_____

_____

_____

_____

_____

_____

_____

_____

Fourteen Personal Competencies Self-Test (Hogan, 2013)

1. _____Be nonjudgmental
2. _____Be flexible
3. _____Be resourceful
4. _____Personalize observations
5. _____Pay attention to your thoughts/feelings
6. _____Listen carefully
7. _____Observe attentively
8. _____Assume complexity
9. _____Tolerate the stress of uncertainty

10. _____Have patience
11. _____Manage personal biases and stereotypes
12. _____Keep a sense of humor
13. _____Show respect
14. _____Display empathy

Evaluating the score:

Add up the points:

61–70 Highly competent

51–60 Moderately competent

0–50 Need more practice

Chapter Review Questions

1. What policies and programs are in place today to assist those with mental illness?

2. What is the Patient Protection and Affordable Care Act? Why is the act controversial?

3. What role do nonprofits play in the field of human services? Why are they important?

4. What have been some modern responses to the issue of crime?

5. What are some challenges that the modern educational system faces?

6. What are the differences among primary, secondary, and tertiary levels of prevention?

7. What are harm reduction models? Why are they controversial?

8. What demographic and cultural shifts have occurred that are dramatically shaping the field of humans services?

9. What are some characteristics of culturally competent programs?

10. What are sociological theories? Why are they important to consider when trying to understand deviant or maladaptive behaviors?

Glossary of Terms

Adult protective services are government-run agencies that attempt to stop elder-related abuse and prosecute the abusers.

Baby boomers are those born between 1946 and 1964, the post–World War II baby boom.

Child protective services are government-run agencies that respond to reports of child abuse or neglect.

Chronic refers to illness or health issues that persist for a long time or are regularly recurring.

Community Mental Health Act of 1963 was signed into law by President Kennedy and drastically altered the delivery of mental health services, including comprehensive community mental health centers, across the nation.

Crisis intervention addresses acute critical situations in the hopes of restoring persons back to their typical level of functioning.

Culture is the full range of human behaviors and patterns and includes a person's values, beliefs, explanatory systems, and behaviors that are learned in the family and within social groups.

Ethnoracial is a way of defining persons based on a blending of one's national heritage and ethnic identity.

Harm reduction models refer to policies, programs, and practices that aim to reduce the harms associated with the use of harmful substances rather than focusing on prevention of the substance itself.

Health maintenance organizations (HMOs) are privately funded agencies in which medical, psychological, optical, and even dental needs may be serviced through a family's insurance plan.

Medicaid is a governmental program that provides medical and health-related services to certain individuals and families with low incomes and few resources.

Medicare is a federal health insurance program that pays for hospital and medical care for older persons and certain disabled Americans.

Macro refers to a level of focus on community organizations and on creating new policies.

Mezzo is a level of intervention that focuses on working with groups and families.

Micro is a level of intervention that deals with individuals.

Patient Protection and Affordable Care Act, commonly called the Affordable Care Act, is a U.S. federal statute signed into law by President Obama with the goal of overhauling the country's health care system by increasing health insurance quality and affordability.

Politics typically refers to government or governing and also includes the practice of trying to influence and gain power over others.

Primary intervention refers to efforts to prevent the occurrence of a disorder or a problem by counteracting circumstances or risk factors that could contribute to or cause the disorder or problem.

Secondary intervention refers to efforts to assist people who have already demonstrated early signs of dysfunction or problematic behaviors or to reduce the duration of the problem.

Social values are ethics based on one's personal and cultural experiences that guide or shape an individual's or a group's behaviors, actions, and belief systems.

Sociological theories are a set of interrelated concepts and ideas that help to explain influences on or causes of human behaviors and actions.

Tertiary intervention is targeted toward a person who already has symptoms of illness or who engages in maladaptive behaviors, with the goal of preventing further damage, reducing further complications, or rehabilitating the person.

Case Presentation and Exit Quiz

General Description

John is a 34-year-old man who is married to Sandy, a 29-year-old stay-at-home mom. John and Sandy have two children. One of the children is disabled; he has a genetic spinal cord deficit and is in a wheelchair. John was recently fired from his job because his employer did not want to offer him the necessary medical insurance to cover his chronic depression. Although John is actively looking for another job, he is concerned about not being able to appropriately feed and clothe his family. In addition, John and Sandy are struggling with the elementary school where their children attend. Their disabled child is being teased and taunted by his classmates. The teacher informed Sandy it may be best to move him to a private school.

Problems That Need Assistance

First, John was fired illegally from his job. He has the right to contact the NAMI and get support, including legal assistance, to sue his former employer. Second,

John and Sandy need to immediately get their basic needs met, including food and possibly shelter. Third, regarding their child who is disabled, their son has a right to be in mainstream classes with typically developing children. John and Sandy have the right to protect their child and can contact the principal and district office to ensure their son receives the same quality and access to safe education as his classmates.

Exit Quiz

1. Under what act was John illegally fired?
    a. Paul Wellstone and Pete Domenici Mental Health Parity and Addiction Equity Act
    b. Patient Protection and Affordable Care Act
    c. Medicare

2. To get their basic needs met, what options are available to John and Sandy?
    a. Medicaid
    b. Local nonprofits
    c. Local social welfare office
    d. All of the above

3. If John and Sandy were working with a case manager, what level of intervention would be most effectively applied?
    a. Primary
    b. Secondary
    c. Tertiary
    d. Crisis
    e. b and d

4. Under which act does John and Sandy's disabled son have rights?
    a. Community Mental Health Act of 1963
    b. New Freedom Initiative
    c. McKinney-Vento Education for the Homeless Children and Youth Program
    d. Education for All Handicapped Children Act.

Exit Quiz Answers

1. a
2. d
3. e
4. d

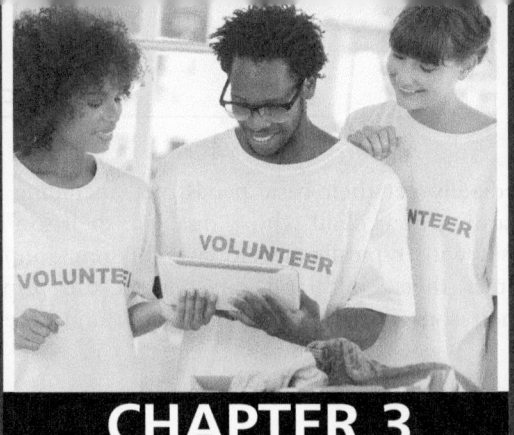

CHAPTER 3

Ethical and Multicultural Issues in the Human Services

INTRODUCTION

The field of human services places a strong emphasis on adhering to specific ethical standards. Recipients of human services are often vulnerable because of the many needs for which they seek help. When people are vulnerable, they may be easily taken advantage of or manipulated. **Ethics** ensure that clients who seek help from human services providers are treated with respect, dignity, and honesty.

WHAT ARE ETHICS?

Ethics are standards of conduct that human services professionals have agreed are vital to appropriate and effective interventions. Although a variety of professional organizations have determined what they consider ethical behavior to be, there is very little disagreement among these organizations. There seem to be some basic ethical standards that cross over among the various human services disciplines.

In general, "ethical issues usually refer to moral imperatives; the 'shoulds' and 'oughts' directed toward protecting the welfare of those who require services of helping professionals and are regulated by the professions. Legal issues refer to the efforts of governmental administrative agencies, legislatures, and the courts to create rules of law which govern the practice of psychology, psychiatry, social work, and counseling" (Herr & Cramer, 1987, p. 156). Sometimes behaviors that are considered unethical are also illegal.

WHY ARE ETHICS NECESSARY?

Although following prescribed rules and standards may seem burdensome and diminish autonomy, in fact, ethical standards benefit human services workers. By knowing and adhering to ethical standards, human services workers are protected from frivolous lawsuits that some clients might file against workers and agencies. Unless clients can prove in a court of law or with a professional organization that a worker engaged in unethical or illegal behaviors, they aren't likely to win such lawsuits. Conservative ethical practice can be a relief to human services workers because they know they won't be liable for sanctions if they follow approved ethical standards.

Ethical standards also protect the consumer. People who reach out to human services workers deserve to receive competent, objective, and fair services. Ethics ensure that people receive services from qualified workers, workers who understand the personal effect they may have on clients, and from workers who provide confidential services that permit clients to be open and trusting.

A third benefit of ethics is that by having the standards written down and standardized there is less opportunity for bickering among helping professionals. Common sense would suggest that if the majority agrees that certain behaviors should be practiced, then those who disagree should have to go along with the majority. Of course, there is always room for changing ethics as new technologies, new problems, and different cultural issues arise. For example, online technology has created an industry where people can access counseling services by logging onto a computer. The ethical standards of the 1980s did not include such services, and so various professional organizations have been discussing this issue and have made certain specific standards regarding the use of the Internet to provide and advertise services. Another example has to do with how workers are to handle the confidentiality standard when working with people who are HIV positive. As HIV is known to be lethal to others, should a human services worker be forced to breach **confidentiality** if he or she finds out that an HIV-positive person is having unprotected sex with someone? These are the types of questions that professional organizations consider and respond to in forming new ethical standards.

As each major mental health, medical, and social welfare professional organization has its own code of ethics, the reader should obtain a copy of the ethical codes of the profession when he or she is sure about what field he or she wishes to pursue as a career. The written standards are often lengthy and would take up many pages to include in this text. Following is a list of many of the various codes of ethics applicable to the field of human services:

1. Code of Ethics, the American Counseling Association (ACA, 2005)
2. Ethical Principles of Psychologists and Code of Conduct, American Psychological Association (APA, 2002)
3. Code of Ethics, National Association of Social Workers (NASW, 1999)
4. AAMFT Code of Ethics, American Association for Marriage and Family Therapy (AAMFT, 2001)

5. Ethical Standards of the National Organization for Human Services, National Organization for Human Services (NOHS, 2000)
6. Code of Professional Ethics for Rehabilitation Counselors, Commission of Rehabilitation Counselor Certification (CRCC, 2001)
7. CCA Code of Ethics, Canadian Counseling Association, (CCA, 1999)
8. Ethical Standards for School Counselors, American School Counselor Association (ASCA, 2004)
9. Ethical Guidelines for Counseling Supervisors, Association for Counselor Education and Supervision (ACES, 1995)
10. Feminist Therapy Code of Ethics, Feminist Therapy Institute (FTI, 2000)
11. The Principles of Medical Ethics with Annotations Especially Applicable to Psychiatry, American Psychiatric Association (APA, 2001)

The National Association of Human Services

As this is a text on human services, we will discuss the creation and purpose of the organizations specifically focused on human services professionals. When the country made a shift to human services generalist positions, a national organization was developed. In 1972, the National Organization of Human Services (NOHS) was created for graduates and students of mental health and human services programs. The name was changed several times: first in 1975 when it was called the National Organization for Human Service Educators, then in 1985 it was changed to the National Organization for Human Service Education, then finally in 2005 to its current and first name, the National Organization of Human Services (Council on Standards for Human Service Education, 2013).

Shortly after the NOHS was developed, an accrediting organization was then formed called the Council of Standards in Human Service Education (CSHSE). This council has created standards that guide human services training programs nationwide. As the field of human services was relatively new on college campuses and within the professional community, it was vital to establish itself as a viable and appropriate field of study with strict standards that were monitored. Table 3.1 presents these standards regarding how human services professionals and paraprofessionals shall be trained.

The CSHSE and the NOHS have created their own ethical standards for human services professionals as well. Table 3.2 presents most of the statements of ethical behaviors put forth by these organizations.

With regard to responsibility toward the community and society, human services professionals should:

1. be aware of local, state, and federal laws and advocate for change in regulations and statues when such legislation conflicts with ethical guidelines or client rights; where laws are harmful to individuals, groups, or communities they should consider the conflict between the values of obeying the law and the values of serving people and may decide to initiate social action

TABLE 3.1	Standards of the CSHSE
1. The primary program objective shall be to prepare human services professionals to serve individuals, families, groups, communities and/or other supported human services organization functions.	
Each educational program shall:	
2. have an explicit philosophical statement and clearly defined knowledge base	
3. include periodic mechanisms for assessment of a response to changing policies, needs, and trends of the profession and community	
4. conduct consistent formal evaluative processes to determine its effectiveness in meeting the needs of the students, the community, and the human services field and to modify the program as necessary	
5. have written standards and procedures for admitting, retaining, and dismissing students	
6. include faculty with both a strong and diverse knowledge base and clinical/practical experience in the delivery of human services to clients	
7. adequately manage the essential program roles and provide professional development opportunities for faculty and staff	
8. include evaluations for each faculty and staff member that reflect the essential roles, and evaluations shall be conducted at least every two years	
9. have adequate faculty, staff, and program resources to provide a complete program	
10. make efforts to increase the transferability of credits to other academic programs	
11. include the historical development of human services	
12. include knowledge and theory of human systems, including individual, interpersonal, group, family, organizational, community, and societal systems and their interaction	
13. address the conditions that promote or limit human functioning	
14. provide knowledge and skill training in systematic analysis of service needs; selection of appropriate strategies, services, or interventions; and evaluation of outcomes	
15. provide knowledge and skills in information management	
16. provide knowledge and skills in human services interventions that are appropriate to the level of education	
17. provide learning experiences to students to develop his or her interpersonal skills	
18. provide knowledge, theory, and skills in the administrative aspects of the services delivery system	
19. incorporate human services values and attitudes and promote understanding of human services ethics and their application in practice	
20. provide experiences and support to enable students to develop awareness of their own values, personalities, reaction patterns, interpersonal styles, and limitations	
21. provide field experience that is integrated with the curriculum	
22. award academic credit for field experience.	

Source: (CSHSE, 2013).

Digital Download Download at CengageBrain.com

TABLE 3.2 Ethical Standards for Human Services Professionals

With regard to responsibility toward clients, human services professionals:

1. negotiate with clients the purpose, goals, and nature of the helping relationship prior to its onset as well as inform clients of the limitations of the proposed relationship
2. respect the integrity and welfare of the client at all times and treat each client with respect, acceptance, and dignity
3. protect the client's right to privacy and confidentiality except when such confidentiality would cause harm to the client or others, when agency guidelines state otherwise, or under other stated conditions and inform clients of the limits of confidentiality prior to the onset of the helping relationship
4. act in an appropriate and professional manner to protect the safety of clients who are suspected to be a danger to self or others to protect the safety of all, which may involve seeking consultation, supervisions, and/or breaking the confidentiality of the relationship
5. protect the integrity, safety, and security of client records and make sure to get the client's prior written consent before sharing client information with other professionals except in the course of professional supervision
6. are aware that in their relationship with clients, power and status are unequal and therefore recognize that dual or multiple relationships may increase the risk of harm to or exploitation of client and may impair professional judgment, but that in some communities and situations it may not be feasible to avoid social contact with the client; and will avoid dual relationships that may impair professional judgment
7. realize that sexual relationships with current clients are not considered to be in the best interest of the client and are prohibited, and sexual relationships with previous clients are considered dual relationships
8. realize that the client's right to self-determination is protected and that clients have the right to receive or refuse services
9. recognize and build on client strengths.

Source: (CSHSE, 2013)

2. keep themselves informed about current social issues as they affect the client and the community and share that information with clients, groups, and the community as part of their work
3. understand the complex interactions among individuals, their families, the communities in which they live, and society
4. act as advocates in addressing unmet client and community needs and provide a mechanism for identifying unmet needs, calling attention to these needs, and assisting in planning and mobilizing to advocate for those needs at the local community level
5. represent their qualifications to the public accurately
6. describe the effectiveness of programs, treatments, and/or techniques accurately
7. advocate for the rights of all members of society, particularly those who are members of minorities and groups at which discriminatory practices have historically been directed
8. provide services without discrimination or preference based on age, ethnicity, culture, race, disability, gender, religion, sexual orientation, or socioeconomic status
9. be knowledgeable about the culture and communities within which they practice, be aware of multiculturalism in society and of its impact on the

community as well as on individuals within the community, and respect individuals and groups, their cultures, and their beliefs
10. be aware of their own cultural backgrounds, beliefs, and values, recognizing the potential for impact on their relationship with others
11. be aware of sociopolitical issues that differentially affect clients from diverse backgrounds
12. undertake the training, experience, education, and supervision necessary to ensure their effectiveness in working with culturally diverse clients.

With regard to responsibility toward colleagues, human services professionals should:

1. avoid duplicating another professional's helping relationship with a client and consult with other professionals who are assisting the client in a different type of relationship when it is in the best interest of the client to do so
2. seek out the colleague when he or she has a conflict with a colleague and attempt to manage the problem and when necessary seek the assistance of supervisors or consultants in an effort to manage the problem
3. respond appropriately to unethical behavior of colleagues, talking directly with the colleague, reporting the colleague's behavior to supervisory or administrative staff or to the professional organization to which colleague belongs
4. keep consultations between professionals confidential unless to do so would result in harm to clients or communities.

With regard to responsibility toward the profession, human services professionals should:

1. know the limit and scope of their professional knowledge and offer services only within their knowledge and skill base
2. seek appropriate consultation and supervision to assist in decision making when there are legal, ethical, or other dilemmas
3. act with integrity, honesty, genuineness, and objectivity
4. promote cooperation among related disciplines to foster professional growth and interests within the various fields
5. promote the continuing development of their profession and encourage membership in professional associations, support research endeavors, foster educational advancement, advocate for appropriate legislative actions, and participate in other related professional activities
6. continually seek out new and effective approaches to enhance their professional abilities.

(National Organization of Human Services, 2013)

Five ethical issues are discussed in the sections that follow: (1) confidentiality, (2) **dual relationships**, (3) self-monitoring and **self-examination**, (4) ensuring ethical competence through **continuing education** and supervision, and (5) multicultural competence. These particular issues were selected because most of the professions emphasize these concerns in their stated standards, and they apply to many different types of human services workers and client populations.

CONFIDENTIALITY

Confidentiality relates to the concept of privacy. Siegel (1979) defines it as "the freedom of individuals to choose for themselves the time and the circumstances under which and the extent to which their beliefs, behaviors, and opinions are to be shared or withheld from others" (p. 251). The ethical standard of confidentiality is meant to reassure clients that they can speak freely to a human services worker without the fear that their confidential information will be disclosed. When clients are open and honest, workers can more effectively meet their needs.

The legal counterpart to the ethical concept of confidentiality is referred to as **privilege**. This is the term used in court actions and "refers to a rule in evidence law that provides a litigant with the right to withhold evidence in a legal proceeding that was originally communicated in confidence" (Swoboda, Elwork, Sales, & Levine, 1978, p. 449). Privileged communication in professional relationships requires mutual trust, such as that between client and attorney, therapist and client, doctor and patient, and priest and church member.

When confidentiality is broken, a professional may be considered to have engaged in unprofessional conduct and may be subject to disciplinary action, such as a suspended license or mandatory education courses on ethical standards. Many states have statutes that consider violations of confidentiality a misdemeanor, and if someone is found guilty, he or she may be imprisoned or required to pay a fine or both (Benitez, 2004, p. 32).

Privacy for people receiving services in any health care organization is such an important issue that Congress passed legislation in 1996 designed to standardize exactly how information might be disclosed by health care providers nationwide, which took effect on April 14, 2003 (Brohl & Ledford, 2012). The **Health Insurance Portability and Accountability Act** (HIPAA) includes four components that aim to streamline communication among health care providers and afford patients more rights. The first component—privacy requirements—creates rights for patients concerning how their health information is used and disclosed by health care providers. It limits what a health care provider can do with a patient's health information without that patient's knowledge and consent. It also sets up standards that require health care providers to keep patient information confidential and secure. While most human services and health care institutions have been practicing under ethical codes requiring the confidential treatment of patient information, this act ensures that all providers in all states adhere to strict privacy standards. The other three components provide standards regarding security of information, how to secure electronic transactions, and how to set up national identifier requirements for health care providers.

Exceptions to Confidentiality

While every attempt should be made to ensure a client's privacy, some situations do require that confidentiality be breached. Situations that have the potential to inflict serious harm or cause destruction need to be revealed.

Mandatory Reporting Standards Since the passage of the Child Abuse Prevention and Treatment Act in 1974, all states in the nation have been required to set up standards for the identification, treatment, and prevention of child abuse. This created **mandatory reporting standards** for professionals who engage in the care or treatment of minors, and the act was amended and reauthorized in 2003 by the Keeping Children and Families Safe Act (P.L. 108-36) (U.S. Department of Health and Human Services, 2010). Mandated reporters may include social workers, teachers, principals, health care providers, counselors/therapists and other mental health professionals, child care providers, and law enforcement officers—and interestingly, in some states, it may also include commercial film and photograph processors. Federal laws also address elder abuse, neglect, and exploitation. However, where and how to report elder abuse varies from state to state, although states are the primary source of sanction and protections related to elder abuse. For example, the elder abuse law in California focuses on the Elder Abuse and Dependent Adult Civil Protection Act (EADACPA), which mandates that the state has a responsibility to protect such persons and that required professionals who intervene with the elderly or disabled adult populations should report suspected instances of abuse to appropriate agencies. Recently, as part of the Patient Protection and Affordable Care Act, the Elder Justice Act of 2009 was enacted in 2010. This act coordinates federal elder abuse detection and prevention programs, including a mandate that owners, operators, and employees of long-term care facilities report suspected elder abuse crimes. In many states, mandated reporters for elder abuse include care custodians, health practitioners, law enforcement officials, clergy members, care providers, advocates, and bank tellers. Also, urban areas usually have agencies specifically designed to manage abuse reports, whereas rural areas depend on the law enforcement agency to manage such reports. Abuse of children, elderly, and disabled require breaching confidentiality.

Duty to Warn Another area in which workers must breach confidentiality and report disclosures to appropriate agencies is when a client poses a serious threat of physical violence against a reasonably identifiable victim or victims. This exception to confidentiality is known as the **duty to warn**. The worker must immediately report such danger to the law enforcement agency. Duty to warn is not applicable when clients pose a danger to themselves but not to others. In cases where clients plan to hurt themselves, workers are not mandated to inform law enforcement officials. However, a worker is permitted to breach confidentiality if it is necessary to prevent an act of suicide or self-harm.

Other Exceptions to Confidentiality Other mandatory exceptions to confidentiality occur when a court order, subpoena, or search warrant is issued, when a coroner requests records as part of an investigation, and when the client

TABLE 3.3 Exceptions to Confidentiality

Exceptions	Follow-through
Suspected physical, sexual child abuse, and neglect	Must report to child protective or law enforcement agencies
Suspected elderly or disabled adult abuse: neglect, physical, sexual, or financial	Must report to adult protective or law enforcement agencies
Duty to warn: someone poses a serious physical threat to another person	Must report to law enforcement agency
Danger to self: someone poses a serious physical threat to himself	Not mandatory to report, although may report to prevent harm
Court order or subpoena	Must disclose to judge
An investigation into the death of a client	Must disclose to coroner
When a client signs a release of information	Must disclose to the person requested by client
Patriot Act of 2001	Must hand over records to FBI, cannot tell client

© Cengage Learning

requests that records be shared. The most recent legal mandate that requires exception to confidentiality is contained in the **Patriot Act of 2001**. This federal legislation prohibits disclosing to clients that the Federal Bureau of Investigation (FBI) sought or obtained personal books, records, papers, documents, and other items of clients as well as requires that such items be provided to the FBI (Benitez, 2004, p. 34). Table 3.3 outlines the exceptions to confidentiality.

DUAL RELATIONSHIPS

Definition of Dual Relationships

Ethical guidelines suggest that human services workers maintain clear boundaries with their clients about the nature of the relationship. Counselors, social workers, probation officers, teachers, and any other types of human services workers are strongly encouraged to keep their relationship with their clients strictly professional. The sole purpose of the relationship should be for the human services worker to help the client meet his or her needs. The reverse should not be the reason—using clients to meet the needs of the human services worker.

The use of the phrase "dual relationship" means that the connection between a human services worker and a client includes two or more types of relationships, and it is strongly discouraged and sometimes illegal, such as in the case of sexual relationships between clients and counselors. This might include any type of social relationship, romantic or sexual relationship, familial relationship, or business relationship. In some areas, especially small, rural towns, this may prove to be difficult because there may be very few human services workers in a community of 500 people, so the chances of relationship crossover would be higher than in heavily populated urban communities. In general, though, human services workers should make every attempt at keeping the relationship with clients solely professional.

Why Should Dual Relationships Be Avoided?

The primary purpose of the dual-relationship ethical standard has to do with the prevention of the exploitation of clients. People who seek the help of human services workers are often vulnerable and therefore may be easy to manipulate. Some human services workers may use their clients to meet their own needs, such as the need to control, need to have someone be dependent, need to have companionships, need for sex and love, or need for money. Although the human services worker may not consciously try to harm or exploit a client through a dual relationship, a client might be emotionally injured if the worker and the client engage in activities outside the helping relationship.

If the relationship were to become personal, the worker might lose objectivity and effectiveness in helping the client. Additionally, if the worker is using the client to meet his or her own needs, then the client's need may become lost and may not be met. Finally, if a personal or business relationship turns sour, the client–worker relationship is also hampered. Several examples of potentially damaging dual relationships are described here.

Examples of Dual Relationships

Example 1   A social worker has been working with a family for six months with three children, ages 2, 6, and 14. They live only with their mother because their father was sent to prison for molesting the 6-year-old girl. The 14-year-old girl is turning 15 and has invited the social worker to her *quincinera*, a coming-out party for adolescent girls that occurs frequently in many Latino families.

Initially, this seems harmless. After all, what needs could the social worker be meeting by attending? How could the family be exploited? Several potential problems might occur. If the social worker attends this affair, how might the 6-year-old girl feel? She may feel that the 14-year-old is getting more attention and feel resentful at the social worker. How will the family explain how they know the social worker to family and friends? They may not have explained the situation to others, and this could prove to be awkward. Also, what if the social worker lets her hair down and has a few drinks and dances with a male guest? How might this affect the professional relationship? If the social worker is a lonely person, she could use this big celebration as an opportunity to meet her own needs. What would you do? Would you go to the *quincinera*, or would you politely decline, informing the family that personal involvement outside the office is not permitted?

Example 2   A male mental health counselor at a substance abuse facility has been working with a woman for about three months. During that time, the woman has cleaned up her act and is working full time. The client, whom the counselor thinks is very attractive, tells him that she wants to end therapy and would like to start seeing him socially. The counselor would be very interested in dating her. So, because she has terminated therapy with him, is he free and clear to do this?

Could any problems occur if they did begin to date? Would it technically be a dual relationship? In fact, most professional associations recommend at least a six-month cooling-off period before a counselor develops a romantic relationship with a former client. The biggest problem in this situation is that she is indicating her feelings for him while he is still her therapist. These feelings that she has for him may be a phenomenon known as **transference**, which occurs frequently between clients and counselors. The client may be attracted to the counselor not because of who he is but because she has attributed characteristics to him based on unresolved issues with a significant other in her life. She may have had a very distant, rejecting father and had never dealt with the pain of this. Her attraction toward the counselor may be an unconscious attempt to have a relationship with a man who will not reject her, to compensate for what was missing with her father.

If the counselor responds to her request, he may at some point reject her, and she would suffer a recurrence of the original wound from her father's rejection. Also, if the client ever needs more counseling, she certainly can't call on him again to help her. Once a relationship turns personal, counselors cannot maintain the objectivity they need. The relationship itself may be the very problem that a client may need further help with, and obviously the previous counselor, who's now part of the problem, could not be impartial. So the correct response if a client tells you they want to date you is, "I feel very complimented that you have feelings for me that way, however, professional ethics are very strict on this matter, and so I must decline your invitation. I am sure you will find someone who can reciprocate these feelings."

Example 3 One of the activities coordinators at a senior center has been interacting with an elderly couple for the past three weeks about their family business. They own several restaurants, and their daughter has recently quit and moved across the country. They need a nighttime hostess part time. The pay is great! The coordinator has been thinking about getting a part-time job to help pay for her son's college tuition. Should she take the job?

This would definitely be a dual relationship and should be discouraged. You may ask, "Why? Everyone benefits." The couple gets a new hostess, and she gets extra money. What could go wrong? As you can guess, things do go wrong. She may turn out to be an incompetent hostess. How would the couple then fire her? Also, how will the coordinator switch roles from employee at night to in-charge program director during the day? Can you picture how awkward this might be?

These three examples provide just a small sample of the potential dual relationships that human services workers might face. In general, keep your relationship with clients professional. Do not engage in activities outside of work with them. Find your romantic partners, friends, and business partners elsewhere. One of the most essential strategies for avoiding dual relationships has to do with continual self-examination of one's values and monitoring of one's reactions toward clients. This requires human services workers to become and stay aware of their emotional needs so as not to consciously or unconsciously use clients to meet those needs. The next section focuses on self-monitoring, self-examination, and being aware of our values and how we can prevent them from negatively affecting our work with clients.

VALUES AND THE NEED TO MONITOR THEM

Human services workers should be aware of their own values. Values usually serve as an internal guide for how to behave and feel about life situations. Human services workers must be aware of their own values so that they do not force them onto their clients.

No one can be completely free of all biases and values. That is certainly true for human services workers. After all, it is their values that influenced them to work in the field of human services.

Ideally, human services workers should work on developing the **self-awareness** necessary to identify any tendency toward dual relationships and other propensities to ignore ethical responsibilities. Human services workers should monitor themselves continually to ensure that clients are not adversely affected by the workers' own personal issues. This means a commitment to life-long self-examination regarding one's own values about life and how people should behave and believe. It is inappropriate for human services workers to decide for clients how they should behave, but rather workers should assist clients in making that determination for themselves.

Values clarification is a process during which a human services worker helps clients figure out their own values and decisions. It is not even considered inappropriate for human services workers to share some of their feelings and values about various subjects, as long as they let the client know that these values belong to the worker and that the client does not need to feel obligated to agree with them.

By merely exposing one's values to the client, the human services worker may be helpful in broadening the client's views, hence giving the client more options to assist him or her in solving problems. Human services workers must be careful to respect the client's values even as they expose their own. The conversation should be more of a values-clarification dialogue rather than a "here's how I think, therefore you should …" lecture. Remember, clients can be very vulnerable and easy to manipulate. They may momentarily agree with the worker's values but later may regret accepting these values when they have a chance to think about it more. They may be afraid to disagree with a professional and institute behaviors that go against everything they believe.

They should be in tune with their own values and biases. It is essential to monitor oneself so as not to impose one's own values onto clients. The more one knows about what one believes to be important, the more one can monitor what is said to clients. All clients deserve to have objective feedback that aims to help clients arrive at solutions that fit their value systems.

When clients' values differ greatly from those of their human services workers, workers need to have the self-awareness and integrity to follow ethical standards and either refer the client to someone else who can be objective or consult with someone to help them deal appropriately with their clients. Some examples of ethical dilemmas involving values are described here.

Examples of Self-Monitoring of One's Values

Example 1 (Self-Awareness Practiced) A psychologist did an intake interview with a new client. The client disclosed that he was gay and was having issues with his partner. This psychologist's religious faith led him to believe that homosexuality was a sin and that homosexuals were beyond hope as long as they continued to live a gay lifestyle. Fortunately, this psychologist's self-awareness about his bias made him realize that it would be inappropriate to continue seeing this client. He referred him immediately to another therapist.

Example 2 (Self-Awareness Not Practiced) A 17-year-old male is brought to a counselor by his parents. They are appalled that their son is gay and want the counselor to straighten him out. The 17-year-old is fine with being gay but feels anxious and depressed about his parents' reactions. His fear at the thought of his parents' rejection nearly brought him to suicide. The counselor tells the boy that being gay is wrong and that if he becomes heterosexual, all his problems will go away. The counselor advises the boy to go through a type of therapy that would be retrain him to be heterosexual. Despite the counselor's awareness of his own opinionated views about homosexuality, he chose to impose his values on his client. He didn't allow for any options. He wasn't self-aware or objective enough to realize that he was overstepping his bounds as a counselor. The damage to his client could be fatal.

Example 3 (Self-Awareness Practiced) A counselor at a free clinic is conducting an intake session with a 15-year-old girl who is pregnant. The girl is not sure what to do. She doesn't know if she should keep the baby, have an abortion, or put the baby up for adoption. The counselor educates the girl on all of these options and helps her examine the pros and cons for each. By the end of the session, the girl has decided to talk with her parents and then come back. The counselor believes that the girl should put the baby up for adoption but never once told her this. She provided all options with equal support. The counselor is aware of her own bias against abortion and against teenage girls keeping and raising babies, but she also knows that it would be unethical to try to persuade the girl in any direction.

Example 4 (Self-Awareness Not Practiced) A different counselor at a birth control clinic sees a 17-year-old girl who is pregnant. The girl is not sure if she wants to keep the baby and is not even sure who the father is. The counselor tells her that abortion is out of the question because it is murder. She also tells her that God will take care of everything and that babies should be with their real moms. The girl should pay for her sin by raising the baby even if it means sacrificing her own adolescence. After all, she committed the sin and now must pay the price. This counselor is obviously way out of line. She has very little awareness about the damage she could be doing to the girl. Her biases are so strong that she doesn't even consider the effect on the client. She is imposing her own values inappropriately. She may think she is giving the best advice but has not examined why she is doing so except that she believes it is best.

The Benefits of Self-Awareness

What we learn from these examples is that human services workers do not always know what is best for all clients. Clients have rights. These rights include the right to examine all the facts, be educated, and be heard by an objective worker before having to make decisions. The more self-aware human services workers are, the greater their ability to be objective and ensure that clients' rights are met. Also, the more self-aware human services workers are, the more likely they are to live successfully and serve as appropriate role models for their clients.

Most formal higher education institutions that teach human services–oriented courses include topics that focus on the importance of self-awareness and self-examination for those pursuing a career in the helping professions. Some programs may emphasize this aspect more than others, but it would be fair to say that self-monitoring and self-development of human services workers are universally valued by educators and professional workers. Therefore, one way to begin the process of becoming aware of oneself and one's needs as a person is to participate in formal education. Textbooks such as this, class exercises, and reaction or reflection papers are common methods for introducing this ethical standard to human services majors. If every course offers just a little bit of opportunity to learn about oneself, then by the end of one's study, the student should have gained a considerable amount of self-awareness.

Of course, human services workers are also encouraged to seek professional counseling or consultation to further the process of self-awareness, especially if problems arise while providing services to clients. This counseling might be in the form of individual, group, marital, or family counseling. It might be for several years or for a couple of sessions depending on the needs of the worker. Many professional workers seek professional counseling periodically throughout their career as the need arises. This is a smart thing to do as it ensures that workers continually monitor themselves as they provide more and more challenging services to a varied client population that may be triggering a multitude of countertransference reactions.

Professional counseling is not required for human services workers. Self-awareness can be gained through personal examination, engaging in meaningful dialogues with coworkers, and reading various books. The vital message is that human services workers should become as aware of their own needs as possible on an ongoing basis so as not to cause any emotional harm to clients.

Critical Thinking/Self-Reflection Corner

- What are some of your values that might conflict with your objectivity with clients?
- What will you do if these values become an issue for you in your work?
- Do you agree that human services workers shouldn't be friends with their clients?
- Would you accept a gift from a client? Attend a wedding?

ENSURING ETHICAL COMPETENCE WITH CONTINUING EDUCATION

Learning about oneself and maintaining ongoing self-monitoring is not the only thing that human services workers must do to meet ethical standards. Ethics also require that professional workers participate in training and education beyond that received in a formal education institution where an actual degree is earned. The field of human services is constantly changing, and human services workers must stay current on new ethical guidelines, new treatment and interventions, and current needs of client populations.

One of the benefits of participating in continuing education for the human services worker is often a renewed feeling of motivation and challenge. After participating in conferences and workshops, counselors, teachers, social workers, and other human services workers usually feel less burnt out. These learning opportunities give them a place to discuss a variety of challenging issues with colleagues. They also increase human services workers' knowledge and skill level, which leads to increased competency when providing services. New ideas help prevent stagnation of thought and behavior.

An additional benefit of continuing education is that some of the situations that human services workers face at agencies aren't taught at colleges and universities. It would be impossible for any one of the programs to teach every possible skill and piece of information. Clients have such a variety of needs, and those needs constantly change; therefore, human services workers must learn about these many needs outside of their college experience.

Many professional associations require 36 or more hours of continuing education in order for counselors, social workers, and doctors to renew their licenses. This indicates the importance of staying current and expanding one's knowledge base beyond the required college curriculum. The reader is encouraged to explore the multitude of continuing education courses available for students and professional workers. They are offered through private organizations, professional associations, and universities and colleges. Many nonprofit and public human services agencies frequently offer training for their own workers and for those who plan to serve internships at the agency. While much of the material covered in these courses may have been taught as part of college curriculum, these training classes usually provide more detailed, practical, and agency-specific knowledge and skills for the participant in an effort to ensure competent practice.

In addition to participating in required continuing education, human services workers are encouraged to consult with colleagues and outside professionals when clients or other activities pose challenges. Many agencies contract with experienced grant writers to ensure that the agency has the best chance at getting funded. When counselors take on clients who have issues in areas in which they have little experience, they often talk with more experienced therapists so they can better serve their clients. Every human services worker from a social worker to a probation officer or a child-care worker must, from time to time, seek the assistance of others to make sure clients are receiving effective services. Ethical standards encourage professional consultations if it means clients will receive competent services. Failure to provide competent service because supervision, consultations, or training was not sought may be grounds for malpractice law suits under the ethical standard of negligence. When in doubt, seek extra knowledge and consultation. The goal is to provide clients with the best standard of care possible.

MULTICULTURAL COMPETENCE

Although many human services practitioners would like to think that current human services agencies offer services free from political and **cultural bias**, this is probably not altogether true. While there has been a trend toward social liberalization since the 1950s (when elimination of forced segregation first occurred), many human services agencies and workers continue to operate within a set of values that does not allow for completely unbiased practice. Admittedly, most human services workers and organizations officially operate in such a way as to demonstrate equality to all their clients. It is politically incorrect to treat people differently because of their gender, race, ethnicity, religion, political orientation, or sexual orientation. Unfortunately, human services agencies and political organizations that establish policies and provide funding to human services institutions sometimes still operate with biases. These biases may take on either obvious or subtle forms of discrimination, such as disparities in services, preconceived notions—**stigma**—about certain populations, and reinforcement of learned helplessness in some populations.

While theories and interventions in practice today are generally effective for working with the majority of clients, a significant number of people who seek services simply do not get what they need. One reason for the needs of some going unmet has to do with the origins of the theories themselves, which were created by educated, middle- and upper-class European American males whose political and cultural values may not be applicable to other cultures' values and ideologies. Although cultural awareness and sensitivity training are now required for many college and graduate degrees, education can only do so much to influence the behavior of human services professionals. Sometimes organizations themselves prevent workers from providing culturally effective services because the **organizational culture** doesn't promote cultural sensitivity. At other times, workers themselves fail to understand or simply disagree with the need to provide culturally sensitive services.

Culture Defined

Culture can be thought of as operating both within and outside of us. At the individual level, it refers to a person's values, beliefs, explanatory systems, and behaviors that are learned in the family and within social groups (Hogan-Garcia, 1999). The United States is home to a variety of cultural groups. Some groups are based on race and ethnicity, such as African Americans, Asian Americans, and Latinos, whereas others are based on religion, such as Catholics, Jews, Muslims, or Protestants. Still others are identified based on age, economic class, sexual orientation, ability, or gender.

At the macro level, culture refers to both specific and unspoken rules under which organizations and institutions, including schools, media, government, workplaces, and mental health and criminal justice systems, operate. The policies, procedures, and practices of these organizations are their culture (Hogan-Garcia, 1999). One could refer to the "culture of the criminal justice system" when attempting to understand practices in a prison.

A major challenge for human services workers is when a client's culture clashes with the culture of the human services agency. Miscommunication and unavailability of services may result in such situations. Educating human services workers about different cultures' values, needs, and priorities and how these may differ from mainstream theories and ideas may help agencies and workers alike provide more appropriate and effective services to all who seek help. Culture may include ethnicity, gender, sexual orientation, age, class, religion, or race. We briefly discuss each of these cultures and some challenges for human services workers.

Gender

While workers may not purposefully engage in gender-based discriminatory practices, they may unintentionally convey narrow ideas about the roles of women and men that may limit their work with clients (Hare-Mustin, 1983; Shields, 1995). The responsibility of every human services worker is to become aware of the importance of gender issues when assessing a client's needs. Of course, gender may not always be a vital issue, but gender-based stereotypes need to be identified and challenged should gender be a factor for a client. It is also very important to resist viewing clients who do not conform to traditional gender roles as being pathological. For example, a soft-spoken man is not necessarily weak-minded and passive. Likewise, not all women who are strong and ambitious have histories of abuse and therefore are out to destroy men. Sexism against men is sometimes overlooked because men have traditionally held power in society. However, human services workers must realize that the roles of men and women are changing. Men and women are almost equal in most areas. Of course, only women can give birth. On average, men are usually physically stronger than women. Beyond those facts, however, men and women are fairly equal. There is no reason that a woman cannot financially support her family. Men can be their children's primary caretakers and take care of a home. Women can be scientists and explore the universe. Men can cry and feel hurt. Men and women are human beings, and that transcends gender.

Critical Thinking/Self-Reflection Corner

- What are some of your behaviors that are typical of your gender?
- What are some of your behaviors that are not considered typical of your gender?
- Have you ever been the victim of sexual harassment? How did that make you feel? Why do you think it happened?

Sexual Orientation

Although society has begun to accept homosexuality in less negative ways than in years past, prejudice and discrimination are still experienced by homosexuals, bisexuals (those who are attracted sexually, emotionally, and romantically to both genders), and transgender/gender variant individuals (those who have surgeries or live as a gender other than the one they were born with). Individuals who identify with one of these sexual orientations are often included in the gay, lesbian, bisexual, transgender (GLBT) community. Fear of discrimination and at times violence has forced many GLBT people to hide their true sexual orientation. Leading such a life is referred to as **being in the closet** and often causes feelings of depression, shame, guilt, and fear. Such people are always vigilant and anxious about having their true sexual preference discovered.

Various social biases create a climate that inhibits homosexuals from living openly. Heterosexism, the belief that the only proper sexuality is between females and males, is probably the strongest bias that influences societal rejection of homosexual behaviors. This belief most likely stems from the Judeo-Christian religious foundation on which U.S. culture is based. These particular religions propose that the Bible and other religious texts teach that homosexuality is wrong in the eyes of God. For many years, homosexuality was thought of as a sin. Later, as science began influencing cultural thought, homosexuality was considered a psychological abnormality. Homosexuality, however, has not been considered a psychological disorder since the American Psychiatric Association removed it as a diagnosis from the third edition of its *Diagnostic and Statistical Manual* (American Psychiatric Association, 1980). Nevertheless, many people still consider homosexuality to be morally wrong. Some people's fear of gay men and lesbians can manifest itself as homophobia, an irrational fear about being around, touching, and liking homosexuals.

Ethnicity

Of course, human services workers should consider cultural values and behaviors that might differ from the mainstream culture when developing interventions for clients whose ethnicity differs from that of mainstream America. The best advice is to listen carefully to each client and family, ask questions about how culture may be influencing a client's needs, and explore options that don't impose conflicting values onto the client. In some situations, it may be necessary to educate clients about cultural conflicts between family members and between societal institutions. Conflicts may occur when one culture sees no problem with a certain behavior that may be considered morally unacceptable or even illegal by mainstream American cultural values. For example, in some cultures, it is permissible to hit children with sticks and other objects, even if they leave marks. While this behavior may be permissible in one culture, it is illegal in American culture, and people who practice such forms of discipline must be told that their behavior must change if they want to continue to live in the United States. Human services workers must explain both the practical side (avoiding jail or losing custody of a child) of assimilating this American behavior, as well as the reason for the American laws about child abuse (psychological and emotional consequences of abuse).

Example of the Need for Cultural Competence with a Latina Client
Child protective services removed the 11-year-old daughter from the home of a Nicaraguan woman after a teacher noticed the child had multiple bruises on her back and legs. The little girl's mother was accused of severe physical abuse. When doctors examined the child, they also found remnants of duct tape on her lips and wrists, suggesting the child's mouth had been taped shut and her wrists bound. When the mother was confronted with the evidence, she openly admitted that she had taped her daughter's mouth and bound her to a chair to control her. She also admitted to having hit the child along her backside with a wooden spoon. The mother stated that the child had been disobedient and was openly defiant. The mother also said that when she was growing up, all children were hit with wooden spoons and were often bound to keep them quiet.

Culturally sensitive intervention with this mother included educating her about U.S. child abuse laws that prohibit such discipline. Her case plan included parenting education, family therapy, and individual therapy during which she talked about her own childhood and her migration experience. A culturally sensitive worker would also explore the environment in which the mother grew up and would not judge her actions without considering the norms established by the community in which she was socialized. On the other hand, a culturally insensitive worker would merely label the woman as an abusive parent and take punitive action against her.

Comparison of Asian American and European American Counselors
Kim, Liang, and Li (2003) studied nonverbal behaviors of Asian American female counselors and those of European American female counselors while working with Asian American clients. Their findings were "consistent with the literature on Asian American communication styles, which indicates that Asian Americans tend to be less expressive and more reticent and restrained in their nonverbal behaviors" (Uba, 1994). The Asian American counselors smiled less than the European American counselors, which supports the observation that Asian Americans tend to value emotional self-control and to avoid openly displaying their feelings, even if those feelings are pleasant ones (Kim, Atkinson, & Umemoto, 2001). Traditional Asian cultures value control over emotional expressiveness even among family members and consider such control a sign of strength (Hsu, Tseng, Ashton, McDermott, & Char, 1985). This behavior is vastly different from mainstream American culture that expects people to openly and directly express affection and other strong emotions to family and friends alike. These and other studies of Asian culture should help human services workers keep in mind the effect free emotional expression can have on their Asian clients and be conscious of not pushing them into doing so. Instead, workers should allow their clients to communicate in ways that are comfortable to them so that they can work through their problems and get their needs met, even if it means taking a more indirect approach than usual.

A Study of Arab Americans A recent study of Arab Americans (Nassar-McMillan & Hakim-Larson, 2003) found some evidence that counseling and other social services for many Arab Americans can be more effective with the support of the community's religious leaders because of Arab Americans' deep religious beliefs. In addition to the support of religious leaders, the study also revealed that the support and endorsement of other community leaders makes it easier for members of the community to use mental health services. Middle Eastern culture is a collectivist one in which community acceptance is important to individuals of the culture. This also differs from mainstream American culture, which values individuality. If community leaders can proactively educate Arab Americans about how mental health services can be used to feel empowered and have better control of life circumstances, then maybe more Arab Americans will use these much-needed services. Unfortunately, human services workers who are not part of the Arab community are often mistrusted (Nassar-McMillan, 1999), which may also be true for counseling and other human services. For the Arab community, physicians, priests, fortune tellers, or other healers traditionally address issues of mental health and the family (Loza, 2001; Al-Krenawi & Graham, 2000). When working with Arab Americans, human services providers should develop a strong rapport based on personal interaction rather than on interpretation or exploration of client issues (Al-Abdul-Jabbar & Al-Issa, 2000). Overall, a multisystem approach that involves religious leaders, medical professionals, family members, and social services is the most effective way to work with this population. Traditional models must be modified to allow for flexibility around timeframe, place of service, and methods of confrontation. Arabs, like so many of us, tolerate neither open criticism nor challenges to the patriarchal position of male family members (Nydell, 1987; Abudabbeh & Aseel, 1999).

African American Issues Probably the most important issue to keep in mind when working with African Americans is racism. Because of their history of slavery and obvious physical differences, many Americans continue to hold negative attitudes toward African Americans. On the other hand, the multitude of abuses and ill-treatment inflicted on African Americans by Caucasians has created distrustful attitudes and stereotypical beliefs toward white people in America. African Americans often feel singled out by police, judges, and others in authority. Unfortunately, their perceptions are often true because institutionalized racism may still exist.

Human services workers should consider these facts when beginning a professional relationship with African American clients. If a client is extremely resistant and distrustful, it may be prudent to involve a trusted minister or someone from the African American community to work with the client. Religious institutions have been a sanctuary for this ethnic group since the days of slavery and continue to be a natural support system for African Americans. Music and athletics have also been trusted and valued institutions for this cultural group, and involving coaches and other role models may be an effective way to work with a client. However, not all African Americans need such traditional support systems. Many middle-class and professional African Americans easily accept mainstream interventions, most likely because they have found ways to circumvent racism and discrimination.

Native American Issues Most Native Americans live in extended families that include, besides their immediate family members, grandparents, aunts (often referred to as mother), uncles (often referred to as father), and cousins (often referred to as brothers and sisters), as well as adopted relatives. As these families relocate away from reservations and to urban settings, they face a constant struggle between sustaining their traditional culture that is built on spirituality, socialization, and language and adopting more mainstream values that emphasize competition and independence. Tribal communities are small and close knit, encouraging dependence within members. These traditions also conflict with mainstream values that encourage children to become independent of their families (Allison & Vining, 1999).

Because many tribes have autonomy within their reservations to intervene using their own traditions, many people whose needs may best be met outside their tribal community do not receive assistance. While autonomy has its benefits, it also has a downside. Communities that live outside government's constraints have difficulty when availing themselves of government-funded resources. When Native Americans do seek services outside of their communities, problems occur because most human services workers cannot speak their language, trained interpreters are rare, and most service providers do not understand Native American culture (Mattes & Omark, 1984).

This section by no means is exhaustive of the cultural issues and traditions that human services workers should understand. It is meant as an introduction, and the reader is encouraged to continue reading the vast literature that discusses the multitude of cultural issues for a variety of ethnic groups.

Religious Issues

The traditional biopsychosocial perspective has recently expanded to include a spiritual component. Many human services workers have found spirituality helpful to clients' overall well-being. In the past, workers may have been reluctant to discuss religion and spiritual beliefs with clients for fear of imposing their beliefs on their clients. Others, however, believe that "addressing spirituality within the therapy is not optional. Human beings are spiritual by nature. If spirituality has no place in therapy then we leave out this part of our humanity and are therefore incapable of best serving the full needs of our clients" (Zylstra, 2006, p. 4). Edward Canda (http://data.socwel.ku.edu/users/canda/, Fall 2009) created an entire course of social work study that he calls "Spiritual Aspects of Social Work Practice." Canda states on his course outline "that social work practice adopts a holistic person-in-environment perspective that requires taking into account the biological, psychological, sociological, and spiritual aspects of human needs, strengths, and experience" (2005). His rationale for creating the course was that "minority spiritual perspectives have been especially neglected given the Eurocentric assumptions common in social work" (Canda, 2005).

CHAPTER SUMMARY

Ethics are guidelines that various professions follow to ensure that consumers of services are protected and that there is some consistency among various workers in the same profession. In the field of human services, there are several ethical standards that ensure that clients can trust workers enough that they will be honest about their problems, such as the standard of confidentiality. However, there are some exceptions to this ethical standard. Usually, if someone is in danger, human services workers must breach confidentiality to protect a potential victim. Other ethical codes deal with the worker's need to maintain professional boundaries with clients, engage in ongoing self-examination and training, and avoid imposing the worker's values onto clients. While there is a growing trend among human services providers to increase cultural sensitivity, there is still room for growth in this area. Most of us would agree that all races, ethnic groups, religions, genders, sexual orientations, ages, and social classes should be treated equally. All of the human services–oriented professions have created standards that mention the need for cultural competence and avoidance of discrimination.

Suggested Applied Activities

Go to the websites of the following professional organizations and find the page that lists each group's ethical standards. Note the similarities and differences among these organizations' standards of practice.

American Counseling Association (ACA) www.counseling.org

American Psychological Association (APA) www.apa.org

National Association of Social Workers (NASW) www.socialworkers.org

American Association for Marriage and Family Therapy (AAMFT) www.aamft.org

National Organization for Human Services (NOHS) www.nationalhumanservices.org.

1. Interview a few people whose race, ethnicity, religion, sexual orientation, gender, age, or class are different from yours. Find out if and how their subculture differs from the mainstream culture. Ask about their experiences with racism, sexism, heterosexism, classism, or religious discrimination.
2. Divide a circle into sections and label each with the name of an ethnic group living in the United States. Describe some of the positive elements that each group contributes or has contributed to the mainstream culture. Divide and label sections of another circle listing the negative aspects of each group.

Chapter Review Questions

1. What is the most important aspect of culturally sensitive human services practice?

2. What is the definition of ethical standards?

3. What is confidentiality?

4. When must a human services worker breach client confidentiality?

5. Why is a dual relationship with a client considered inappropriate?

6. Give three examples of dual relationships.

7. Why is continuing education important?

Glossary of Terms

Being in the closet refers to homosexuals who hide their sexual orientation from society.

Confidentiality is an ethical standard promising that disclosures made by clients to human services workers stay private.

Continuing education is postgraduate training and courses for human services workers once they have begun working in their profession.

Cultural bias is making judgments that are based solely on a person's background and ethnicity.

Dual relationships are those that come about when a human services worker develops another relationship with a client that is outside their professional one.

Duty to warn is an exception to the promise of confidentiality whereby workers are obligated to take appropriate action when clients appear to be posing risk of serious physical harm to themselves or to others.

Ethics are moral guidelines created by various professional associations that set standards for how human services workers should behave with clients.

Health Insurance Portability and Accountability Act (HIPAA) standardized the way information might be disclosed by health care providers.

Mandatory reporting standards were created after the enactment of the Child Abuse Prevention and Treatment Act and the Elder Abuse and Dependent Adult Civil Protection Act to set a nationwide standard requiring that all instances of suspected physical, sexual, financial abuse and neglect of children, elderly, and disabled adults be reported to the appropriate authorities.

Organizational culture refers to the accepted policies, rules, and behavior under which an organization operates.

Patriot Act of 2001 was enacted after the terrorist attacks of September 11, 2001, in order to give the government authorities access to clients' records and disclosures without the knowledge or permission of the client.

Privilege is the legal counterpart to confidentiality that allows a litigant in a court proceeding to withhold evidence if it was communicated in confidence.

Self-awareness is workers' ability to have insight into how their own needs, feelings, and values affect their actions and behaviors, especially regarding their clients.

Self-examination is a process of looking honestly within one's own motives and reactions in an attempt to understand and resolve any emotional or psychological issues.

Stigma is a negative label given to a person because of an affiliation with a particular group, religion, culture, or lifestyle, or because of a physical or a mental disability.

Transference occurs when a client attributes qualities and emotions to a helper based on interpersonal patterns experienced with significant others from his or her past.

Case Presentation and Exit Quiz

General Description and Demographics

Mark works at a juvenile diversion program funded by the county probation office, federal grants, and private donations. Mark has his bachelor's degree in human services. His typical duties include running counseling groups for first-time offenders and substance abusers, conducting intake interviews with new clients, and providing crisis intervention services when necessary. He also conducts educational groups about drug and alcohol abuse. His title is group counselor I, and his supervisor is a licensed marital and family therapist.

Mark recently interviewed a new client. The client, Jason, is a 15-year-old boy who was caught selling marijuana at school. As this was Jason's first arrest for anything, the judge ordered him to participate in a drug-diversion program for one year instead of sending him to jail. If Jason does not complete the program, he will be subject to jail time.

Jason has always been a popular, above-average student. He has many friends and likes to hang out at the beach. He lives with both of his parents and his 17-year-old sister, Heather. Although he and Heather have been smoking pot for the past three years, their grades have not suffered because of it.

Jason and his parents have their arguments, especially about what time Jason must be home at night. Naturally, Jason wants to stay out as late as Heather, but his parents believe he is too young to be out until 1 a.m. Jason also argues with his parents about doing chores around the house, but what 15-year-old doesn't?

Specific Problems

During Mark's interview with Jason, Jason reveals that he's been cutting himself for the past three months. Jason has razor marks all up and down his wrists. Mark asked him if he wanted to kill himself. Jason said that sometimes he does, especially when his parents fight with him and with each other. Jason says that when he's at home he prefers to stay in his room and listen to music because it drowns out his parents' constant bickering. Sometimes, when his mother drinks, she throws things, usually at his dad. But once, she threw a plate at Jason that cut his head open. When they went to the emergency room to get his head stitched up, Jason wanted to protect his mother so he told the doctor that he was fooling around at a party and unintentionally cut his head.

Another time when Jason's mother was drinking, she became enraged because Jason hadn't taken out the trash, so she scratched him on his neck so deeply that Jason started to bleed. Although it was quite painful, he didn't cry. He understands that his mom has a drinking problem.

Jason tells Mark that he gets into fistfights with kids at school when they look at him "the wrong way." He and his friends like to fight; in fact, the next time they're at the beach they're going to beat up this guy who keeps surfing on their territory. They have a plan to surround him and then drag him into the water and hold him under until he almost drowns. Mark asked what the other kid's name was, but Jason didn't know.

As Jason tells Mark about his life, Mark begins to feel inwardly nervous. Mark really likes Jason, and because Mark also loves to surf, he feels he can easily relate to Jason. Also, at one time Mark's mother had a drinking problem, although she's been sober for quite a while. Mark feels that if Jason's mother gets help, she can stop drinking. Mark feels very guilty about reporting the incidents with Jason's mother to child protective services. After all, the emergency room doctor never reported anything. Also, Mark believes that 15-year-old boys can be so obnoxious that their parents can't help but take out their frustrations on them.

Jason invites Mark to his 16th birthday party, which is coming up in a few weeks. Jason says that it will be great. It will be at the beach, with lots of food, drinks, and chicks. It sounds good to Mark because he would probably be at the beach anyway.

Exit Quiz

1. Mark is mandated to
   a. report Jason's suicidal feelings to the police.
   b. report Jason's use of pot to the police.
   c. report Jason's intention to hurt the intruding surfer to the police.
   d. all of the above.

2. If Jason's mother agrees to undergo personal counseling for her drinking
   a. Mark must still report the acts of physical violence against Jason to child protective services.
   b. Mark may hold off reporting the acts of physical violence against Jason as long as his mother shows improvement and stops drinking.
   c. Mark may breach confidentiality and tell the other parents in the group about what Jason's mother did.
   d. none of the above.

3. If Mark goes to Jason's 16th birthday party, he is
   a. helping the trust-building phase of a counseling relationship.
   b. engaging in a dual relationship.
   c. engaging in acceptable, ethical behavior.
   d. all of the above.

4. Because Jason told Mark that he sometimes wants to kill himself
   a. Mark must guard this secret.
   b. Mark may talk to Jason's parents about this.
   c. Mark must not tell his supervisor about this.
   d. none of the above.

5. Mark is not familiar with self-mutilation. To engage in good ethical practice, Mark should
   a. read books about the problem.
   b. talk to his supervisor about it.
   c. attend a conference on the subject.
   d. all of the above.

6. If Mark were to tell Jason's parents that they should get divorced, he might be
   a. exposing his values.
   b. imposing his values.
   c. exploring Jason's values.
   d. all of the above.

7. The fact that Jason felt close enough to Mark on his first visit to invite him to a birthday party might indicate that Jason experienced
   a. delusions of love.
   b. clarification of his values.
   c. transference toward Mark.
   d. none of the above.

Exit Quiz Answers

1. c
2. a
3. b
4. b
5. d
6. b
7. c

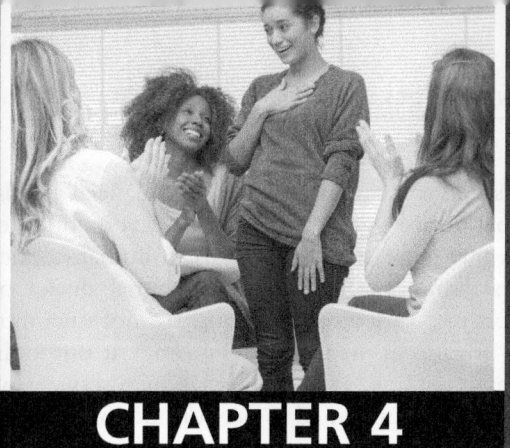

CHAPTER 4

Human Services Workers

INTRODUCTION

Listing every possible human services job title would be difficult. Jobs in human services vary by city, county, and state. Even educational requirements change depending on the supply of and demand for human services workers and the specific needs of a community. For example, in 1997, the Los Angeles Mental Health Association conducted a study of the needs of clients with mental health problems in Los Angeles, a city that's home to millions of people of various cultural and ethnic backgrounds (Mental Health Association of Los Angeles, 1997). The study found that there were simply not enough mental health workers, social workers, and case managers to handle the needs of the population, especially those of the large Spanish-speaking and Vietnamese-speaking communities. To help meet those communities' needs, the city created a high-school program that trained students of various ethnic backgrounds interested in careers in human services to meet the needs of people in their communities. A contrasting example might be the use of psychiatrists to provide counseling services (a function not typically provided by that profession) in rural areas where there are few, if any, licensed master-level therapists. Additionally, given the increasing prevalence of older adults, there is a tremendous need to have more skilled human services workers enter the field of gerontology. Unfortunately, there is currently a looming workforce shortage in aging services, and sadly, many of those already working with older adults have limited or inaccurate knowledge.

This chapter details some of the careers in human services and their educational requirements. You will get a fairly good idea about the types of job opportunities and the specific duties associated with each position. We have tried to showcase people who work in public and nonprofit agencies and deal with social welfare issues such as financial needs, child abuse issues, housing, criminal justice needs, mental health, and educational needs.

A few general job functions in human services are defined to assist you in understanding the vast array of actual duties performed by human services workers in a variety of positions. It's not uncommon for human services workers to engage in many of these duties at one point in their careers. Because of the generalist approach used by human services workers, many of the functions listed will be performed as part of one job title. In other words, human services workers wear many hats while serving clients. The Southern Regional Education Board (SREB, 1969), a consortium of community colleges in 14 southeastern states, first proposed some of the positions and responsibilities discussed throughout this chapter. We've also added other functions to supplement SREB's list.

JOB FUNCTIONS OF HUMAN SERVICES WORKERS

Administrators and Assistants

Someone must run an agency. These people are usually interested in the field of human services, but they don't want to work directly with clients. Agency administrators and assistants focus on program development, fundraising, grant writing, scheduling, and community representation. They often collaborate with administrators of other agencies, politicians, and executive board members. They coordinate various agency programs.

Another duty in the administrative area involves data managing. Most agencies have one or more people who collect data on how many people use the agency, costs, and other statistics. Often, surveys are conducted by **data managers** with former clients to gather information that can be used during an agency evaluation.

For example, an adult reentry program on a college campus needs to keep track of how many students visit the center and what their needs are. The data manager develops a form that advisors and counselors complete after each visit with a student. These forms are given to the data manager and input into a computer program. In this way, the data manager has ongoing information about where the agency stands in terms of usage and needs.

Advocates

Human services workers who speak on behalf of clients to ensure that other agencies and people treat them appropriately are advocates. This advocacy might be with city, state, or federal legislators as well.

Examples of advocates include a staff member at a battered women's shelter who helps a client file a restraining order in court and a family therapist who writes a letter to a school department for a Spanish-speaking family whose child needs an evaluation for a learning disability.

True Stories from Human Service Workers

Administration in Human Services Agencies

Most nonprofit agencies employ administrative workers who engage in a variety of tasks. Four real-life examples of duties performed by agency administrators are presented. The functions of administrators serving in the following agencies are highlighted: a center that helps individuals struggling with issues related to their sexual orientation/identity, an agency that helps victims who have been sexually assaulted, an agency that provides shelter and other services for homeless families and individuals, and an agency that provides a variety of services to individuals struggling to overcome substance abuse.

Example 1: The program manager at the Center of Orange County describes his tasks as including evaluations, follow-up with staff, and a lot of writing for grants, newsletters, and the press. At times he also sees individual clients, runs groups, goes out to the community and does workshops, and networks. This administrator epitomizes the generalist worker attitude.

Example 2: The supervisor of client services at Sexual Assault Victim Services in Santa Ana, California, states that her duties include grant writing, agency reporting, writing reports for the human resources department, and keeping track of services for clients in order to provide three reports to the state every year. These reports consist of the age groups, gender, ethnicity, cities served, and services provided to each client.

Example 3: The assistant to the director at an agency in Santa Ana, California, that serves individuals and families who are homeless describes her duties as including daily administration support and little tasks such as making sure the newsletter is ready and out for delivery. She also performs relational tasks such as checking with the case manager, the bookkeeper, and the community.

Example 4: The program director at Heritage House, a drug and alcohol program in Costa Mesa, California, states that she is responsible for overseeing the running of the program and conducting and attending meetings. She is also in charge of hiring, training, monitoring, and in some cases terminating staff. The director monitors the residents and makes sure all the regulations are followed. She verifies that things are flowing and writes letters of recommendation, evaluations, and grants. Every day is different, and it all depends on what needs to be done, whether it is driving the women, conducting some of the sessions, or simply filling in wherever there is a need. This worker also shows the generalist attitude.

Behavior Changer

Clients who have debilitating behavioral problems may best be helped by receiving a very direct approach from human services workers. These clients can be either children or adults and may have a variety of issues, including those who are disabled, mentally ill, and residents in treatment programs, in school settings, or in correctional facilities. **Behavior change specialists** focus on eliminating, decreasing, or increasing certain behaviors and use such approaches as positive reinforcement and response cost or extinction (Kazdin, 2001) to work with clients to change a behavior.

> ### True Stories from Human Service Workers
>
> #### *Advocates' Responsibilities*
>
> Those who work in human services have long been acting as advocates on behalf of their clients. Many political issues have encouraged agencies to help clients fight for their rights in a world in which people in certain situations, such as those who have been raped or who are dealing with unwanted pregnancies, can be stigmatized and treated insensitively by society.
>
> Advocates at the Sexual Assault Victim Services may accompany clients to hospitals, law enforcement agencies, district attorneys' offices, court proceedings, or other agencies. There are also three paid advocates who work for the district attorney's office that help with these duties.
>
> Client advocates at the Whittier Pregnancy Care Clinic in Whittier, California, have a variety of responsibilities such as offering pregnant women options and emotional support and assessing community referrals for appropriateness.

For example, a hyperactive first-grader wins a happy face sticker every time she stays seated for an entire five minutes. Another example of reinforcing desired behavior might involve a hospitalized, mentally ill patient who believes he is unable to care for himself. Every time he brushes his teeth, takes a shower, or puts his clothes on in the morning he receives a point that he can trade in for privileges, such as buying sodas or candy.

Another example demonstrates a method used to discourage unwanted behavior: a teenager in juvenile detention earns a two-day pass to visit her parents after going two months without receiving any warnings or violations.

> ### True Stories from Human Service Workers
>
> #### *Focus on Changing Behaviors*
>
> Those who work with clients to change their behaviors often have a captive audience, that is, clients in residential facilities or students in a classroom. Patients in mental hospitals, inmates in prison, students in school, and residents of a diversion program or other 24-hour live-in facility are often involved in behavior modification programs.
>
> A counselor at a home for abused children shared some of the ways she works with children to change their behavior. She tries to give them consequences that communicate that they did something wrong without replicating the shame and rejection experiences they had with their parents, because for these kids it is easy to perceive anything as more abuse, deprivation, or rejection. She has the child practice positive behaviors or has the child make amends to a person he or she has hurt—usually together so the shared activity will strengthen their relationship. This has the added benefit of giving the child an accomplishment to be proud of. The agency uses a philosophy called "love and logic" when it comes to working with kids' behaviors.

Brokers

Often, a human services worker cannot provide the exact service that a client needs. Brokering allows workers to connect clients with someone who can better meet their needs. A broker serves as a go-between, connecting a client to another human services worker. Brokers must know a community's resources thoroughly.

For example, a therapist acts as a broker when, in treating a woman for depression, he discovers that his client is being beaten by her husband and provides names of shelters for battered women to her client. A probation officer takes on the role of a broker when she notices that one of her probationers suffers from panic attacks at job interviews and refers him to a therapist.

A teacher who hears that the father of one of his students wants to learn to speak English and who tells him about English-as-a-second-language classes at a local adult-education center is also being a broker.

Caregivers

At times, human services workers provide clients with direct care. Caregivers often provide transportation, food, shelter, medical assistance, or attention.

Examples of caregiver responsibilities include a worker at a senior center who serves clients their lunch, a case manager at a welfare office who provides a client with bus tickets and food stamps, and a worker at an HIV/AIDS clinic who makes home visits to provide critically ill patients with nurturance and support.

Caseworkers

This function epitomizes the generalist role of human services workers. Caseworkers manage all of the various needs of their clients and perform a multitude of duties.

Child protective workers are one example of caseworkers. They contact clients to verify that parenting and drug-awareness classes are being attended, that their homes are clean and have appropriate and sufficient food and heat, that they're working, and that visitations with their children who are in temporary foster care are taking place.

Probation officers, another type of caseworker, meet with clients to make sure they are working, that their drug tests are coming back negative, and that they're not involved with people who will get them into trouble. If a client is in crisis because of a failed relationship, a probation officer may offer support and refer the client to a counselor. Casework is so important to the human services profession that an entire chapter (Chapter 11) is devoted to case management.

Consultants

Some human services workers may have specialized expertise and might work as an independent contractor on specific issues with an agency. Consultants who are specialists in a certain area might work at an agency that provides services to other agencies that need a consultant's expertise.

A nonprofit agency that needs to submit a grant proposal to receive money may hire a consultant who has grant-writing skills to teach the agency's administrative staff how to write grants by working with them closely on the current proposal.

A consultant who specializes in gang prevention may be called in to an elementary school that's having trouble with gang membership among its sixth-grade students. The consultant may set up a program aimed at diverting these children from gang affiliation before they enter junior high school.

A counselor at a local clinic may call on a consultant when a new client seems to have multiple personality disorder. No one at the clinic has treated this disorder, so a therapist from the private sector is asked to consult with the supervisors and the counselor about how to proceed.

Crisis Workers

Many agencies deal with clients who have problems that need immediate attention. Without some resolution, these problems could lead to serious impairment in functioning. The crisis worker attempts to calm the client down, assesses the problem and needs, offers a different perspective on the situation, and connects the client to appropriate resources.

Crisis workers may work for suicide hotlines, conducting telephone interviews and attempting to get callers to calm down and to promise to get professional therapy.

A case manager at a drug rehabilitation center becomes a crisis worker when a client is struggling to stay sober. The case manager provides emotional support, allows the client to vent, and then offers a new perspective on the issues.

In a very different example, an academic advisor at a local community college assists a student in crisis after receiving a failing grade on a test. The advisor offers suggestions about how to retake the course so that the "F" is replaced on the transcripts.

Because crisis management is needed in almost every agency, it will be covered in detail in Chapter 6.

Evaluators

As most human services agencies are funded through grants, there is a need to assess the effectiveness of the program in order for the funding agency to continue the funding. Evaluators are trained to make a thorough assessment of the continuing need for a nonprofit agency and whether the program has been utilized effectively.

For example, the United Way has given a $25,000 grant to a community drug-education program for first-time teenage offenders. An evaluator visits the agency and studies the data collected over the past year. The evaluator looks at how many teens attended the groups, what the rates of success have been after attending the groups, and what is being done to increase the success rate. This process requires that agencies maintain detailed records and statistics.

Educators

Most human services workers who deal directly with clients perform educational functions. Educators disseminate information that will assist clients in making better choices, understanding how clients' problems developed, or understanding how to manage stress.

For instance, an educator will conduct a parenting class for pregnant teens to help prepare them for the birth of their baby and show them how to succeed as new mothers.

Another example of an educator is a worker at a clinic for HIV-positive patients who provides a client with information on how HIV/AIDS is spread after that client's blood test came back negative.

A client advocate at the battered women's shelter becomes an educator when she holds discussions with shelter residents about the battering cycle and how women develop battered women's syndrome.

Fundraisers

In large, nonprofit agencies, staff may be hired to raise money by holding various events, such as charity balls and donation drives. Fundraisers may work for an agency full time or be hired periodically for fundraising campaigns. Of course, many nonprofit agencies utilize administrative staff to conduct fundraisers rather than creating a separate job title for a fundraiser. Larger nonprofits such as the Easter Seals or the United Way usually have fundraiser positions.

Grant Writers

Although executive directors often write grants for their agencies, specialists are sometimes hired to prepare documents aimed at acquiring funds from various institutions to provide money to the agency for a specified period of time. Grant writers are in high demand because it is essential for the funding of nonprofit agencies.

Outreach Workers

Outreach workers conduct presentations to community groups or make visits to people's homes rather than having them come into their office or agency. This is done because some people are resistant to visiting an agency, especially a government agency. Other reasons for outreach are that some people don't have transportation or the time to go to an agency for services. At other times, it is more convenient for the agency because one outreach worker can reach multiple clients at one time.

One example of outreach work is done by community organizations that offer various services such as counseling, education, or medical care that are invited by a local factory to set up booths in its parking lot. The factory workers are given an extra 30 minutes from work to visit some of the booths. Each agency can talk to the people and assess any needs, explain what services are available at its agency, or make referrals to appropriate agencies.

Another example involves an outreach coordinator from a community college who visits high-school seniors to tell them about various majors, careers, and how to enroll in that particular school.

A final example of outreach work is done by a community worker at a free clinic who visits 10th-grade health classes to talk about birth control and sexually transmitted diseases.

Therapists

"Therapist" is a broad term that can include a number of functions. It usually involves some type of intensive work to help an individual resolve a serious impairment in functioning. A therapist may help with physical or psychological problems.

For instance, an occupational therapist works in a convalescent home to help stroke patients relearn how to use their hands by getting them work on projects, such as ceramics, painting, or knitting. A recreational therapist at a psychiatric facility teaches schizophrenic patients how to play card games, billiards, and ping pong. A psychotherapist provides long-term counseling to a client who has difficulty functioning at work because of panic attacks that are related to being sexually abused as a child.

Critical Thinking/Self-Reflection Corner

- Do you think it is more efficient for workers to be trained in one duty and then perform that duty exclusively or for workers to be trained in many duties and perform them all when necessary?
- What types of duties can you foresee yourself performing on the job?
- Which of the previously mentioned duties would you be least interested in performing and why?

EDUCATIONAL REQUIREMENTS FOR HUMAN SERVICES WORKERS

Human services workers may be employed at a variety of levels, often depending on the extent of formal education, experience, and other forms of training. The higher the education level, the more responsibility one has and the more money one makes. A brief summary of what defines various educational levels is provided in the sections that follow. Specific careers for each level are then described.

High-School Diploma

This is the least educated human services worker. It does not mean that this type of worker is insignificant or useless. In fact, due to economic efficiency, many programs employ this level of worker and train the person on the job. Jobs for this person are considered entry level, and these workers are considered to be paraprofessionals.

Associate's Degree

Most community colleges offer courses that lead to an associate's degree of arts (an A.A.) or science (an A.S.). Students receive this type of degree when they complete a two-year course at a community or junior college. Community and junior colleges frequently offer associate's degrees in human services and offer certificates in drug and alcohol counseling, domestic violence advocacy, and gerontology.

Recently, the National Organization of Human Services, in collaboration with the Council for Standards in Human Services Education and the Center for Credentialing and Education, has developed a new certification in human services. The Human Services Board Certified Practitioner requires the applicant to take an exam and must have earned a degree from a regionally accredited college or university or a state-approved community or junior college at the technical certificate level or above. The applicant must also have completed the required post-degree experience. This certification was created to strengthen the visibility and credibility of human services careers and the unique and valued role of human services professionals. Anyone interested in applying for this certification should seek information at www.nationalhumanservices.org (National Organization for Human Services, 2013).

True Stories from Human Service Workers

A Human Services Worker Shares Her Experiences Working in Human Services After Obtaining a Two-year Degree

The career path of Stacy Day began when she completed her two-year degree in mental health in 1996 from Wayne County Community College in Detroit, Michigan. Her first job was at a nursing home as a social work assistant. Her duties included ensuring that each resident's social needs were being met. She often contacted family to communicate these needs. She also consulted with residents' doctors. She described the pay as low, but the job was rewarding. Her next job was at Wyandotte Hospital as a mental health assistant on a geriatric psychiatric unit where she earned substantially more money and felt it was equally as rewarding. At this job she performed patient care, conducted educational groups, and did much more. She loved that job. Her next job provided more benefits. She worked as a forensic security aide at the Center for Forensic Psychiatry in Michigan. She worked with criminally insane patients. Her job was to chart their behavior to ensure they couldn't beat the system. Once she moved to North Carolina she decided to continue her education to become a certified nursing assistant so she could continue helping people (Day, 2010).

This story highlights the advantage that certifications hold for human services workers. While there are jobs for those who secure an associate's degree, certainly certification in domestic violence, chemical dependency, gerontology, or a similar field will increase one's marketability and income. Depending on the region and availability of human services workers with a bachelor's degree, human services workers with a two-year degree may find themselves in competition with those with a higher level degree. In heavily populated urban areas, many candidates may seek employment for a human services worker position, and the agency will probably offer it to the one with a bachelor's degree (everything else being equal). However, in small towns and rural areas, a two-year degree may be enough for securing that same position when competition does not exist. Hiring a human services worker is not always about the degree obtained but often about whether the individual is competent and experienced.

According to the *Occupational Outlook Handbook* (2013), employment of social and human services assistants with high school or a two-year degree is expected to grow by 28 percent from 2010 to 2020, faster than the average for all occupations. There should be good job prospects, as low pay and heavy workloads cause many workers to leave this occupation. The median hourly wage of a social and human services assistant was $13.56 in May 2010. The description provided in this handbook states that social and human services assistants help people get through difficult times or get additional support and help other workers such as social workers. It goes on to say that without additional education, advancement opportunities are limited. *Salary Wizard* (2013) reported that the median expected salary for a typical human services worker in the United States is $23,217 annually. This basic market pricing report was prepared using their Certified Compensation Professionals' Analysis of survey data collected from thousands of human resource departments at employers of all sizes, industries, and locations as of June 2013. The *Houston Chronicle* reports that human services assistants earned a mean $30,710 a year in 2011 (Locsin, 2013). Keep in mind, though, that some of these workers may have had a bachelor's degree, which does tend to increase one's salary.

Bachelor's Degree

To earn a bachelor's degree, students must fulfill course requirements of the college or university they attend. Students typically choose a specific major, such as human services, psychology, sociology, or history, and then take courses specific to that major. The time it takes to complete a bachelor's degree after already completing the equivalent of an associate's degree is usually at least two to three years, depending on how heavy a course load a student takes on each semester. Students can earn a bachelor of science (BS) or a bachelor of arts (BA) degree, depending on their major. Both are considered equivalent in terms of hiring potential for most jobs. Some bachelor's degrees may allow a person to receive certification by various professional associations. For example, to qualify as a certified social work case manager, a human services worker must

> ### True Stories from Human Service Workers
>
> #### Job Description for Human Services Worker
>
> Following is an example of an actual job description for a human services worker at the bachelor level: "Provides assistance to individuals with disabilities or who need assistance with daily tasks. Provides training in life skills. May work in social service facilities and programs such as group homes, mental health centers, youth service agencies, and adult care center. May require a bachelor's degree in area of specialty and 0–2 years of experience in the field or in a related area. Familiar with standard concepts, practices, and procedures within a particular field. Relies on limited experience and judgment to plan and accomplish goals. Performs a variety of tasks. Works under general supervision. A certain degree of creativity and latitude is required. Typically reports to a supervisor or manager" (*Salary Wizard*, 2013).

be an active member of the National Association of Social Work (NASW); hold a bachelor of social work degree (BSW); have one year of postgraduate, paid, supervised work experience and hold one of the following: National Association of Social Work (NASW) Accredited Bachelor of Social Work (ACBSW) credential or a current state BSW-level license (NASW, 2006). In addition to a certified social work case manager, human services workers with a BSW may also be eligible for certification in the areas of children, youth, and family; health care; alcohol, tobacco, and other drug diversion programs; and school social work.

Recruiter.com (2013) lists a variety of human services careers on its website. Some of the careers listed that require a bachelor's degree include the following:

> **Child, family, and school social workers** provide social services and assistance to improve the social and psychological functioning of children and their families and to maximize the family well-being and the academic functioning of children.
>
> **Residential advisors** coordinate activities in residential facilities in secondary and college dormitories, group homes, or similar establishments.
>
> **Social and community service managers** plan, direct, or coordinate the activities of a social service program or community outreach organization. They oversee the program or the organization's budget and policies regarding participant involvement.
>
> **Social and human services assistants** assist in providing client services in a wide variety of fields, such as psychology, rehabilitation, or social work, including support for families.
>
> **Substance abuse and behavioral disorder counselors** counsel and advise individuals who abuse alcohol, tobacco, or drugs or have other problems such as gambling and eating disorders.

Master's Degree

Earning a bachelor's or an associate's degree is referred to as undergraduate education attainment. When students earn a master's degree, they have moved to graduate-level education. To enter a master's degree program, students must have already earned a bachelor's degree. Many graduate programs also require students to take graduate record exams, complete a thorough autobiography, and supply letters of reference. In human services, the most common master's degrees are a master of science (MS) or master of arts (MA) in counseling, which would qualify you to become a licensed marital and family therapist or professional counselor; a master of social work (MSW), which could lead to licensure as a licensed clinical social worker; an MA or MS in psychology; and an MA or MS in sociology. These graduate-level programs can take from two to four years to complete. Students who earn a master's degree are usually considered professionals and are eligible for more challenging and responsible positions than those with only associate's or bachelor's degrees.

Students often wonder about the difference between an MSW and an MS in counseling. Both degrees allow people to be licensed counselors and practice on their own or in a variety of agencies. Licensed clinical social workers, licensed marital and family therapists, and licensed professional counselors may be employed as psychotherapists or as social workers. Some agencies may prefer one over the other. The coursework differs in the various programs. MSW programs usually have courses that focus on program development and community assessment, whereas counseling programs usually focus primarily on mental health counseling issues. Because licensing requirements differ from state to state, students should investigate the specific requirements for licensure in their state of interest. Another master-level license available in some states is the licensed professional counselor (LPC). This requires a master's degree in counseling.

Locsin (2013) describes two master-level careers in human services:

Social workers are arguably the professionals most often associated with human services who either help people cope with everyday problems or treat mental, behavioral, and emotional issues. Locsin goes on the say that child and family social workers look after the welfare of children at home or in school, and as of May 2011, they averaged $44,410 annually according to the Bureau of Labor Statistics. Health care social workers help the sick, injured, or disabled understand their medical conditions and find helpful resources such as support groups or home health care. Their average salary was $50,500 per year. Finally, mental health social workers help those struggling with mental illness or substance abuse, and their annual salary was listed at $42,650.

Counselors: These professionals treat emotional, mental, and social problems through individual and group therapies. They listen to their clients discuss their problems, diagnose disorders, and offer strategies for changing unproductive behaviors and making decisions as well as offer strategies for coping with difficult situations. They averaged $42,590 a year in 2011. Substance abuse counselors develop treatment goals and plans for eliminating addictions, and their average salary was $42,590 as well. Rehabilitation counselors help those with physical, mental, or emotional disabilities live independent lives by offering coping strategies and resources for equipment and community services and their average salary per year was $37,710.

Keep in mind that these salaries are a nationwide average. The income will fluctuate depending on the state and city in which one works.

Doctoral Degree

When students earn a doctoral degree, they usually receive a doctor of philosophy (PhD) in psychology, counseling, sociology, or a similar field, a doctor of psychology (PsyD), or a doctor of social work (DSW) degree. These degrees may allow students to become licensed psychologists in some states. Many people who hold doctoral degrees also teach at colleges and universities. Doctoral programs may take three to six years to complete. Students usually select a specific area of study that interests them and must complete either a dissertation (a thorough research study in written form) or a thorough clinical paper. Both these papers may be as long as 100 pages. They may officially be called "doctor."

Some people earn an EdD, which is a doctor of education. These programs vary from university to university. After completing an EdD program, students may gravitate toward the field of psychology or education. In some states, a person may sit for the psychologist licensing exam with an EdD. Persons interested in pursuing careers as school principals and other school administrative positions may opt for the EdD as well.

Medical Degree

Human services workers with medical degrees are psychiatrists. Psychiatrists attend medical school and then specialize in psychiatry. They must become certified medical doctors before they can practice psychiatry. Medical school may take from 6 to 10 years. Psychiatry focuses on learning about the physiological causes of mental disorders and various treatments to minimize symptoms of these disorders. Typically, psychiatrists emphasize the use of medications to assist people in leading better lives. Sometimes, psychiatrists engage in more drastic forms of treatment such as brain surgery or electroconvulsive therapy (sometimes referred to as electric shock therapy).

The Bureau of Labor Statistics (2012) reported on the income differences for individuals with various educational attainments. This includes all occupations, not just human services. Table 4.1 presents these differences.

TABLE 4.1 Education Pays

Unemployment rate in 2012 (%)	Degree	Average weekly earnings
2.5	Doctoral degree	$1,624
2.1	Professional degree	$1,735
3.5	Master's degree	$1,300
4.5	Bachelor's degree	$1,066
6.2	Associate's degree	$785
7.7	Some college, no degree	$727
8.3	High-school diploma	$652
12.4	Less than high school diploma	$471
All workers = 6.8%		All workers = $815

Source: Bureau of Labor Statistics (2012).

Digital Download Download at CengageBrain.com

Critical Thinking/Self-Reflection Corner

- How do you feel about continuing your formal education at a college or university?
- Are there any specializations or certifications that you are interested in obtaining?
- What are your concerns about applying for graduate school?
- Can you see yourself working as a licensed professional?
- How much responsibility do you see yourself accepting in your career?
- At what level of education do you think you will feel most satisfied?

HUMAN SERVICE AGENCIES AND JOBS BASED ON EDUCATIONAL ATTAINMENT

Social Welfare Agencies

Two-Year Degrees Positions in social welfare agencies that require some education beyond high school include social workers in group homes for abused and neglected children or for disabled people and in nursing homes for elderly people and those unable to live independently. These workers are often caretakers, supervisors, and crisis managers. They may take clients on outings, prepare food with clients, or provide an understanding ear for someone who's lonely. They usually work with professionals in a multidisciplinary team approach.

In addition to social service agencies, there are many nonprofit agencies, such as shelters for the homeless, sanctuaries for battered women, hospices for the terminally ill, and rehabilitation facilities for alcoholics and drug users. These shelters often have a staff of people who do not necessarily have impressive academic credentials but who do have a lot of life experience and possibly have been in situations similar to the people they are now working with and therefore are effective in gathering intake information, conducting phone interviews, managing cases, and providing data management.

Organizations such as Easter Seals, the United Way, the American Heart Association, and the Ronald McDonald House also use workers to greet people who enter a facility, to work on pamphlets and outreach programs, or to collect data. Some organizations use minimally trained workers to supervise field trips and other outings for children, developmentally disabled people, or the elderly. The worker may also help serve food at senior centers or assist Alzheimer's patients at daycare centers. While this is not an exhaustive list of possible job opportunities, this may give you an idea of what is available for people who, at most, have an associate's degree.

Bachelor's Degrees Having a bachelor's degree makes it easier to find better-paying jobs in social welfare agencies. Most communities have county- or state-run agencies for families and single parents with children as well as for the elderly and disabled people who need financial and social services.

In some social service departments throughout the nation, having a bachelor's degree might permit someone to work in the area of child protection. These workers provide case management, advocacy, and crisis management, and they may be asked to testify in court. Their first priority is to act in a child's best interests, which may or may not be to reunite parents with their children who might have been taken from their home because of abuse and neglect. The social worker may make referrals to other agencies and professionals if a family or an individual has a need which can be met through counseling, parenting classes, and drug-education classes.

Adult protective services also offer bachelor's-level positions that involve working with elderly and disabled adults. In addition to being a case manager, adult protective workers might also act as an **ombudsman** who visits nursing homes to ensure that the residents are receiving appropriate services. This worker might also serve as a **conservator** for individuals who are disabled when families cannot do so. Social welfare programs might employ someone at this level who would conduct financial need assessment and provide general case management to assist families in finding work, enroll in college, and find housing and child care.

Generalist skills are definitely needed to deal with issues related to child abuse, poverty, drug addiction, spousal abuse, and criminal activities. These workers must be able to communicate effectively with different types of people from a variety of backgrounds.

Nonprofit social welfare agencies often employ bachelor's-level workers to perform functions that public agencies might not deem appropriate. Using paraprofessionals in nonprofit agencies is cost effective and is more widely accepted than in county or state facilities where money is not as big an issue as it is for nonprofit agencies. The bachelor's-level worker might serve as client advocate, case manager, intake worker, or group counselor. They often conduct educational groups. For example, in a home for teen mothers, a bachelor's-level worker might conduct groups for the teens about parenting, nutrition, and how to utilize community resources. At a battered women's shelter, this level of worker might run groups related to child care, how to reenter the workforce, and how to access legal assistance or financial assistance.

Master's Degrees Once a human services worker attains a master's degree or above, duties and responsibilities increase. More job opportunities exist, more money can be made, and more autonomy on the job is available.

These people might serve as supervisors in financial assistance programs and work as administrative personnel in the federal, state, or county welfare systems. They often work in group homes for abused children as therapists, they conduct investigations into child abuse and elderly abuse, and they maintain caseloads of families who may be trying to adopt. Sometimes they work in hospitals and provide crisis management and counseling to medical patients.

The MSW is a flexible degree that is recognized nationwide. It allows the worker to perform a variety of duties and work in many settings. People who hold master's degrees may sometimes serve as an executive director at a nonprofit agency where the functions include administration of the program, grant writing, fundraising, and meeting with community board members and other community representatives who may have an interest in the agency.

The master's-level social worker may also provide supervision for interns at shelters and develop new programs and policies. They may also serve as mental health counselors, which is discussed in the section on mental health.

Some master's-level social workers are employed in nonprofit programs in hospitals and serve as a link between the patients and their families. They also assist with referrals and discharge plans. Much of a social worker's function has to do with connecting people with community resources to meet a variety of needs.

Doctoral Degrees People with a doctoral degree have more choices in occupations and typically have greater earning potential than those with lesser degrees. In the field of social welfare, those with doctoral degrees may work as psychologists for group homes, serve as expert psychological evaluators in regard to custody disputes, and serve as managers and directors of various programs. Some choose to serve as lobbyists to help change legislation. Others may choose to spend their time in grant writing and other community activities.

Mental Health Agencies

Two-Year Degrees Although the community mental health centers of the 1960s employed nonprofessionals to provide crisis management services, current hiring practices in government-funded **mental health agencies** tend to emphasize the employment of workers with at least a master's degree. In facilities that work with people dealing with substance abuse and chemical dependency, certified chemical-dependency workers may be hired. This certification can be achieved at the paraprofessional level after two years of college. These positions can pay well and offer the worker the opportunity for challenging duties such as group counseling, educational group presentations, and individual counseling. Many community colleges offer courses that will qualify students to apply for certification not only in chemical dependency but also in gerontology and domestic violence.

These human services workers are often employed at nonprofit agencies, where they provide group and residential counseling and do intake work. They may provide guidance, solve problems, and help with everyday crises. Some agencies that typically hire such workers include juvenile halls, battered women's shelters, and group homes for developmentally disabled people.

Bachelor's Degrees There are probably not many positions available for counselors with only a bachelor's degree in county mental health facilities. Some agencies may still employ this level of worker if there is a great need for counselors and not enough master's-level therapists are available to handle the caseload. Some agencies may employ a bachelor's-level worker if he or she is working toward a master's degree. Typically, bachelor's-level counselors are employed more in nonprofit agencies than in government-funded mental health institutions.

Because nonprofit agencies must function with very little money, it is not uncommon for counselors at these agencies to conduct individual and group counseling, especially for people in crisis. Often, these workers are working toward a master's degree, but not always. Sometimes, they attend special training programs to become certified in a specialty such as domestic violence or sexual assault intervention. The focus of these counseling sessions is to resolve immediate crises and receive education. Sometimes, a worker at this educational level may serve as a coordinator of a program within the agency and provide outreach and informational services.

Master's Degrees Community and county mental health and behavioral health services often hire therapists who hold master's degrees in counseling or social work. Whether or not a license is required would vary from state to state. These counselors provide all basic counseling, psychotherapy, and crisis management services to the clients who utilize county services. These clients are often very emotionally disturbed individuals who also need the services of a psychiatrist who prescribes the medication.

While students are working toward an MS or MA in counseling, psychology, social work, or some other related field, they often work in nonprofit settings as part of their licensing internship. Here, they have an opportunity to provide in-depth counseling and psychotherapy and receive supervision from a licensed therapist as a way of earning hours toward their own license. The benefit for the worker is gaining experience and hours. The benefit for the clients is receiving therapy at reduced fees in comparison to what it might cost to see a licensed therapist in a private setting. However, many nonprofit agencies hire

True Stories from Human Service Workers

Career Opportunities for Workers with Bachelor's Degrees

Some agencies might even hire someone who has not even quite earned a bachelor's degree based on the person's experience at the agency. The following human services worker served one of her required internships at a group home for abused children and was hired as a paid employee while still working on her bachelor's degree. She describes some of her job responsibilities below.

"As a residential support counselor at a home for abused children, I was hired even before I graduated with my bachelor's degree in human services. I pick children up from school, hang out with them, help them with homework, and do something fun with them. I may spend time with the children and their parents or talk with the parents alone. Sometimes crisis situations arise. I don't do therapy but instead try to empower the children and focus on making better choices. I use reality therapy and stay in the here and now."

The next example is a personal story by one of this text's authors, Kristi Kanel, which illustrates how an internship turned into a full-time job that later led to a position with a county mental health center, where she worked while pursuing a master's degree in counseling.

"My third internship was at a nonprofit organization called the Free Clinic, where I conducted support and educational groups on birth control and sexually transmitted diseases. When a job opening for a counseling services coordinator became available, I applied. Although other applicants held master's degrees, I was hired because of the experience and training I received at the clinic while completing my bachelor's degree in human services and because of the good rapport I had with the director.

"As I recall, the pay wasn't very much, but the experience was invaluable. It allowed me to transition from my college job as a clerk at the department of motor vehicles to a real human services job. This job gave me experience beyond that of an intern. In addition to running groups, I learned how to coordinate volunteer schedules and responsibilities, how to manage data, how to write grants, and how to provide outreach services. This job was an entry-level position that gave me more credibility when I applied for my next human services position as a mental health worker with County Mental Health. Although I only had a bachelor's degree, I was hired because of my experience at the Free Clinic and also because I was working toward a master's degree and I could speak Spanish—a definite advantage, especially in Santa Ana, California.

"My duties at County Mental Health included running groups at a day-treatment program for severely mentally ill patients, conducting intake interviews, and providing case management for the patients. While there, I learned how to diagnose and make treatment plans."

---

licensed therapists to provide counseling as well. Also, these agencies often use these licensed therapists as supervisors and administrators. Of course, some of the supervisors might also hold doctoral degrees, and they may be the directors of the agencies. Individuals who don't wish to obtain a clinical license may choose to merely coordinate and administer programs. Across the nation, there are several types of master's-level licenses. As discussed previously in this chapter, some typical ones include licensed clinical social worker, licensed marital and family therapist, and licensed marriage counselor. In addition to acquiring a master's degree, these counselors usually need to complete 3,000 hours of supervised experience and pass a written and sometimes oral exam through the state's licensing board.

As with most of the nonprofit agencies that have been discussed, the worker at this level often serves as a primary counselor, psychotherapist, case manager, supervisor, and manager. He or she may be the executive director of a program as well. Depending on a person's desire, he or she may conduct fundraisers, write grants, provide outreach, and serve as a liaison with other programs. This person may testify in court at times. The worker at this level might run a batterers treatment program and be involved in all aspects of the program.

Doctoral Degrees Workers who hold a doctoral degree may choose to work in public mental health clinics, private practice, HMOs, or nonprofit agencies. They often acquire a license as a psychologist. Whatever the setting, they typically engage in the provision of psychotherapy, group and family counseling, and psychological testing. They are qualified to treat almost any client population and are usually paid more than a master's-level therapist. Some doctoral-level workers prefer to serve as supervisors and administrators at clinics and hospitals. They may be more likely to work for facilities such as the veteran's hospital or prisons because these are often used as internships in doctoral programs. Although they can't prescribe medication, they often consult with physicians about appropriate medical treatment for their clients.

True Stories from Human Service Workers

Master of Science in Counseling Leads to More Challenges, Pay, and Status in Mental Health

"I'm going to continue to share my chronology of employment beginning at county mental health, where I worked for four years. During the first two years, I was working toward the 3,000 required hours to become a licensed marital and family therapist (MFT). Once I completed my master of science in counseling and completed 3,000 hours of counseling required to sit for a licensing exam, I became a licensed MFT. I was then promoted to mental health specialist. In addition to earning more money, I also performed slightly different duties. I now provided individual psychotherapy to all types of clients. I was qualified to diagnose and conduct emergency evaluations in the community. I could also supervise MFT interns as well.

"I was offered a position as a therapist at a managed-care facility where my salary increased considerably. At this HMO, I provided individual, family, marital, and group therapy for a variety of clients. My hours were more flexible, and the pay was good. During this time, I returned to school to work on my doctoral degree in counseling psychology. Once I earned the doctorate, I opened a private practice as an MFT but was able to increase my fees because of my advanced degree. I also contracted with many managed-care insurance providers at that time, and I earned more money for my services than I had received at either the private HMO or the public county mental health facility."

Correctional Facilities

Two-Year Degrees A good example of this type of position would be the counselors at juvenile detention facilities. These workers generally do not need advanced degrees. They conduct group counseling and crisis management for the inmates at correctional facilities for youth.

Many interns and paraprofessionals work as group counselors in halfway houses. They may also provide drug-awareness classes if they are certified chemical-dependency counselors. Sometimes they provide case management services at diversion programs and residential homes as well.

Bachelor's Degrees In many probation departments, workers with bachelor's degrees may be hired as deputy probation officers. They may supervise inmates who are working out in the field (cleaning up the highways). They may also assist probation officers in monitoring cases. Some probation departments may even hire a worker at this level as a probation officer. These duties include case management, counseling, and crisis management for the probationer.

In addition to probation work, a worker with this education may also work at a juvenile hall as a counselor, case manager, or supervisor. Some police departments have positions available at this level in gang prevention and drug education. Outreach work and field crisis management may be duties in these positions.

As with the entry-level worker, this worker may provide case management and crisis management for residents at halfway houses. They may also conduct outreach educational services for diversion programs. Counseling would most likely be limited to group counseling at diversion programs with teens or with residents in the halfway house. They may also be involved in grant writing, fundraising, and data management.

Master's Degrees The department of probation may employ master's-level workers, some of whom may be licensed therapists or social workers, while others may have master's degrees in sociology or criminal justice. These workers often serve as probation officers and supervisors. They provide case management services, crisis intervention, and some law enforcement activities when the probationer violates the terms of probation. At this level of education, administration and management duties are frequent as well.

Doctoral Degrees Psychologists hold a special place in the court system. The courts often require that people undergo psychological evaluations in order to stand trial, to gain custody of children, or to be deemed disabled. They are qualified to conduct a variety of tests such as the Minnesota Multiphasic Personality Inventory (MMPI) in their evaluation of people. Some psychologists provide counseling services in correctional facilities as well. No doubt, some doctoral-level workers serve as probation workers, probation supervisors, and administer nonprofit diversion programs.

Specialized Education Programs

Two-Year Degrees Workers at this level might serve as a classroom aide, perhaps a bilingual aide in a variety of specialized education programs. There may also be positions at this educational level for workers to assist with data management at community colleges and state universities. Some outreach duties might also be available. Tutoring opportunities might be available in some school systems as well.

Many human services workers enjoy working in recreational, after-school programs, such as the Boys and Girls Clubs, the YMCA, and other organizations for children and teens. These are viable careers and require some human services generalist skills. While the pay may not be great, these are worthwhile programs.

Some programs are designed to assist youth considered to be at-risk, such as those involved in gangs, drugs, or at risk for pregnancy. These agencies may be funded through public monies or may be nonprofit. Positions may be available for those with, at most, community college-level education, depending on the function of the agency. Some agencies may provide residential living for pregnant teens and need counselors, case managers, and caretakers. Others need outreach workers that can educate the at-risk populations.

Bachelor's Degree It is possible for workers at this level to work as kindergarten through 12th grade (K–12) classroom teachers, preschool teachers, special education teachers, and resource specialists. However, many schools require a graduate degree for a resource teacher who works with learning-challenged students K–12. Community colleges and state universities often hire workers at this level to provide guidance counseling to at-risk students, to work as resident advisers in dorms, or to provide orientation for new students. Administrative positions, such as data management and program coordination, might also be available.

Master's Degrees With a master's degree, a person might provide counseling, either personal or academic, to students. This worker might be a school psychologist or a guidance counselor. Many schools employ master's-level social workers to be on campus to aid in the detection and resolution of child abuse issues. As stated earlier, many schools require a graduate degree for employment as a resource specialist.

There are a variety of programs on college campuses that utilize master's-level workers. These range from psychological counseling, to coordination of programs, to student retention management. Some universities offer specific master's-degree programs in student assistance at the college level.

Doctoral Degrees With a doctoral degree, people are able to become professors at community colleges and most universities. They may choose to work as deans, coordinate various student programs, and serve as counselors at a college as well. In the K–12 system, many people with doctoral degrees become school principals. Some may serve as school psychologists, too.

CHAPTER SUMMARY

Careers in the human services are varied and include positions that require minimal college education to graduate degrees. Human services workers often work in social welfare agencies, mental health agencies, correctional facilities, and the educational system. The duties performed by human services workers may be specialized, such as performing data collection, or general, such as performing case management functions. While most human services workers deal with similar types of populations and work in similar settings, those with higher education usually perform the most challenging jobs and earn higher pay than those with lower educational attainment.

Suggested Applied Activities

After learning about various careers and their duties, you may be feeling overwhelmed with regard to deciding on a career. To help clear up any confusion, you might want to take a few minutes to answer the questions in the Brief Career-Decision Inventory to see where you stand at this point. These reactions may change once the text and course are completed.

Brief Career-Decision Inventory

1. If I worked directly with clients, what specifically would I like to do?

   _____

   _____

2. What type of program or service might I like to create in the community?

   _____

   _____

3. How do I feel about engaging in fundraising activities, grant writing, or managing data?

   _____

   _____

4. Do I want more than an associate's degree?

   _____

   _____

5. Do I want more than a bachelor's degree?

   _____

   _____

6. Do I want to work toward a doctoral degree?

   _____

   _____

7. Do I want to work in a government-funded agency or a nonprofit agency? What are the advantages of each?

8. Do I want to provide counseling-type services?

9. Do I want to provide more general case management?

10. Do I want to educate others?

Chapter Review Questions

1. What are some of the differences in responsibilities between human services workers who hold associate's or bachelor's degrees and those who hold master's or doctoral degrees in the field of social welfare, mental health, corrections, and education?

2. What duties would a social worker typically be engaged in on a regular basis?

3. What types of duties comprise a large part of a mental health worker's day?

4. What skills and duties do teachers often perform?

Glossary of Terms

Behavior changer specialists eliminate, decrease, or increase specific behaviors and improve functioning using positive reinforcement and extinction methods.

Conservator is designated by the county department of social services to make financial and personal decisions for someone who has been assessed by the courts as incompetent to care for him- or herself.

Data managers input information into computer systems, analyze it, and create effective data management at an agency for purposes of statistical collection and accountability for program evaluation.

Mental health agencies provide therapy, crisis management, and case management to clients with psychological and behavioral disorders.

Ombudsman is a person whose primary function is to monitor the conditions of residential facilities where the elderly and the disabled reside. They work with county and state officials to ensure that proper treatment is provided.

Case Presentation and Exit Quiz

General Description and Demographics

Glen, age 52, and his wife of 20 years, Karen, age 50, have a daughter Jenna, age 18, and two sons Jacob, 15, and Eric, 10. The family lives in a very nice neighborhood, and both parents work full time in administrative positions. Both parents have medical insurance and pay very little out-of-pocket expenses for medical, dental, and eye care.

Recently, Glen's father died, leaving his 75-year-old mother, Emma, a widow. Glen's siblings live in another state but do visit their mother occasionally. Both of Karen's parents have died several years ago. Emma still lives in the house she raised her children in and lives off her late husband's and her social security checks.

Jenna was supposed to graduate from high school this year but has been ditching classes recently and may have to go to summer school if she doesn't graduate in the spring. Jenna is quite popular and has always been an average student.

Jacob started high school this year and seems to have adjusted well. He is involved in sports and hangs out with his friends most of the time at an Internet cafe.

Eric is doing well in school but has recently gained about 20 pounds. He likes to play video games most of the time rather than play outside with friends.

Problems That Need Assistance

Emma has been showing symptoms of Alzheimer's disease for the past 10 years. She cannot remember her grandchildren's names and at times forgets her son's name. Her husband used to take care of her when he was alive, but now she lives alone and her children are worried about her. She sometimes forgets to eat and bathe. She is often found sitting alone in her living room, smelling of body odor. Her son pays her bills and takes her to the doctor's appointments.

Glen and Karen have begun to have arguments about Emma's care. Karen thinks the other siblings should put more effort into Emma's care, but Glen believes that because he lives locally he should shoulder the bulk of the responsibility, especially as his brothers and sister have been uninterested in their mother's care. Glen has always been very attentive to his mother's needs, which has created resentment between Emma and Karen for many years. Karen and Glen have been growing apart since his father's death and can barely speak without arguing.

Jenna has been using crystal methamphetamine for the past five months and has been hanging around with friends who do the same, instead of her former friends who don't use drugs. Her parents just found out about her drug use after she stayed away from home for two days straight without calling them. When her parents confronted her and threatened to take away her car, cell phone, and all other privileges, Jenna said she needed help to stop using drugs. This was the reason she was ditching school and not passing her classes.

Jacob has also gotten into trouble. He and his friends stole a car to go joy riding. Although the car belonged to one of his friend's parents, they were all arrested.

Eric has been feeling depressed lately. He says he eats because he's sad and has had thoughts of suicide but has not tried to kill himself.

Services Provided for Each Family Member

Glen took his mother to her family doctor and explained her worsening symptoms. The doctor referred Glen to an Alzheimer's association and prescribed his mother medication to attempt to slow down the progression of the disease. Glen called the Alzheimer's association and spoke with someone about his mother's behaviors and about the family's lifestyle. The worker recommended that Glen explore the possibility of having his mother attend a special daycare program and live with him at night. A worker was assigned to visit his mother's home to assess her level of functioning. Another worker came to visit Glen and Karen to talk about caretaking responsibilities. They gave Glen and Karen information about the progression of Alzheimer's disease as well as information about respite care that provides workers who can stay with an Alzheimer's patient when caretakers need a break.

Karen doesn't want Emma to stay with them, but Glen does. Karen sets up an appointment with a licensed marital and family counselor to help them deal with this major difference of opinion and potentially life-altering decision. At their first session, the counselor recommends to Karen and Glen that he should urge his siblings to get involved with their mother's life and perhaps share caretaking responsibilities. Glen is resistant, but the counselor points out that at a time when their children are getting into trouble, he and Karen need all the support and help they can get.

After hearing about Jenna's drug problem, the counselor refers all of them to a facility that offers drug-education classes and group counseling for Jenna and her parents. The counselor also gives them a list of appropriate 12-step programs and then schedules regular marital counseling sessions for Karen and Glen.

Jenna and her parents enter an outpatient drug-treatment program paid for by the family's medical insurance. Jenna attends groups five days a week, and her parents will be going to group and family therapy once a week for the next 12 weeks. A psychiatrist evaluates Jenna and prescribes antidepressants for her. The program emphasizes changing behaviors through parental reinforcement of appropriate behaviors and parental removal of privileges after negative behaviors.

Jacob and his parents go to court where he is put on probation and must attend a diversion program if he wants to stay out of jail. Jacob must also meet with his probation officer once a month and stay away from other criminal offenders. Jacob's probation officer monitors his progress in school and makes sure Jacob doesn't associate with anyone who has had problems with the law. Jacob must also attend group counseling and classes at a community services agency.

Eric visits his pediatrician who sets him up with some nutritional guidelines and an exercise program. He doesn't feel the need to see a counselor yet. Karen and Glen's counselor has suggested that they keep a close eye on his suicidal feelings and encouraged them to bring him in to see her if he doesn't feel better soon.

Exit Quiz

1. Which service provider has the highest level of education?
    a. Glen and Karen's counselor
    b. Jenna's group counselor
    c. Eric's pediatrician
    d. Jacob's probation officer

2. Jacob's probation officer is serving as
    a. a data manager
    b. a caseworker
    c. an advocate
    d. an educator

3. The model at Jenna's substance abuse program encourages workers and parents to serve as
    a. outreach workers
    b. therapists
    c. behavior changers
    d. brokers

4. Karen and Glen's counselor most likely holds a
    a. PhD.
    b. MS
    c. BS
    d. MD

5. What function does Emma's family doctor serve when he referred Glen to an Alzheimer's association?
    a. broker
    b. administrator
    c. evaluator
    d. grant writer

6. Which organization is most likely to use volunteers and paraprofessionals primarily?
   a. pediatric clinic
   b. probation department
   c. Alzheimer's association
   d. Jenna's psychiatrist's office

Exit Quiz Answers

1. c
2. b
3. c
4. b
5. a
6. c

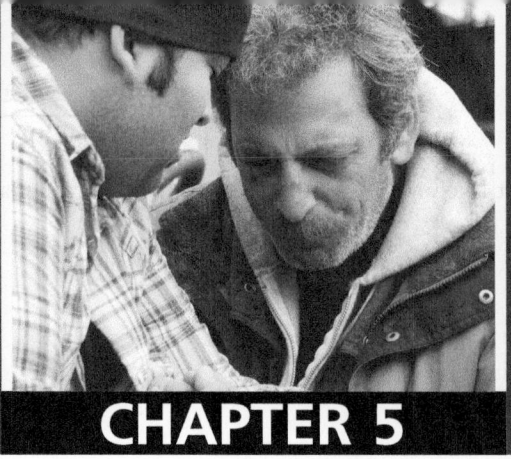

CHAPTER 5

Basic Counseling Skills, Personal Characteristics of Human Services Workers, and Theoretical Approaches in Counseling

INTRODUCTION

All people undoubtedly benefit from clear and sensitive communication styles. However, in the field of human services, the need for effective communication skills is vital in order to maximize beneficial outcomes for clients. Even if a human services worker does not work directly with clients, he or she will be interacting with colleagues and learning how to present his or her point of view clearly to others, which is always helpful to anyone.

In addition to acquiring effective communication skills, human services workers must also develop and strengthen certain personal qualities. The personhood (the overall way in which a person relates to others and to himself, including personal characteristics such as warmth, sensitivity, etc.) of a human services worker can be his or her best resource when dealing with people in need.

Developing a good, solid working knowledge of a variety of theories related to counseling is also vital to becoming an effective human services worker, as these theories offer strategies for understanding people in need and interventions for how to help them. The lack of such knowledge, or even outdated knowledge, can actually do more harm than good; keeping updated on theories and related skills and strategies is therefore critical.

The first part of this chapter presents specific communication skills that are essential to being an effective human services worker. Following the discussion on communication skills are some personal characteristics that are considered vital for human services workers.

The second part of this chapter presents a variety of counseling theories and the corresponding intervention strategies for each, including a section on evidence-based practice.

PART I: EFFECTIVE COMMUNICATION SKILLS OF HUMAN SERVICES WORKERS

The idea that there are certain methods of interacting with others that enhance trust and promote open sharing has been supported by many. Books such as *Effective Helping* (Okun, 1992), *Basic Attending Skills* (Ivey, Gluckstern, & Ivey, 1997), and *Helping Relationships and Strategies* (Hutchins & Cole, 1992) all indicate that professionals in the field of helping others have formulated ideas about how to proceed in an organized, effective manner. Of course, caring about people and wanting to help them fix problems is important; however, providing intuitive feedback and advice may not be enough to actually help people. If that were all that was needed, you could simply find a caring and intuitive friend or family member to talk to, but that is not always enough to solve people's problems. Also, many people do not have the support of family and friends and need outside intervention when facing problems.

General Goals of Effective Communication

Certain communication methods and interaction strategies have been shown to be effective in helping people work through their problems. To successfully work with people in overcoming their problems, a sense of trust must be developed that allows clients to open up and speak honestly about their problems. If clients do not feel comfortable sharing their problems with a counselor, then their problems will remain unresolved. Effective strategies both for establishing trust between a counselor and clients and for helping clients work through problems will be covered later on in this chapter. But first, let's briefly review the goals of effective communication.

Goal One: Create a Sense of Trust A human services worker must help people talk about their problems to assess their needs and create appropriate interventions. Because people often feel that their problems are personal and are perhaps ashamed of them, human services workers must work to establish a relationship in which the clients can openly speak about their problems.

The first steps to creating trust include the following: When speaking with a client for the first time, maintain a calm demeanor and comfortable eye contact, nod your head to let the client know you are listening carefully, and remain nonjudgmental, no matter what the client is saying.

Goal Two: Create a Sense of Empathic Understanding In addition to developing trust, clients must believe that their human service worker understands their problems and therefore is able to help them. If workers do not seem to "get" their clients' problems, how could the worker do anything to solve it? Empathy is the ability to walk in someone else's shoes and attempt to see the person's world as they see and experience it. Like anything else, this is a skill that can be developed over time by spending time with people from other culture's and traveling to new places as well as taking time to read the literature about the causes of dysfunction. These activities often help to increase insight and sensitivity into what people deal with in their daily lives. The key, though, is to have healthy empathy and not experience compassion fatigue, which results from the stress of caring too much. Particularly as human services professionals who listen to stories of fear, pain, and suffering of others and who may feel similar fear, pain, and suffering, it is critical that when working with people, you do not lose your sense of self, that healthy boundaries are maintained, and that regular self-care is practiced. People who feel they have been empathized with tend to feel a greater sense of safety and acceptance.

Some examples of empathic statements include, "I can see how this is painful for you." "I hear that since your husband left you, finances have been difficult." "Your fears about relapsing are understandable as you had been using for over 10 years."

Goal Three: Allow Clients to Explore and Clarify Their Thoughts Clients don't always express themselves in an organized manner. Human services workers must often help clients verbalize what they're trying to say to better assess their clients' needs. Certain communication strategies provide an arena for clarifying and exploring a problem.

Examples of comments and questions that can help the clarification process include: "How does it make you feel as you think about losing your job?" "So I hear you saying that after your son tore your book in front of you, you became so angry that you hit him with your belt." "What do you feel about your husband giving you a black eye?"

Goal Four: Instill Confidence in Your Ability to Help Your Clients Clients also need to believe that their human services worker is knowledgeable and confident so that when clients get feedback, suggestions, and information about other resources they will accept and put all that information to use. Certain comments and observations help establish a confidence-building rapport: "I have recently attended a seminar about marital infidelity and the speaker provided many examples of couples who have been successful in reuniting." "I know of a great support group for women who have survived date rape. Let me give you their phone number." "Perhaps you could contact the district attorney's office about getting a restraining order."

> ## True Stories from Human Service Workers
>
> ### Building Trust in the Real World
>
> The following comments are from two human services workers who share their views about building trust with clients. Although they do not consider their primary role as being a therapist, they still emphasize the goals previously discussed.
>
> One of the workers who works at a group home for abused children shares her communication methods: "My focus in working with these kids is on building relationships. I am not a therapist, and I do not do therapy with the kids. However, I believe it is therapeutic just to establish a relationship with the kids and be someone they can trust. Showing **empathy** for these kids helps them learn to soothe themselves when they are overwhelmed or upset. It helps the kids feel safer with their own feelings."
>
> Another worker who is a nurse manager and client advocate at a pregnancy care clinic says that "no deep psychological counseling is done here. Emotional support is given when the clients are in crisis, and appropriate feedback and education is given for each client's unique situation."
>
> These examples illustrate how basic counseling skills are used by various human services workers.

Specific Effective Communication Skills

The skills detailed in this section are presented in order from basic to more advanced; however, they are not necessarily used in this order while interacting with a client. Beginning workers will probably be most comfortable with the first few skills, and as workers become more experienced, they will be comfortable incorporating other skills in their client interactions.

Active Listening Active listening is the basis for all effective communication between a helper and a client. The difference between simply hearing and listening to what someone says is considerable. Active listening requires a listener to concentrate solely and without distraction on what someone is saying at the moment; that means putting aside personal problems and daydreams. It also means hearing beyond what the person is saying—trying to understand deeper levels of meaning when appropriate and encouraging the person to say more. In our everyday conversations with family and friends, this is not how we usually listen. Often, people are so wrapped up in their own problems and concerns that when someone is talking to them, they barely let the other person get out a statement and are ready to add something about themselves.

Because people are unaccustomed to listening in this manner, active listening may seem odd or unnatural at first. In an average conversation, one person says something, then the other gives a suggestion, discloses something that may be related to what the first person said, or tells the other person not to worry because everything will be all right. The result may be feelings of frustration and lack of validation. Human services workers must learn to interact in a way that assures clients that they are being heard, understood, and are allowed to explore problems or needs thoroughly. The personal concerns of a human services worker should not be part of these interactions.

Active listening includes a variety of skills that have been studied by many professionals in the field. When Rogers (1970) was first conducting his research on the therapeutic effects of encounter groups, he found that many therapeutic benefits resulted when group facilitators used active listening techniques. Additionally, he discovered that certain qualities (discussed later in this chapter) of group facilitators influenced therapeutic outcomes.

Some active listening skills that contribute to effective communication are discussed here.

Using Minimal Encouragers   Using **minimal encouragers**, though simple, is the foundation of active listening in all interactions. Minimal encouragers are both verbal and nonverbal signals that indicate the listener is interested. When you feel that the person you are talking to is really interested in the conversation, you are motivated to keep talking. Likewise, when you feel that your words aren't being heard, you're more apt to quit talking. Being interrupted, having a completely new topic brought up, or simply being ignored does not usually make people feel good about themselves nor does it encourage them to keep talking. Effective communication encourages clients to keep talking and makes them feel that what they are saying is important.

One technique that encourages conversation is head nodding. When people are truly interested in what you are saying, they tend to unconsciously nod their heads. In addition, maintaining good eye contact says, "Go on, I'm with you, and want you to continue." Of course, adding a few "uh-huhs," "I sees," or "ohs," along with attentive body language, also lets clients know you're involved in what they are saying. In American culture, the "basic listening posture is a slight forward trunk lean with a relaxed easy posture" (Ivey et al., 1997).

Critical Thinking/Self-Reflection Corner

- Have you ever been bored while someone was talking to you, having no interest in what the person is talking about?
- How easy is it to drift off and stare into space?
- How often have you drifted off during class, or while reading this text?
- What did you do to bring yourself back to listening and paying attention?
- Have you ever felt someone shut you out? How did that make you feel?
- Can you think of someone in your life who makes you feel listened to? What does that person do to make you feel like truly heard and understood?

Verbal Following   The next level of active listening is to focus on what clients have already said instead of "topic jumping" (Ivey et al., 1997). One way to let the clients know that you are listening and understanding them is to paraphrase, reflect on, or question what a client has just said. There is usually no need to bring up new topics or issues. Following a client's lead will get you to the relevant problems. This will create a climate of understanding and empathy that assures clients that their experiences are understood, both emotionally and intellectually. Here are two examples of **verbal following**. In each example, two possible responses are given to show poor and effective verbal following.

Scenario 1

Client: "I'm pretty bummed out because I didn't study hard enough and I got a D on my exam. My parents are going to be mad, and I'm not going to be able to go out this weekend."

Poor response: "Who's your favorite teacher?"

Better response: "It sounds like you understand why you didn't do well on the exam and are concerned about your parent's reaction to your grade."

Scenario 2

Client: "I forgot to bring in the paperwork to verify my income level. I really need the food stamps today. How are my kids going to eat?"

Poor response: "When is the last time your kids have seen a doctor?"

Better response: "I can see it's really important for you to make sure your kids eat today."

Paraphrasing This can be done either by restating in your own words what you heard your client say or by clarifying what was said in the form of a question. This technique can clear up confusion or ambiguity and thus avoid misunderstanding and confirm the accuracy of what was heard. It is not parroting or repeating exactly what the client says, but the goal is to share with the client what you heard (Kanel, 2015). This allows clients to either correct any misunderstandings or confirm that both of you are on the same page. As you become more sophisticated and skilled, try to develop this skill and paraphrase at deeper levels. When Carl Rogers was first developing his theory about empathic understanding, he expressed a desire to understand the exact meaning of what a person was communicating. He believed that this could clarify a speaker's message and help others understand some of the complicated details that are often missed (Rogers, 1970).

The following example of **paraphrasing** and clarifying statements contains a poor response and an effective one.

Client: "My son upsets me so much. He stays out too late and refuses to do his homework. I don't know how to get him to cooperate."

Poor response: "Your son upsets you so much. He stays out too late and refuses to do his homework and you don't know how to get him to cooperate." (This is merely parroting the client verbatim).

Better response: "It sounds like you just can't find a way to get your son to adhere to your curfew rules and schoolwork which makes you upset" (puts client's comments into own words).

Reflecting Emotions Listeners use **reflection** to reflect the affective part or emotional tone of a client's message. It is a powerful tool that can create an empathic environment (Kanel, 2015). Reflection says to the client, "Your feelings are understood and it is ok to continue talking about them and feeling them." Expressing feelings openly has been considered a characteristic of effective coping and should be encouraged when possible (Caplan, 1964). Reflection is most effective when it simply emphasizes the emotional aspect of a client's spoken and unspoken emotions. Here is an example of reflection. While one response is too wordy, the other is simple and more effective in keeping the client in touch with his feelings.

Client: "My wife left me this past weekend, and I can't stop crying. I can't eat, sleep, and don't feel like going out at all."

Poor response: "I hear that you've been crying since your wife left you and don't feel like doing anything" (doesn't encourage client to focus on his feelings and may distract him from his feelings).

Better response: "It sounds like you are hurting a lot" (encourages client to focus only on feelings of sadness).

Asking Open-Ended Questions Sometimes you can guide the flow of a conversation by asking questions based on information already given by a client. As with paraphrasing, you should not topic jump but instead ask questions to help clients explore more of what they have already said. The key here is asking pertinent questions to which the client will relate. "**Open-ended questions** provide room for clients to express their real selves without categories imposed by the interviewer. They allow clients an opportunity to explore themselves with the support of the interviewer" (Kanel, 2015). It is useful to ask questions that begin with "what" or "how" because these types of questions allow clients to explore their ideas and feelings without being defensive. Asking too many close-ended questions might make clients feel that they are in a police interrogation, and so questions that begin with "do," "did," "why" are often avoided in client interviews. It is a good idea to communicate by combining paraphrases, reflections, and open-ended questions. This will reduce defensiveness and increase trust and **openness** on the part of the client. Here are examples of effective and ineffective questions.

Client: "I'm scared to apply for graduate school. Where should I go? How do I know if I can make it?"

Helpful response: "What would you like to learn at graduate school?" (allows client to explore her motivation).

Helpful response: "What are you scared of exactly?" (allows client to explore her fears).

Poor response: "Do you want to make more money?" (might have the effect of client answering "yes" or "no." How is this even relevant?).

Poor response: "Why do you want to go to graduate school?" (This almost sounds like the worker doesn't believe the client should go to graduate school and may make the client feel like she must justify herself. It might create a less defensive response by the client to ask, "What are some reasons you would consider going to graduate school?).

Providing Feedback Once you clarify and understand a client's needs, you need to provide your client with **feedback** that is based on objective observation and thoughts about the client's needs. During the verbal-following stage of communication, you are formulating ideas about the problem. This is often referred to as assessment. Once you believe you have something to offer your client in terms of help or assistance, you can begin to communicate various ideas in a nonjudgmental manner. Sometimes this feedback is very supportive and easy for a client to accept. At other times, feedback must include candid appraisal of certain behaviors' consequences, for both the client and others who may also be affected (Hutchins & Cole, 1992). This can be more difficult for some clients to accept, and so it must be presented in a way that allows clients to maintain dignity and save face.

Feedback can range from validation of a client's behaviors to confrontation of discrepancies in a client's behaviors and words. Some feedback is educational and provides information about which a client was misinformed or ignorant. An effective form of feedback is to try to help a client perceive a situation in a new way that may make the situation seem more solvable. Cognitive approaches to counseling emphasize this type of feedback (Kanel, 2015).

Sometimes, feedback comes in the form of direct suggestions about how to solve a problem or meet a need. This may be a referral to another agency, an assignment that encourages a client to try a new behavior, or one that highlights the benefits of reconnecting with family or friends. The key to all forms of feedback is to offer it without judgment. The focus should be on creating a climate that lets a client hear the feedback as being helpful and in the person's best interest. The following are examples of appropriate feedback.

Client: "I know I should quit drinking so much, but my life is so stressful that I need the wine to fall asleep. I'm not happy, but I just don't know how to reduce stress but still keep my job and manage my kids' social world."

Helpful feedback: "Perhaps you could make a list and prioritize your activities. Maybe some days you could put off one of the least important activities until the next day."

Helpful feedback: "Many people drink as a way to medicate depression and reduce stress. In fact, alcohol is a biochemical depressant and can actually worsen depression. Although it seems to work at first, at some point, too much alcohol consumption often has the effect of increasing stress because it affects the body negatively. Also, it's probably not good to depend on alcohol to sleep. Would you consider seeing a physician about your depression and stress?"

Other Things to Consider

While these tactics provide a solid foundation from which to communicate with people, sometimes you will have to adapt these approaches depending on the need, level of ability, and cultural background of the client(s) you are working with. For example, in some cultures it is not respectful to look someone directly in the eyes. Another example is working with older adults who suffer from Alzheimer's disease. One common symptom of this disease is significant memory loss. Often, a person will be confused about dates and events, such as thinking it is April when it is really February. In such cases, it is recommended that

compassionate communication, which is connecting with people in loving, kind ways, be used. In the context of dementia, it is encouraged that you do not ask questions about recent memory or attempt to correct memory if it is wrong. If the client thinks his or her daughter is a friend from college, the daughter is advised not to explain how that is not possible, but to merely respond by saying something like "What a great time that was mom."

Personal Characteristics of Human Services Workers Perhaps more than in any other profession, the personhood of human services workers is integral to becoming a competent practitioner because the nature of the work demands close interaction with others. As human beings, we are all full of emotions and needs. These emotions can, however, become overwhelming and needs might be unmet. When people find themselves in such difficulties, extensive research (Gibb, 1970) has shown that they tend to respond more openly to practitioners who interact appropriately and possess certain traits.

Rogers (1970) also studied the effectiveness of various client-counselor interactions. Additionally, he examined the ways in which clients respond to various personal qualities of a counselor. Based on his findings, Rogers proposed that there are certain qualities—genuineness, acceptance, and empathy—in order for therapeutic change to occur. What follows are descriptions and examples of each of Rogers's conditions for positive, therapeutic change.

Congruence or Genuineness **Congruence** and **genuineness** both mean that interactions with clients must be sincere, allowing you and your client to openly express feelings, thoughts, reactions, and attitudes that are present and relevant to the relationship. Displaying authenticity also serves as a model of a real human being who also struggles with life (Corey, 2005). Of course, no one is expected to be authentic 100 percent of the time, but it is a quality worth developing. On the other hand, authenticity does not mean sharing your every thought and feeling, but only those that are relevant for the situation, as the following example illustrates.

Client: "I am so sad. I'll never get over my father dying."

Appropriate response: "I was sad too when my father died and never thought I'd get through it. Thankfully, I did though, and I think you can too" (response is relevant to client's experience, validates feelings, and comforts feelings of hopelessness).

Unconditional Positive Regard and Acceptance **Unconditional positive regard and acceptance** mean that interactions are "not contaminated by evaluation or judgment of the client's feelings, thoughts, and behavior as good or bad" (Corey, 2005). When clients feel accepted and worthy of being understood, they may be more inclined to speak honestly and reveal the real issues and problems. As a result, they have a better chance of being helped and receiving the most appropriate interventions, as exemplified in the following example.

Client: "I am so ashamed to tell people that I'm HIV positive and that I got it because I use heroin. If I got it through a blood transfusion, people wouldn't be so weird about it."

Appropriate response: "No matter how you got the virus, you are deserving of the same respectful service and treatment as anyone with a serious disease" (response shows no judgment of the client or the disease).

Empathy Rogers (1958) also found that clients must be assured that their frame of reference is understood from their own point of view—viewing a situation from their perspective. Empathy assures clients that their problems are really understood. Consider the following interaction:

Client: "I didn't really do anything that bad, my parents are just overreacting. I just smoked pot once, and now everyone's making a big deal out of it. Like no one else has smoked a joint before. I don't need counseling."

Empathic response: "Sounds like everyone else thinks smoking pot is a big deal, but for you, it's just not that horrible. After all, a lot of kids smoke pot." (Response lets client know the situation is being viewed as the client sees it, even if it is a big deal.)

Concreteness Carkhuff and Berenson (1967) have identified four basic traits that seem to facilitate effective client-practitioner relationships. The first three, like Rogers's, are empathy, respect and positive regard, and genuineness. To those, they have added concreteness, which refers to the ability to respond accurately, clearly, specifically, and immediately to your clients. Carkhuff and Berenson made significant contributions to the field of human services by conducting their studies using applied research, which demonstrated that the quality of client-practitioner interactions had a greater effect on the outcome than the educational level of the practitioner. Therefore, paraprofessionals can be just as effective as professionals if trained to develop these traits and communicate them to clients, as the following scenario reveals.

Client: "I am so overwhelmed. I need to go to court, apply for welfare, enroll my kids in a new school, get the restraining order, and now I find out I have to help clean the shelter and cook too. How am I going to do all of this?"

Appropriate response: "There is much to do, so let's prioritize the tasks. As you are safe for now, the restraining order can wait until later. It would be good to ensure your kids are enrolled in school, so why don't we go to the school and get that done, and then while we are out, we can stop off at the welfare office. When we return to the shelter, we can set up your cleaning and cooking schedule and have you start some groups. Tomorrow, we'll go to court and file all necessary documents."

Developed Sense of Well-Being Bugental, a proponent of the existential-humanistic counseling approach, addressed the need for therapists to have a **developed sense of well-being** when he asked, "How can someone who's messed up himself help someone else get un-messed up?" (1978). This does not mean you must be problem free, but you are expected to seek help with your problems to be able to maintain emotional stability while working with others, as illustrated in the scenario that follows.

Janice has been feeling increasingly tired. When she arrives at her office, she feels angry and resents having to talk to her clients. She realizes that something is wrong. At lunch, she goes to the gym to try to work out her feelings. As she still feels very negative, she calls her health insurance to get a referral for a counselor. Janice sets up an appointment and discovers during the first session that her anger stems from her mother-in-law's interference with the raising of Janice's child. Her husband hasn't helped the situation, so Janice discusses this with her husband, who talks to his mother, which leads to an honest conversation between Janice and her mother-in-law. Janice feels better and returns to work with a refreshed outlook.

Self-Awareness **Self-awareness** can help you recognize whether you need help yourself. That means paying close attention to who you are, what values you have, what your emotional needs are, and how you interact with others. Self-awareness makes the helping profession unique in comparison to other fields in which this quality is not necessarily encouraged. Besides being aware of your own values and needs, you must also be aware of cultural biases and other values and attitudes that influence your thinking so as not to inappropriately impose these biases on your clients. Human services workers should be able to recognize "the strong set of Western assumptions underlying helping theories and techniques, and realize that helpers from non-Western cultures may have altogether different perceptions of their problems and what to do about them" (Okun, 1992).

For example, John has been interning at the YMCA. In a session the other day, a girl confided that she was pregnant. John became enraged and told her to quit having sex, because she was too young. John was brought up to believe that people, especially teenagers, should not have sex unless they're married. Obviously, John was not being aware of his own values when he spoke with the girl. As he has such strong beliefs, he should be very careful when working with clients who might believe it is all right to have sex, whether or not you're married. He must also try to understand why he gets so angry about this issue or he may take out his own feelings on his clients, which would be inappropriate and irresponsible.

Flexibility Generally speaking, all people have multiple needs and can be unpredictable—more so for those who seek out human services. Therefore, human services workers must learn **flexibility** and allow for modifications in assistance plans when appropriate. While a structure is helpful, and in many circumstances necessary, you should not rigidly implement your intervention plans or expectations. Things happen to people that make changing the rules at times necessary. For example, many people who use human services must rely on public transportation to get them to their appointments. Someone might be late for an appointment because the bus was running late. The worker might need to allow the person to still be seen despite his being tardy. Flexibility simply means to learn how to "roll with the punches" by keeping in mind that people are not always consistent and by being realistic about an intervention's results, which might not turn out as you expected. Preparing alternative plans and keeping an open mind about new methods or ideas are imperative for working effectively with clients.

For example, Maria's friend Claudia gets called into work unexpectedly, just 10 minutes before Maria's social work appointment. Maria doesn't drive and was depending on Claudia to drive her to her social worker's office. Maria now has to take a bus, which doesn't leave for 45 minutes. As she realizes that there's no way she can get to her appointment on time, Maria calls her social worker to tell her about what happened. Her social worker makes another appointment for the next day and suggests that Maria always have available an alternate plan, such as various bus route schedules, in case this happens again. The social worker also says that she'll allow this to happen once but doesn't want last minute calls about appointments to become a habit.

Openness   Closely related to flexibility is openness, which means having an open mind to different views and behaviors, to learning something from and about clients from the clients themselves, and to making mistakes and learning from them. Having a nondefensive attitude when getting feedback from clients and coworkers is also part of this openness. Human services workers must freely admit when they are wrong or need to improve. Making mistakes is inevitable, and making an effort to learn from your mistakes sometimes even makes them worthwhile. The field of helping is ever changing, and therefore human services workers must remain open to changing and learning. The need to be perpetually learning is acknowledged by most human services agencies and professions. Most agencies and licensing boards require ongoing, continuing education and in-service training for human services workers. This is what makes the field dynamic and interesting.

The following interaction is an example of a human services worker's open attitude:

Client: "Last week you told me that you would have a hard time taking back your husband if he had cheated on you. That made me feel really bad, like I was doing something wrong by getting back together with my husband."

Appropriate response: "I'm sorry. I sure didn't mean to make you feel that way. I was trying to impress on you how much I admire your strength for being able to cope with something very difficult."

Knowledgeable and Resourceful   Although it is important to care and be genuinely concerned about your clients, it is also necessary to be knowledgeable and **resourceful** so that you have the best information on how to work with your clients and about other places for them to get help. Some of this information is usually based on research studies or anecdotes from workers who have many years of experience serving people. Recipients of human services are entitled to be served by workers who put thought into interventions rather than merely offering intuitive and spontaneous advice. In addition to acquiring knowledge about client needs and interventions, human services workers should develop a list of resources by actively seeking connections with the rest of the human services world. This involves using a collaborative approach. Human services workers should want to give their clients access to as many resources as are available to assist them with whatever problems they may have. Human services workers should use all available resources and knowledge to meet as many of a client's needs as possible. This is part of the eclectic and integrative, generalist attitude discussed in Chapter 1. Here is an example of such an attitude.

Client: "I tried going to the grief group at the hospital, but I can't relate to anyone. They are all old and all their spouses died of heart attacks and cancer. My son was five when he got run over. No one there understands what I'm going through."

Resourceful response: "I can see why that group may not work for you. Your loss is very devastating, and you need a very special group. I have read about a group called, Compassionate Friends. They only take members who have lost a child. I think you might do better in that group."

Caring Professionalism Another quality that human services workers should develop is **caring professionalism** in which they demonstrate both their knowledge and their humanity to their clients. This attitude allows workers to present information and give feedback to their clients in a way that doesn't make their clients feel like they are just another case.

Helping people based on research and the experiences of others is part of being a professional. Human services workers must be both professional and real. This can take years to develop. Beginning human services workers often feel awkward when first trying to be professional. Many times these workers approach clients as they would their own friends and family. Learning to set boundaries as a professional may initially seem as if you're being uncaring; however, clients deserve to receive services from a professional who can objectively help them with their needs.

For example, the first author conducted a research study of Latinos in Southern California that revealed that the vast majority prefer counselors who are very professional and give a lot of advice. The study participants didn't want their counselors to get too personal (Kanel, 2002). These results are particularly interesting because Latinos are known for having very warm and personal relationships. There is even a word for it in Spanish: *personalismo*. This suggests that while people want friendly and personal disclosures from family and friends, they might not want this from people whose professional services they need.

Desire for Self-Preservation Finally, the important quality of **self-preservation** involves finding a balance between work and a satisfying personal life outside of work. Human services workers deal with people on a regular basis who have severe problems. It is not easy to listen to these problems daily, and stress and even burnout are not unusual. Hearing about trauma and injustices may cause human services workers to feel traumatized themselves. Therefore, it is vital for human services workers to take care of themselves emotionally and physically so they can handle the stress that comes with the job. Having a life outside of work that is healthy and active can help reenergize you for work. Self-preservation involves leaving your clients' problems at work and seeking help when you need it. Overusing alcohol and drugs are not optimal ways to handle stress. Burnout can be avoided by seeking out personal relationships that are fulfilling and healthy and by exercising and doing fun things.

The following example profiles a human services worker who has found a healthy balance between work and play. Judy regularly jogs and rides her bike after work and on weekends. She also reads novels for fun. When she goes out to dinner, she may have a glass of wine, or might just have water. Judy is not perfect, but she does try to eat nutritious food when possible. Although she cares for her clients, she does not think about them after work hours. Someone asked her if she feels guilty about having fun when she knows her clients are suffering. She said, "Absolutely not! I would feel more guilty if I thought about them all day and didn't take care of myself. I wouldn't be worth anything to them if I was depressed."

The Critical Thinking Box invites you to think about how human services workers are held to a different standard regarding their personal qualities than those in other professions.

Critical Thinking/Self-Reflection Corner

- Do you think people who work in human services should be held to a different standard of self-development than those in other professions, such as doctors, lawyers, and businesspeople? Why?
- What are some ways in which you take care of yourself to ensure that you don't burn out and deplete your energy?
- Should human services workers be required to work through their own problems with a professional therapist? Why?

PART II: THEORETICAL APPROACHES TO COUNSELING

Evidence-Based Practice

Toward the end of the 20th century and into the 21st century, designing and implementing evidence-based practices have become valued in public, nonprofit, and private human services agencies.

Evidence-based practice encourages helpers to draw on research, theory, practical experiences, and a consideration of client perspectives and then pick the best option at the moment using the best information available (Department of Mental Health, 2013). This approach is exactly what effective human services workers must do. As was discussed in Chapter 1, integrative, eclectic, and multidisciplinary practice is vital for effective helping.

While most of the theories to be discussed in the following sections have been shown to be effective based on tradition, belief, and anecdotal evidence, evidence-based practices are based in theory and have undergone scientific evaluation. Because of financial constraints in mental health agencies, it is not surprising that administrators would be most satisfied with practices that have been shown through scientific studies to be most effective.

What are evidence-based practices? Typically, these are interventions for which there is consistent scientific evidence showing that they improve client outcomes (Drake et al., 2001). Sometimes, the research involves using medications for certain populations, and at other times it may involve skill training for family caregivers. Using comparison groups often helps scientists review studies and make conclusions that allow others to examine the same evidence.

The Agency for Healthcare Research and Quality has identified levels of scientific evidence, which is used to score evidence-based practices. Three levels have been used: (1) level A indicates good research-based evidence with some expert opinion; (2) level B indicates fair, research-based evidence, with substantial expert opinion to support the recommendation; (3) level C indicates a recommendation based primarily on expert opinion with minimal research-based evidence (Drake et al., 2001). They also suggest that there may be limitations to evidence-based practices as well. For example, research evidence demonstrates that assertive community treatment reduces hospital use for clients diagnosed with schizophrenia, but evidence is less clear regarding employment for these clients and differences among various ethnic groups and other diagnoses (Drake et al., 2001).

An example of an evidence-based practice research project that focused on assertive community treatment (ACT) using dialectical behavioral therapy is provided by Burroughts and Somerville (2012). They tried to focus on the effectiveness of this model for those with borderline personality disorders (BPD) as it has been demonstrated that ACT is effective with those suffering from schizophrenia. Additionally, dialectical behavioral therapy has been proven to be effective with BPD, so they set out to prove that combining these two approaches would help keep those with BPD out of the hospital as 40 percent of those with BPD have frequent psychiatric hospitalizations (Geller, 1986; Swigar et al., 1991). Dialectical behavioral therapy draws from a cognitive behavioral framework and emphasizes skill development. It focuses on validating the experience of the client, treating the client's parasuicidal urges, and increasing compliance, therapeutic alliance, and the process between acceptance and change (Linehan, 1993). The five modes of treatment in this approach are skills training groups, individual therapy, telephone consultation, case management, and consultation meetings (Feigenbaum, 2007).

Borntrager and colleagues (2013) provide another example of the importance of evidence-based techniques. They found that in the treatment of trauma-exposed youth, many clinicians use interventions that have not been shown through research to be the most effective. Of most interest is the fact that 100 percent of evidence-based protocols for trauma included exposure-based techniques. Exposure techniques involve having the client face the trauma through a virtual computer-based program, visualization, verbalization, or a simulated real-life experience such as flying on a simulated airplane. In their study of trauma-exposed youth, only 14 to 22 percent received any type of exposure therapy. This may have been due to the fact that a majority of clinicians fear that exposure will harm their clients or may evoke anxiety and stress, despite its known effectiveness. This example highlights the importance of increasing our knowledge of evidence-based practice so that our clients will receive treatments that have been studied and shown to be effective in alleviating symptoms and problems.

We now turn to traditional approaches to counseling that have been used to help human services workers understand and intervene with a variety of client populations.

Human services workers at all levels should be familiar with the best-known of these theories and strategies so they can be used in a client's best interest. Familiarizing yourself with these various approaches and implementing them when appropriate is largely based on the generalist approach and an eclectic point of view.

Some theoretical models may be more appropriate for certain clients than for others. We begin our discussion with an approach that is considered to have been the impetus for most modern-day counseling theories and strategies.

Psychoanalysis

Sigmund Freud is credited with having developed the first of the **psychoanalytic theories** in an attempt to understand how symptoms and deviant behaviors serve a psychological function for individuals. Freud proposed that all humans are born with certain instincts that need to be expressed. These instincts reside in the part of the psyche that Freud called the **id**. The instincts, often called **libido** or eros (sexual and pleasure drives) and **thanatos** (aggression and death drives), are considered primitive drives and include all the impulses, fantasies, wishes, and feelings people have (Brenner, 1974; Guntrip, 1973; Freud, 1966). Freud suggested that as we grow, we develop another aspect to our personality structure, the **ego**, which is our sense of self. As children's egos develop, they begin to understand that a separate reality exists outside of their own drives, needs, and feelings. While the id operates under the pleasure principle, the ego operates under the reality principle and is vital for healthy functioning. A weak ego may hinder an individual's ability to approach the world realistically and thereby hamper that person's ability to manage daily stress and problems. By about four years of age, children begin to develop another part of their personality, the **superego**, commonly known as a conscience. At that point, children begin to internalize the demands and societal boundaries that their parents, teachers, religious leaders, and other authority figures have placed on them (Guntrip, 1973).

Freud postulated that problems may occur when the demands of the id are in conflict with the internalized boundaries of the superego. A person may have impulses (the id) to assault someone, but if that person has internalized the parameters of appropriate behavior (the superego) such aggressive urges will not be acted on. Conflicts between the id and the superego can make people feel threatened and anxious. To abate those negative feelings, Freud suggested that the mind represses these conflicts. This concept of **repression** relates to another concept that Freud postulated—the **unconscious**. Freud believed that the bulk of our mental lives resided in a part of our mind not readily available to conscious scrutiny. To manage our daily lives, Freud believed that we bar from consciousness (in other words, repress) psychological and emotional knowledge and experiences that would cause us overwhelming anxiety and shame and prevent us from functioning normally. In addition to basic repression, Freud theorized that we engage in other behaviors—**ego defense mechanisms**—that help us cope with unmanageable feelings of threat and conflict and that are believed to operate outside of conscious awareness. These behaviors allow the ego to manage reality without the burden of anxiety (Brenner, 1974; Strachey, 1966).

Some of the ego defense mechanisms that we humans use are defined here.

- **Projection** is used to attribute to others qualities and actions that are considered unacceptable to yourself. For example, a husband might accuse his wife of having an affair when in fact he is the one who has been unfaithful.
- **Denial** is used when a problem is too threatening to acknowledge. Refusing to recognize and get treatment for a health problem is one example of denial that can have serious consequences.
- **Minimization** is used to turn a serious problem into a minor one, such as the battered wife who says that her husband isn't being abusive since he hasn't broken any of her bones.
- **Rationalization** is making excuses for behavior or thoughts that might be deemed unacceptable or justifying situations to avoid feelings of shame such as when someone doesn't get the job he or she applied for and the individual tells people that he or she didn't really want that job anyway. Another example might be when the wife of an alcoholic excuses the drinking by saying that her husband drinks only because his job is stressful.
- **Reaction formation** is denial of a certain desire or impulse while responding vehemently to an opposite impulse or desire. For example, a new mother who has thoughts of drowning her baby instead overindulges the baby in front of other people.
- **Regression** is used to cope with an intolerable situation by returning to an earlier and safer level of functioning. For instance, a five-year-old who's been toilet trained for three years starts wetting herself after her baby brother is born. Unconsciously, she feels threatened by the attention her parents are giving to the baby and reverts to an earlier stage of development to get the attention and comfort she feels she has lost.
- **Intellectualization** is used to distance yourself emotionally from a difficult situation. A rape victim who calmly and unemotionally describes the attack in full detail is using this defense.
- **Compensation** uses strengths to make up for difficulty or an inability to do something, such as an athlete who becomes paraplegic and gets actively involved in wheelchair sports.
- People use **displacement** to direct feelings away from the threatening object that's causing the emotions and toward a safe one instead. For instance, a husband who's angry with his boss comes home and yells at his children and his wife instead.
- **Sublimation** is a healthy, socially acceptable way to express psychological energy and drives. For instance, a woman takes out her frustration with rush-hour traffic by playing a rigorous game of tennis (Brenner, 1974; Corey, 2005).

The Critical Thinking Box asks the reader a few questions related to the use of ego defense mechanisms.

> **Critical Thinking/Self-Reflection Corner**
> - What are some examples of ego defense mechanisms that you use or that you observe others using? When have you used them?
> - How do these defenses help you or others cope with difficult situations?

Freud also proposed that people develop through certain stages that he called **psychosexual stages**. He believed that if children are overindulged or deprived during these stages of development they could become **fixated** at that stage and develop personality problems in adulthood.

Oral Stage This is Freud's first stage of psychosexual development. In infancy, the basic source of pleasure is the mouth. All needs should be met during infancy. When infants are appropriately nurtured, they will feel safe and develop a sense of trust in the world. When basic needs during this phase are not met adequately, individuals may grow up to have issues with dependency and trust.

Examples of appropriate behavior at the oral stage are babies who, as soon as they learn to crawl and walk, begin sticking everything—even inedible things like dirt—in their mouths. Also, when babies cry, they are given a bottle or pacifier to quickly stop their crying.

Anal Stage As toddlers, children need to learn how to be independent and empowered, but they also need boundaries. While infants don't usually have boundaries placed on them, children at this age begin to hear and understand the meaning of "no." Freud believed that at this stage, much of the instinctual and psychological energy revolves around toilet training. Parents of two- and three-year-olds can verify that this is a truly difficult time because toddlers are learning to assert their independence. If needs are not met adequately at this stage, children may grow up burdened by shame and doubt. Freud claimed that those who are fixated at the anal stage often develop obsessive-compulsive personality disorders.

Normal behaviors at this stage are toddlers who fly into a tantrum when they can't have a toy that they want. They often insist on feeding themselves and refuse to hold their parents' hands when walking up stairs.

Phallic Stage At the phallic stage, development moves from biological to social. Preschoolers learn to engage in relationships and begin to develop a sexual identity. This is accomplished primarily by interacting with their parents. Primitive sexual and aggressive drives need to be repressed, and children need to internalize socially appropriate behaviors. Problems during this stage might lead to faulty superego formation, difficulties with sexual identity, and primitive sexual longings.

Appropriate behaviors observed at this stage may be a four-year-old girl who asks a boy in her class to play house, where she's the mother, he's the father, and a third classmate is the baby. A three-year-old sees his mother and father sitting close together on the sofa and sits between them.

Latent Stage   During the elementary school years, if repression of a child's primitive drives was accomplished in the previous stage, children are basically free from mental conflict and engage in the process of learning new skills and social behaviors.

Examples of typical behaviors during the latent stage may include a fourth-grade boy who feels proud when he learns how to do long division or a third-grade girl asks if she can sharpen pencils for her teacher.

Genital Stage   In adolescence, teenagers should be developing mature ways of relating to others and turning primitive energy and instincts into socially acceptable behaviors, such as being responsible sexually and having a mature work ethic.

Appropriate behaviors at the genital stage are seen when an eighth-grade girl asks a boy to dance at a school prom or a 17-year-old boy kisses his girlfriend at the end of a date (Brenner, 1974; Corey, 2005; Guntrip, 1973; Strachey, 1966).

Object-Relations Theory

Object-relations theorists, while still proponents of Freud, focus more on the impact the relationship between a mother or primary caretaker (**object**) and her baby has on a child's psychological development. **Object-relations theory** proposes that, rather than being controlled by instincts, a person develops a self-concept and a procedural code about how to have relationships. When children are traumatized or endure unhealthy parenting practices during the first three years of life, they may become deficient in relational skills and develop inappropriate or unrealistic self-concepts (Gabbard, 2000; Guntrip, 1973).

Margaret Mahler's (Mahler, Pine, & Bergman, 1975) emphasis in object-relations theory was on the stages during a baby's first three years of life. She proposed that the inability to move from one stage to another may develop into **personality disorders** in adulthood. Mahler's stages of development are described in the following sections. Notice that both this theory and Freud's model do not contradict each other. Object-relations theorists use these stages to determine when people begin to develop their own self-concepts and to learn to relate to other people.

Autistic Stage   Infants live in their own world of feelings, impulses, and drives. For them, life is about survival. **Normal (infantile) autism** occurs during a baby's first three or so months of life. If infants are not nurtured sufficiently so that they can move on to the next stage, deficits may develop in emotional relationships with others. They may be distrustful and may have difficulty receiving realistic feedback about their self-identity. This may lead to a schizoid, paranoid, or antisocial personality disorder.

Appropriate behavior for babies at this stage is, for instance, not crying when strangers hold and kiss them.

Symbiosis   During **symbiosis**, an infant (at about three months) begins relating to others, primarily the mother or primary caretaker. All of an infant's needs are met by the mother, and a sense of total relatedness to the object (mother) develops. It is as if the two are connected and live as one. This phase should last until children are about two years old, when, as toddlers, they begin the process of becoming independent.

Children who do not move on from this stage may, as adults, feel incomplete when not involved in an emotionally intense relationship and even may worry about being abandoned. Fixation at this stage might also result in borderline personality disorder. Adults with this disorder have great difficulty managing relationships, emotions, and impulses. They often feel empty, have intense fears of abandonment, and may have suicidal thoughts.

A 14-month-old who cries when her mother leaves for work or a nine-month-old who will only calm down and go to sleep when his mother puts him to bed are both examples of normal behavior at this stage.

Separation/Individuation From ages two through four, children learn how to experience themselves as separate individuals who must get along with other separate individuals. At this stage, children need to receive validation and empathy for who they are. Children who do not receive proper validation may become fixated at this stage. As a result, they may continue searching for validation and empathic response throughout their lives. Individuals who don't receive appropriate validation during the **separation/individuation** stage may lack a sense of cohesive self-identity, which can develop into narcissistic personality disorder. Those with this disorder are, typically, obsessed with self-acceptance and self-affirmation and appear self-involved and to lack empathy. They often have difficulty developing intimate relationships and may use others only to meet their own needs (Gabbard, 2000).

The Critical Thinking Box encourages the reader to explore whether early stages of development are observable in his or her own life.

Critical Thinking/Self-Reflection Corner

- Do you believe that people can be fixated in an early stage of development and that this fixation can determine their personality in adulthood?
- Have you noticed any of your own or anyone else's personality traits described in Freud's or Mahler's stages?

The Neo-Freudians

Neo-Freudians, most of whom were students of Freud, offered another theory to explain internal conflicts that can lead to psychological problems. Alfred Adler, Karen Horney, Harry Stack Sullivan, and Erich Fromm proposed that children, rather than being instinct-powered and preprogrammed, are instead beings who, aside from such innate neutral qualities as temperament, are entirely shaped by their cultural and interpersonal environment. A child's basic need is for security, acceptance, and approval from significant adults. The quality of interaction with these adults determines adult character structure (Yalom, 1980).

Adler emphasized that the ways in which people perceive their interactions with others greatly influence how they feel and behave. He proposed that every person has a unique, **individual psychology** that is determined by mistaken beliefs and faulty logic. Adult behavior that is considered deviant may result from distorted perceptions developed in childhood. Adults with mental health problems may be discouraged because they can't find ways to feel secure and accepted in childhood. Adler believed that understanding each person's own frame of reference is vital to understanding that person's unique lifestyle and choices. He used a **phenomenological** approach to understanding people and a cognitive approach to affecting change in their behavioral patterns. Adler introduced a more integrative way of dealing with people that continues to be practiced today by human services workers.

Implications of Psychoanalytic Theories for Human Services Delivery
The psychoanalytic models offer human services workers a theoretical basis for understanding clients. Many of these concepts can be used in counseling or providing other service. In terms of a typical human services worker practicing psychoanalytic therapy, there are some limitations. This type of therapy usually involves a long-term commitment, is costly, and should be limited to clients who have enough ego strength to handle the stress of uncovering painful emotions and to those who have enough money to pay an analyst for several years. This is not to say that counselors, social workers, probation officers, and other human services workers cannot successfully put to use some of these models' ideas and techniques. If these methods are used, workers will most likely modify their interventions to fit the needs of their clients. The idea of gaining **insight** into a person's unconscious is the main goal of psychoanalysis, and this is done by having the client talk freely about whatever comes to mind during a session. Many human services workers provide an opportunity for their clients to talk openly and freely about their problems. Although the goal may not be to uncover unconscious conflicts, the idea of a client talking to a human services worker was introduced by the psychoanalytic theorists.

Adler's model of providing encouragement and focusing on a client's strengths is probably used more often by typical human services workers. His model can be modified to benefit clients who are in short-term treatment because, unlike Freudian and object-relations psychoanalysts, Adler focused on the conscious mind and conscious goals. This focus is more amenable to short-term interventions.

Existential/Humanistic Approaches

While Freud was developing his psychoanalytic model for understanding people, a group of philosophers and novelists were establishing their views about the human condition. Existentialism is a philosophy that examines the meaning of being human. It examines the basic core of the human condition and how that condition influences behavior and emotions. Existential-humanistic theories focus on conflicts that flow from an individual's confrontation with certain **givens** of existence. These "givens are the intrinsic properties that are a part, and an inescapable part, of the human being's existence in the world" (Yalom, 1980, p. 8).

Irvin Yalom's Model Yalom, a well-known existential therapist, focused on four ultimate givens: death, freedom, isolation, and meaninglessness. He believed these concerns create conflicts within humans. In *Existential Psychotherapy* (1980, p. 10), Yalom states that awareness of these concerns leads to anxiety when an individual realizes that he or she is alone to make choices and then must accept responsibility for the consequences of those choices. To cope with this existential anxiety, many people use psychological defense mechanisms that can create dysfunction and unhealthy behaviors and restrict a full existence in which people can realize their full potential. Instead of facing anxiety and making choices based on will, people may instead seek an ultimate rescuer to make those decisions for them. Although anxiety may be reduced, the cost, according to Yalom, is an inauthentic existence, depression, and a feeling of psychological deadness.

In Yalom's *The Theory and Practice of Group Psychotherapy*, he describes how to assist clients by having them engage in **group therapy** that focuses on the existential givens (Yalom, 1985). Yalom's group therapy model also provides a detailed understanding of the group therapy process as experienced by individual group members and by the group as a whole. Group therapy is used frequently in many human services settings, and many use Yalom's model. Rather than talking to clients one at a time in private sessions, Yalom's approach has group members talking directly to one another while the therapist serves as a relationship-building facilitator among members. Of course, the therapist also speaks to clients about what they are talking about but is encouraged to disclose more than what a typical therapist might in individual therapy.

Carl Rogers's Approach Rogers's **person-centered model** followed existential theory more closely than it did the psychoanalytic theories and heavily emphasized the concepts of self-awareness and human growth and potential. Rogers believed that humans behave in symptomatic ways because they suffer from blocks to this growth. He also believed that people would be able to actualize their potential by forming a relationship with a genuine, nonjudgmental, and empathic person.

Rogers also considered group participation to be very beneficial for many clients. He described the values of groups in *Carl Rogers on Encounter Groups* (1970), in which he shows how his original ideas about the necessary and sufficient conditions of therapeutic change can be used in a group therapy setting.

Although Rogers is known for these conditions of change, he has also written about the humanistic basis of becoming a person in *On Becoming a Person* (1961). Rogers's works all focus on the positive elements of humans and encourage all of humanity to communicate respectfully with one another. In his later years, Rogers's writings and presentations focused on world peace and race relations (1987). He believed that his approach to counseling could be implemented in a variety of situations, not just therapy.

Reality Therapy William Glasser developed his approach in the 1960s when he was involved in treating teenage girls in the Ventura, California, correctional facility. He found that the long-term psychoanalytic models and the humanistic self-examination models weren't effective for this population. Rather than examining anxiety derived from being aware of core human conditions, Glasser focused on changing deviant behavior into responsible behavior. However, his model did incorporate many of the existential and humanistic concepts such as stressing that people have choices and are responsible for their behaviors and emphasizing the importance of an authentic therapeutic relationship.

Glasser believed that people not only need to develop a relationship with someone who cares about them but that they also need to care about others. He also suggested that people need to contribute something meaningful to society, concepts first introduced by Adler and other existentialists. Glasser believed that all behavior is an individual's best attempt to meet those needs. When people have not learned how to meet those needs responsibly, they meet them through irresponsible and sometimes deviant behaviors. In **reality therapy**, he explained that a strong client-therapist relationship based on honesty, trust, humor, and boundaries allows clients to move toward appropriate, responsible behaviors and feel more in control of their world (Glasser, 1975).

Implications of Existential-Humanistic Theories for Human Services Delivery Existential and humanistic-based therapies can be either long or short term, depending on a client's needs. Clients who have the time and money to examine their identities and how they fit into the world may benefit from long-term existential therapy. Most clients, however, can benefit from a genuine, nonjudgmental relationship that focuses on helping clients find answers to a specific problem through clarification and empathic understanding. Reality therapy concepts are very effective for people who want help correcting their irresponsible behaviors, especially if those behaviors have landed them in jail.

One of the biggest impacts these approaches have had on the human services is the use of group counseling as a prevalent form of intervention. Group counseling is a cost-effective and valuable way for clients to learn about their relational skills. Most residential treatment facilities, hospitals, and outpatient clinics conduct group therapy sessions on a regular basis. Prior to Yalom and Rogers, group therapy only referred to a bunch of clients sitting in the same room with one therapist who basically conducted individual therapy with each member while the others watched.

Behavioral Approaches

Behavioral theories usually include several models for understanding both animal and human behavior. Two particularly relevant models for those in the human services are B.F. Skinner's **operant conditioning** model and Ivan Pavlov's **classical conditioning** model. Both models provide concepts that explain behavior and allow for treatment of deviant behaviors.

Operant Conditioning B.F. Skinner's name is virtually synonymous with operant conditioning. He conducted many experiments with rats and pigeons in an effort to understand how to encourage and discourage behavior. In *Walden Two* (1948), Skinner introduced many of the concepts that he later expanded on in *Science and Human Behavior* (1953). Skinner's laboratory work with animals has been applied to people who have a variety of problems.

The basic premise of Skinner's theory is that all behavior is learned through reinforcement and any behavior can be extinguished by removing the reinforcement. A **positive reinforcement**, usually a reward or some positive stimulus, encourages a behavior to continue. Sometimes the reinforcement is the removal of a negative stimulus after a desired behavior is performed, this is called **negative reinforcement**. Along with increasing desired behaviors, this model also suggests that an individual will cease exhibiting undesirable behaviors if positive reinforcements cease to follow the behavior. Also, behavior will extinguish if the person suffers a **response cost**, the removal of a positive stimulus, after an undesirable behavior. Sometimes this theory is referred to as behavior modification.

Classical Conditioning This model introduced the idea that certain states of arousal, such as anxiety and cravings for sex, nicotine, drugs, and food, may result from learning through association. Ivan Pavlov (1927), a Russian physicist, famous for his experiments with dogs, demonstrated that when the dogs were presented with food (**unconditioned stimulus**) they would salivate (**unconditioned response**). In this part of the experiment, no learning had taken place, just a reflex response, in this case, salivation. Pavlov then gave the dogs food while ringing a bell (**neutral stimulus**) and found that they also salivated. Then Pavlov tried ringing the bell without presenting the food, and the dogs salivated, even though there was no food. This reaction he called a **conditioned response** (salivation) to a **conditioned stimulus** (the bell). His theory suggests that people learn certain arousal states because an unconditioned stimulus has been paired with a neutral stimulus. For example, a person may become afraid of the dark after having a traumatic experience as a child when the electricity went out. Another example might be a person who desires cigarettes because as a teen other kids told him he looked cool when he smoked.

Joseph Wolpe (1990) used Pavlov's theoretical model as the basis for his treatment of phobias. Wolpe's treatment, called systematic desensitization, pairs anxiety-evoking stimuli with relaxation to create what he called **reciprocal inhibition**. In commonsense terms, his treatment works on the theory that a person cannot be relaxed and anxious at the same time. If a person with a particular fear is exposed to the feared object or event while being deeply relaxed, that person will no longer feel as much anxiety when confronted with the feared situation. Consider how many people take warm baths to relieve stress. It is hard to be stressed out while in a nice, warm bath.

Implications of Behavioral Theory for Human Services Delivery The behavioral models can be effective with many clients with whom human services workers might work. They work especially well with students in classrooms, inmates in correctional facilities, and patients in hospitals because workers have almost complete control over positive reinforcements and response costs in these settings. The focus for these clients is to eliminate undesirable behaviors and increase more socially appropriate behaviors.

Pavlov's model is useful for clients with phobias and certain addictions and is sometimes used with pedophiles. When people are given unpleasant stimuli while engaging in socially unacceptable behavior, they eventually begin associating the unwanted behavior with the unpleasant experience. Using this model to treat, for example, a child molester may involve that person receiving an electrical shock when he becomes aroused by looking at pictures of children. Likewise, alcoholics may be given the medication Anabuse, which causes vomiting when mixed with alcohol. If an alcoholic begins associating drinking with becoming violently ill, then the desire to drink will vanish. As far as phobias are concerned, a person may be put in a deeply relaxed and comfortable state and then presented with the fear-producing object. The person becomes less fearful by associating what was feared with a pleasant experience.

Cognitive Approaches

This approach to understanding people suggests that behavior and feelings come from the ways in which people think about their life situations. If their perceptions are distorted or unrealistic, people will generally suffer from emotional and behavioral problems. In this view, people experience feelings of shame, guilt, anger, depression, and anxiety because of their perceptions about things that happen.

Approaching people from a cognitive model first began with Alfred Adler, who suggested that people first think, then they act, and then they feel. Adler focused on helping people change their distorted and mistaken beliefs. He said that the way people remember their childhoods is more important in determining adult problems than what actually did happen (Adler, 1959).

Cognitive theory became very popular in the 1970s and 1980s and is still widely used by therapists. In *Reason and Emotion in Psychotherapy* (1962), Albert Ellis presented his main idea: All people are capable of both rational and irrational thinking. Ellis believed that emotional disturbance was rooted in blame and irrational, unrealistic thoughts and beliefs. In his book, he suggested methods that could change people's irrational beliefs and therefore automatically eliminate many emotional problems.

Donald Meichenbaum, among others, followed Ellis in developing stress inoculation training and cognitive behavior modification (Meichenbaum, 1985; 1986). Aaron Beck is another cognitive therapist who developed a model for understanding and treating depression. According to Beck, people often use specific cognitive distortions that lead to emotional disturbances (Beck, Rush, Shaw, & Emory, 1979).

1. Arbitrary inferences involve jumping to conclusions that aren't supported by evidence or facts.
2. Selective abstraction is used to form a conclusion based on an isolated detail of an event that doesn't take into consideration the total context.
3. Overgeneralization bases extreme beliefs on a single incident. Such a distortion can lead to racism and other prejudices.
4. Magnification is perceiving a situation as being worse than it really is.
5. Personalization is believing that someone else's unrelated behaviors have something to do with you.
6. Polarization views something as being at one extreme or another—all or nothing (Beck et al., 1979).

Cognitive therapy can be used with clients who are old enough and have the cognitive faculties to talk about their thoughts. Typically, young children and people with brain disorders have a difficult time using this model. Cognitive therapy can be used in short-term interventions, making it practical and cost effective. The goal is to help clients change their perceptions into ones that are more realistic and rational. This approach can be used by most human services workers in any situation where someone is thinking unrealistically. As with many therapies, cognitive therapy is most effective when clients are sincerely trying to change their thoughts to more rational ones. Of course, the more experience you have in helping people think more rationally, the more effective you will be with your clients.

Family Therapy

These theories attempt to explain people's problems by examining them in the context of their family unit. Instead of looking only at the person who is behaving symptomatically, attention is focused on the dysfunction within the entire family. In the 1950s and 1960s, Murray Bowen (1992) and R.D. Laing and Aaron Esterson (1977) researched various aspects of pathological families extensively. They were all interested initially in families in which a member of the family had been labeled as schizophrenic. Their research involved observing communication patterns between patients and their parents and between parents both in the presence of the patient and alone. Prior to these studies, overbearing and overprotective mothers were thought to cause schizophrenia. The possibility that a chemical imbalance might cause the disease hadn't been fully explored. The research conducted by Bowen, Laing, and Esterson concluded that the patterns of communication observed in families of schizophrenics were also seen in families with no history of schizophrenia, making their findings useful for all families in treatment.

Families with a member identified as schizophrenic were further studied by Bateson, Jackson, Haley, and Weakland (1956) and Wynne, Tyckoff, Day, and Hirsch (1958), all of whom concluded that a family works together to a unique balance, and that the behaviors of any one family member make sense in the context of that family's rules and roles.

These studies also suggest that a family is a **self-regulating** mechanism in which rules are established to preserve the continuing essence of a particular family. Many times, family members with symptoms or other deviant behaviors are responding to obsolete rules or a lack of clear and appropriate rules. For example, a teenage girl may attempt suicide because her family rules prohibit her from having any social life. She may see suicide as her only way out. Another example might be a wife who develops agoraphobia (fear of leaving the house) in response to her husband who prevents her from having access to household expenses, from participating in raising their children, and from having a say in their social life. She may unconsciously believe that agoraphobia is the only way to take back some control of her life. In both of these examples, the family's rules are faulty. If the rules were to change, the symptomatic family member might not need to go to such extremes.

Family therapy is particularly well suited for many human services, allowing workers to take into consideration various cultural differences in family units and work sensitively to overcome cultural traditions that may be creating problems for certain family members.

Family therapy approaches are helpful in educational facilities, in social service and mental health settings, and within correctional agencies because most clients were raised in a family setting, continue to be involved in one, or were denied appropriate family care and are dealing with issues of neglect and abandonment. Family therapy approaches encourage brief intervention aimed at taking all family members into consideration. Those who want to explore the various family therapies in detail should examine the works of Murray Bowen (1992), Virginia Satir (1983), Salvador Minuchin (1974), Jay Haley (1976), Carl Whitaker (1976), and Cloe Madanes (1981).

CHAPTER SUMMARY

Because the primary role of human services workers involves human interaction, certain skills are considered vital for effective job performance. Table 5.1 summarizes the qualities and communication skills that human services workers need to develop over the years.

Most of these communication skills emphasize communicating genuine empathy and acceptance of clients' feelings and views about their situation. Skills such as active listening, feedback, and reflection help show clients such empathy. In addition to various communication skills, human services workers must also possess

TABLE 5.1 Qualities and Effective Communication Skills

Personal Characteristics	Effective Communication Skills
Congruence and genuineness	
Unconditional positive regard and acceptance	Using minimal encouragers
Empathy	Verbal following
Concreteness	Paraphrasing
Developed sense of well-being	Reflecting emotions
Self-awareness	Asking open-ended questions
Presence of mind	Providing feedback
Flexibility	
Openness	
Resourcefulness and knowledgeable	
Caring professionalism	
Desire for self-preservation	

Digital Download Download at CengageBrain.com

certain personal qualities that can increase their effectiveness. Some of these qualities include warmth, self-awareness, flexibility, openness, and self-confidence. Human services workers are encouraged to develop both effective communication skills and their own personhood as they begin helping others.

In addition to knowing how to intervene with clients in need, human services workers should have an understanding of why their clients have problems. The intervention strategies utilized by human services workers are also largely based on these causality models.

Effective human services workers should know about all of these theories and methods of intervention. They utilize this knowledge with clients and employ whichever model and intervention strategy that makes the most sense with any given client. This eclectic and integrative practice often leads to effective practice. Theories of causality may be primarily biological, psychological, or social and may be spiritual in nature. Generalist human services practice accepts that all theories may be useful with some clients. Table 5.2 summarizes the various theoretical approaches.

TABLE 5.2 Psychological Models of Causality

Therapy Model	Approach to Problem	Implications for Intervention
Psychoanalytic theory (Freud)	Anxiety results from conflict between the id and the superego and between pleasure and death instincts, and from fixation during psychosexual stages of development	Useful as a theoretical foundation in understanding serious disorders and clients who are very low functioning or who have had long-standing problems
Object-relations theory	Deficit in relationship skills from an inability to move through normal stages of development	Due to the length of time it takes, clients must have financial resources, time, desire, insight, and be able to cope with painful psychological material
Neo-Freudians (Adler)	Mental health and social problems come from being discouraged; people are motivated by social urges so involvement with others in friendship, intimacy, and contributing to society is necessary to overcome feelings of inferiority; how a person perceives life experiences determines adult personality	Can be used with many types of clients; can be short term or long term; there is latitude in implementing this model, whose focus is on conscious goals and providing encouragement, making it useful in a variety of human services settings
Existential-humanistic theory	Anxiety and defense mechanisms result from awareness of core human conditions, such as aloneness, meaninglessness, freedom, and death; people must fulfill their potential or live restricted, inauthentic lives	May be either a long-term or a short-term approach; its philosophical approach allows techniques to be flexible; may also help clients who have trouble finding meaning in life and who fail to accept responsibility for their behaviors
Person-centered model	Lacking self-acceptance, living closed and restricted lives, and looking to others for direction come from blocks in the natural growth process and the absence of an empathic, accepting, and genuine relationship	Basic attending skills, such as active listening, reflection, and paraphrasing, are essential for communicating with clients; applicable to all relationships, including parent-child, teacher-student, counselor-client, warden-convict, etc.

(Continued)

TABLE 5.2 Continued

Therapy Model	Approach to Problem	Implications for Intervention
Reality therapy	Problems created by the inability to feel cared about and worthwhile; irresponsible behavior is an attempt to have those needs met	Useful for motivated clients to understand how past influences affect current behavior; a short-term model can be effective for clients who are irresponsible and have socially unacceptable behaviors, such as criminals, juvenile delinquents, substance abusers, and those who are physically and sexually abusive; the focus is on changing behavior, now!
Behavioral theory	Belief that all behaviors are learned through reinforcement (operant conditioning) or association (classical conditioning) and can be modified by changing reinforcements and associations	For clients whose environment can be controlled and who have specific behaviors that need to change, such as children, inmates, patients in a hospital, and clients in residential facilities; also used for clients suffering from illegal behaviors (pedophiles, drug addicts, etc.)
Cognitive therapy	Problems and deviances come from illogical and irrational thinking	Can be implemented with clients with minimal intelligence and verbal skills; can be short term and cost effective; can help with stress management, crises, depression, and dysfunctional behaviors
Family therapy	Problems and other dysfunctional behaviors stem from families whose rules and roles do not allow for normal development, where faulty communication exists, and where members' behaviors that contradict family stability are counteracted	Can be used especially with clients from cultures that have traditional rules and roles; helps understand why a family discourages change and how deviant behaviors are inadvertently reinforced

Digital Download Download at CengageBrain.com

Suggested Applied Activities

1. Find a partner to play the role of a client or simply ask someone to talk with you. Let the person know you are interested in listening to whatever he or she wants to talk about for about five minutes. As the person talks, maintain good eye contact, nod your head, and say "uh-huh" every half minute or so. After the five minutes, ask the person if he or she felt heard and did it seem that you were paying attention to the conversation.

2. Find a partner to role-play an interaction between a counselor and a client. As the client talks, try to restate what you heard. Try to reflect feelings or information. Remember, the goal is to understand your client's experience. Do not try to solve any problems. Don't give advice. Just try to understand the problem or the client's needs.

3. In another client-counselor role-playing exercise, ask five close-ended questions in a row. For example, "Do you feel angry?" "Do you want to cry?" "Did you tell anyone?" "Why did you do it?" or "Does it make you want to get back at him?" Ask your role-playing partner for feedback about what it feels like to be asked those types of questions. Next, try asking

open-ended questions. A simple trick is to reword the first set of questions by beginning each with the words "what" or "how." For example, "How do you feel?" "What does it make you want to do?" "What did you do?" "What made you decide to do it?" "How do you feel toward him?" Then find out if these questions make your partner feel any different.

4. During your everyday social interactions, pay attention to how people listen to each other. Can you observe people interrupting each other in the middle of a thought or sentence? Do people ask questions that allow the speaker to continue with his or her thoughts? Make a list of the types of things people actually say to each other. Are any of these things similar to the types of communication skills presented in this chapter?

5. List the various theoretical approaches. Next to each approach, describe a problem someone might have that would best be treated using that approach. You may even use yourself as an example. Try to think about real issues that affect you or someone else when completing your own list.

Chapter Review Questions

1. What are the three active listening skills?

   _____

   _____

2. In what way are open-ended questions more effective in helping clients open up than close-ended questions?

3. What personal characteristics are human services workers encouraged to develop that differentiate them from other professions?

4. What is empathy?

5. What do the concepts of authenticity and genuineness mean when referring to qualities of human services workers?

6. How might you show someone that you are verbally following them?

7. Describe the id, ego, and superego.

8. What are the typical tasks and relationship processes that take place during the oral, anal, and phallic phases of development?

9. How do Mahler's phases of development differ from Freud's?

10. With which population would Glasser's reality therapy be most useful? Why?

11. What is the central focus of operant conditioning?

Glossary of Terms

Active listening involves not only hearing what clients say but offering feedback and helping them explore more about what they are saying.

Behavioral theories explain human behavior as resulting from reinforcements and associations in the environment. All behavior is learned and can be extinguished. Self-esteem and cognitive function influence people in adulthood.

Caring professionalism indicates to clients, "I care about you and your needs, but I am a professional and the nature of our relationship is professional. I will be friendly but not your friend."

Classical conditioning uses a neutral stimulus to elicit a response when the neutral stimulus is paired with a stimulus that naturally leads to a response in an organism.

Cognitive theory points to irrational thinking as the cause of emotional disorders.

Compassionate communication is a form of nonviolent communication that promotes trust, respect, and kindness.

Compensation is an ego defense mechanism used to replace or make up for inabilities or disabilities with abilities.

Conditioned response is a state of arousal or a behavior that occurs in reaction to a conditioned stimulus.

Conditioned stimulus is anything that is paired with an unconditioned stimulus to elicit a response.

Congruence and genuineness involve being real and genuine in the moment.

Denial is an ego defense mechanism used to cope with an unbearable reality that denies the actual existence of a problem.

Developed sense of well-being requires human services workers to take care of their own emotional needs and actively deal with any life struggles so that they may be fully available to their clients.

Displacement is an ego defense mechanism used to channel strong emotions away from a threatening object that is eliciting those feelings and toward an unrelated, safe object.

Ego is, according to Freud, the part of the personality that operates under the reality principle. It allows people to function realistically.

Ego defense mechanisms are behaviors that allow people to function by pushing anxiety related to conflict into the unconscious mind.

Empathy involves being able to put yourself in another person's shoes and understand that person's emotional and cognitive experience of a situation.

Feedback provides clients with an assessment of their problems. It can be both supportive and confrontational but should always be based on an objective assessment and presented in nonjudgmental terms.

Fixated at a stage of development occurs when a person receives too much or too little gratification and therefore remains stuck at that stage.

Flexibility is being open to adopting and modifying new ideas and behaviors and to learning new ideas.

Givens are the core human conditions with which all people must struggle and that often lead to anxiety. Yalom focused on four givens: death, freedom, isolation, and meaninglessness.

Group therapy involves more than two clients and one or two facilitators who mediate among group members as they share personal information related to their lives and others.

Id is the part of the personality, according to Freud, that contains basic instincts, impulses, fantasies, wishes, and feelings.

Individual psychology was how Adler referred to his neo-Freudian model of psychotherapy. Its focus is on how each individual perceives his or her own experiences and creates a unique style of life rather than focusing on being determined by instincts and specific phases of development.

Insight is the goal of psychoanalysis in which a person gains understanding and self-knowledge of unconscious feelings that have created psychological symptoms and dysfunctions.

Intellectualization is an ego defense mechanism used to remove oneself emotionally from the reality of a difficult situation.

Libido is the pleasure instinct, according to Freud, and is also called eros.

Minimal encouragers are verbal and nonverbal cues that let clients know that their human services worker is interested in hearing what they are talking about. Head nodding and a forward-leaning posture are two examples.

Minimization is an ego defense mechanism used to view a problem as being less significant than it is in reality. .

Negative reinforcement uses a negative stimulus to eliminate or decrease a behavior.

Neo-Freudians are a group of theorists and clinicians who focus on social and cultural factors to determine personality development.

Neutral stimulus is something that does not create a response.

Normal (infantile) autism, according to Mahler's object-relations developmental theory, is the phase in which infants live in their own world of impulses, drives, and instincts and exist only to survive.

Object (in object-relations theory) usually refers to the mother, father, or primary caretaker who is the significant being in a child's life.

Object-relations theory focuses on how children develop personality traits and patterns in relation to how their mother (object) relates to them during their first three years of life.

Operant conditioning uses positive or negative reinforcement to increase or extinguish a particular behavior.

Open-ended questions begin with what and how and allow for further exploration of what a client is saying. Clients feel less defensive answering these types of questions.

Openness is a nondefensive approach that actively seeks new information with the realization that there is always something new to learn.

Paraphrasing is used to restate what a client is saying to make sure that the practitioner and the client are understanding each other.

Person-centered model, founded by Carl Rogers, relates human growth to certain characteristics such as empathy, genuineness, and acceptance.

Personality disorders typically create dysfunction in a person's life especially in regard to relationships. People who suffer from these disorders are considered deficient in many social skills and have unhealthy self-concepts.

Phenomenological approach attempts to understand people from their own personal frame of reference rather than a preconceived theory.

Positive reinforcement is usually a pleasurable stimulus/reward that is given in response to a desired behavior.

Projection is an ego defense mechanism used to attribute qualities and actions to others that are considered personally unacceptable.

Psychoanalytic theories attempt to explain human behavior by focusing on early childhood experiences, conflict between parts of the personality, and instincts.

Psychosexual stages, according to Freud, are specific stages that people experience as they grow from infancy to adulthood. During these stages, psychological and sexual energies must be mastered. Failure to do so may lead to personality disorders later in life.

Rationalization is an ego defense mechanism used to excuse or justify certain behaviors or situations.

Reaction formation is an ego defense mechanism used to reject an unacceptable desire or impulse; the person using this defense is vehemently repulsed by that impulse or desire.

Reality therapy, created by William Glasser from his work with juvenile offenders, focuses on taking responsibility for and facing the reality of your own behaviors.

Reciprocal inhibition is based on Wolpe's idea that evoking a relaxation response while exposing a person to a feared object will eliminate the anxiety related to the object. If a client could be trained to relax and then be exposed to fear-evoking stimuli while relaxed, the relaxation would inhibit the anxiety.

Reflection is the use of verbal and nonverbal cues to reflect back a client's emotions.

Regression is an ego defense mechanism used to revert to an earlier and safer level of functioning.

Repression is used to push painful memories or anxieties out of conscious awareness and into the unconscious mind.

Resourcefulness is the ability to work collaboratively to learn about all the agencies and services that are available to help out and meet the needs of clients and requires the use of active problem-solving methods.

Response cost removes a pleasurable stimulus or reward in response to an undesirable behavior.

Self-awareness is the recognition of your own feelings, thoughts, values, and behaviors and how they affect people around you, as well as the awareness of your strengths and the areas in your life that need improvement.

Self-preservation gives you the ability to protect yourself from harm (and job burnout) by regularly monitoring your emotional well-being and doing what is necessary to stay healthy.

Self-regulating means to maintain one's own state of homeostasis and stability.

Separation/individuation is the final phase in Mahler's model during which children begin experiencing themselves as separate individuals and developing a stable, integrated sense of self.

Sublimation an ego defense mechanism used to channel psychological energy and drives into socially acceptable outlets.

Superego, or the conscience, according to Freud, is the part of the personality that responds to the world according to a set of internalized morals, societal demands, and commands.

Symbiosis is the second phase in Mahler's theory, during which an infant develops a strong sense of relatedness to the mother or primary caretaker who meets all of the infant's needs.

Thanatos is the aggressive drive that Freud believed is often in conflict with the pleasure drive.

Unconditional positive regard and acceptance of clients allows them to believe that feelings, thoughts, or behaviors are not being judged.

Unconditioned response is an emotion or behavior that is a natural reaction to a stimulus.

Unconditioned stimulus can be anything that leads to a reflex or natural response.

Unconscious is the part of the mind that contains most of our mental life and is not readily available to the conscious mind. It is speculated that this mental material may flow out of the unconscious mind through the process of psychoanalysis.

Verbal following keeps the focus of a conversation on what a client is saying rather than jumping from topic to topic.

Case Presentation and Exit Quiz

General Description and Demographics

The client presented in this counseling session is a 23-year-old woman, named Gloria, who entered a battered women's shelter last night. Gloria has been married for six years. She has two children, a three-month-old baby girl and a four-year-old son, both of whom are with her at the shelter because she has no relatives living in the area. Her family lives in Mexico, and she rarely communicates with them since she's been married. Gloria married a U.S. citizen whom she met in Mexico. He brought her to the United States and began beating her two months into their marriage.

The abuse escalates when he is drinking. Gloria has had bruises around her eyes and on her ribs. He even beat her while she was pregnant, and yesterday he attempted to choke her. She was so afraid that he might kill her that she finally told a neighbor what's been happening. The neighbor gave her the number of a battered women's shelter. Gloria called the shelter, and an intake worker made arrangements to get her and her kids to the shelter while her husband was at a bar. Gloria speaks English, but not fluently. Her client advocate speaks some Spanish. The following conversation takes place the next morning and is the first that Gloria and her advocate have had.

Interview between Gloria (G) and her client advocate (A.)

A: What happened yesterday that made you call our hotline, Gloria?
G: My husband, he choked me bad.
A: How are you feeling now?
G: I am scared.
A: What scares you?
G: He might try to find me and kill me.
A: That does sound scary.
G: Yes, he told me he will kill me if I leave.
A: Uh-huh.
G: He gets drunk and is very mean. I hope he doesn't find me here.
A: It sounds like you believe he might look for you and hurt you.
G: Yes, he told me many times that I am his now, and that I won't be allowed to stay in the United States if I leave him.
A: I can see why you would be afraid then. I am not sure if that is true, but we have an attorney who comes here weekly, and we could find out about that if you like.
G: That would be good.
A: Are you saying that you want to leave your husband?
G: I want our family together so the children can have a father, but I ...
A: This seems like a difficult decision for you.
G: Yes, my family told me not to marry him because he would be a bad father. He was known to have a bad temper in our town in Mexico. My mother told me I should stay in Mexico.
A: So even before you got married, your family didn't really think he was right for you.
G: I am ashamed to tell anyone that he beat me. They will think it is my fault.
A: Unfortunately, many people don't understand these types of situations. I don't think it was your fault at all. Nobody deserves to be mistreated. It is a crime to beat one's wife.
G: But I don't keep my children quiet enough, and sometimes I don't want to be close with my husband.
A: It is hard to keep children quiet all the time, especially a baby.
G: My husband says he will take the children from me. I cannot live without them. I love them so much.
A: You sound like a good mother.
G: My husband says I am a bad mother and that the children love him the most.
A: What do you think about that?
G: I don't think so. My son is afraid of his father.
A: How do you mean, afraid?

G: He told me he is scared when papa comes home.
A: Has your husband ever beat your son?
G: He yells at him, but has not hit him yet. He hits me instead because I don't raise our son right.
A: I am sure glad he hasn't hurt your son. But I am scared that your husband could get violent with your children. Your husband might have a serious problem with his anger and with the need to be in control.
G: I think you are right, but my husband, he does love us. Sometimes he is nice and brings us to the park, and we eat McDonalds. My son loves that.
A: That is good that your son has some good times with his father. It is important that children have a father and a mother in their lives. It is not good for children to watch their father hurt their mother. It could affect them later in life. Many children who see violence in the home repeat it as adults.
G: Of course, I saw my father beat my mother, and I was afraid. But I thought it was normal.
A: It is very common. About one woman out of three lives with a man who mistreats her. But it is not normal, and it is against the law. Your husband needs professional help to stop doing it.
G: But I don't want him in trouble with the law. He needs to work.
A: It is your choice to decide whether you want to report it to the police. If you do, the court will most likely make your husband go to group counseling and get educated about his problems. Here at the shelter, you will have a chance to learn more about this problem and how you want to handle it. I am so glad you are here with your children. You will all be safe from violence while you are here. You can talk to an attorney and other women who have gone through this. Try to focus on getting help for your family while you are here. We will take it one day at a time. You have at least 45 days to make decisions.
G: Thank you. I need to go feed my baby now, but I will see you later. You have been so much help.
A: Good, I'll see you in group at 10 a.m.

Exit Quiz

1. When the advocate says words like "seems" and "sounds," she is
   a. providing direct feedback
   b. asking open-ended questions
   c. clarifying and paraphrasing
   d. unsure of what to say

2. When the advocate tells Gloria that she is glad that her son hasn't been hurt, the advocate is
   a. showing professional caring
   b. crossing the line between being a professional and being a friend
   c. lacking empathy
   d. all of the above

3. An example of a reflective statement is
   a. Uh-huh.
   b. Are you saying that you want to leave your husband?
   c. How are you feeling?
   d. That does sound scary.
4. When the advocate tells Gloria that it is good that her son has some good times with his father, the advocate is demonstrating
   a. lack of empathy
   b. lack of congruence
   c. unconditional positive regard
   d. lack of flexibility
5. Including an attorney to help this client is an example of the advocate being
   a. lazy
   b. resourceful
   c. uncaring
   d. incongruen
6. When the advocate asked questions related only to what Gloria said in the session, this is an example of
   a. the advocate's inability to develop empathy
   b. lack of trust between Gloria and the advocate
   c. verbal following
   d. lack of creativity

Exit Quiz Answers

1. c   3. d   5. b
2. a   4. c   6. c

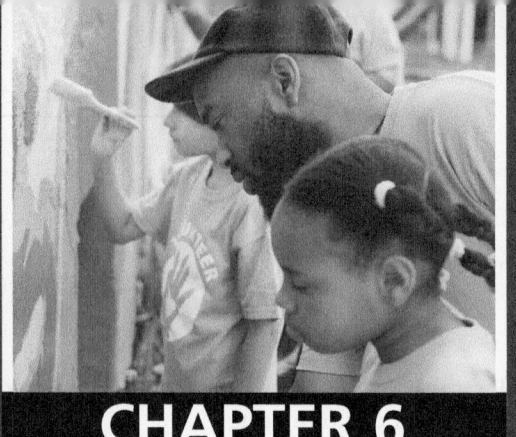

CHAPTER 6

Crisis Intervention, Suicide Prevention, PTSD, Community Disasters and Trauma Response, and Military Trauma

CRISIS INTERVENTION

Crisis intervention is a short-term counseling approach. However, human services workers do not necessarily have to be serving in the position of counselor to provide crisis intervention, which can be conducted by many types of workers, including social workers, correctional officers, and school personnel, in a variety of settings. This is because crises occur regularly in the lives of most people. In providing crisis intervention, workers must assess the client's presenting needs, offer some new perspectives on the problem, and help the client decide on the interventions that will be most helpful in effectively managing the crisis. Sometimes human services workers refer clients to outside agencies and workers, and at other times the crisis can be managed in-house without input from others. An important part of the assessment phase is determining how much intervention will be provided by the worker doing the assessment and how much will be provided by others.

Crisis intervention focuses on identifying the precipitating event (a situational or developmental stressor) and how clients' perceptions of this event have led to negative, painful feelings and impairment in functioning. Once the nature of the crisis has been identified, the crisis worker then offers new ways of thinking about the situation and offers new coping skills. The usual duration of crisis intervention is no more than six weeks. Many agencies and facilities follow this model and offer 45-day-treatment programs.

The ABC Model of Crisis Intervention

The **ABC model of crisis intervention** (Kanel, 2015) offers a helpful guide for conducting short-term, problem-focused counseling.

A: Basic Attending Skills   These interactions include active listening, paraphrasing, reflection, and open-ended questions (discussed in Chapter 5). Such questions create a sense of safety and trust that encourage clients to discuss their problems freely and openly. The crisis worker wants to develop a strong relationship with the client rather quickly to ensure that the client accepts the counselor's suggestions and referrals.

B: Identifying the Problem   To properly design an appropriate intervention, counselors must understand what triggered the crisis, how the client perceives and feels about the situation, and the areas in which the client is having trouble functioning. Once the nature of the crisis is appropriately identified, the crisis worker must offer the client new ways of thinking about the situation. Often, this requires education, cognitive restructuring, and empowerment. Once clients perceive the crisis differently, they will be better able to accept various coping solutions offered by the worker because the client will be feeling better. Crisis theory suggests that feelings of distress are closely linked to how a person perceives the situation, so if the perceptions are changed, the emotions will be changed as well.

C: Coping   Solutions may be offered during this stage and may include suggestions such as keeping a journal, exercising, going to **support groups**, connecting with other human services workers, and working on assertive communications and stress management (both of which will be described in Chapter 10).

Crisis intervention is provided for many problems because it is immediate and useful in assisting people to function in as many areas as possible in their lives. It is cost effective and encouraged by most agencies. It can be conducted by phone, such as when a client calls a suicide hotline, or in person during a normal office visit. It can last as long as two hours, such as when someone is severely suicidal and may need to be hospitalized, or be resolved in 10 minutes as is often done in residential living facilities, such as when a resident has a conflict with another resident and a worker steps in to help resolve the conflict.

Crisis intervention is commonly used to assist individuals who are suffering from depression and suicidal thoughts. Additionally, it is useful when someone is struggling with posttraumatic stress disorder (PTSD) caused by some type of trauma such as a manmade disaster, a natural disaster, personal victimization, or military combat. Each of these situations will be examined next. Although crisis intervention is utilized in dealing with all of these issues, there are other interventions that may be specific to the particular trauma or the reaction to a trauma. Personal victimization issues are discussed in Chapter 9 while suicide prevention, combat-related PTSD, and community disasters are explored in this chapter.

SUICIDE PREVENTION

The first part of suicide prevention is assessing someone's **suicide risk** level. The goal of **suicide assessment** is to determine whether a client is actually intending on doing himself or herself harm, and the ability to conduct this type of assessment is vital for human services workers who have direct involvement with clients. Once the risk level has been determined, an intervention strategy for prevention is implemented.

Not every client who feels suicidal will openly disclose this to a human services worker. These thoughts and feelings must often be explored in connection with other complaints and presenting issues. Some typical statements made by clients who may be suicidal include

"Life's just not worth living anymore."

"Why should I bother to try? Nothing ever goes my way."

"I wish I could just sleep and never wake up."

"I have to find some way to get out of my depression." (Sometimes a person's depression lifts because they have decided to kill themselves as a way out of it.)

"I'm so alone, and no one cares if I live or die."

Of course, some people actually say, "I think about killing myself." When a client discloses one of the previous statements, suicide assessment is a good idea, especially whenever someone states that he or she feels very depressed. Other factors that may make someone at risk for killing or harming themselves include living alone, drinking alcohol excessively, taking drugs, attempting suicide in the past, knowing someone who has committed suicide, and suffering from chronic physical pain.

Stages Used in Suicide Assessments

Assessing for suicide risk is usually done in stages (see Table 6.1). Human services workers who suspect that a client may be thinking about suicide must first ask whether this suspicion has merit. The stages progress logically from first thinking about suicide, to making a **plan**, to identifying what **means** are needed to carry out the plan, and to wondering what, if anything, can persuade a client from carrying out the plan. While many risk factors are associated with committing suicide, the following are the essential factors that human services workers must assess to determine an effective intervention strategy. Remember, the goal of a suicide assessment is to gather enough information to understand the risk level of a client at the time of the assessment. Once the risk level is assessed, the best intervention plan can be implemented.

TABLE 6.1 Stage Response Risk-Level Intervention

Stage	Response	Risk Level	Intervention
1. Is there suicidal ideation?	No	Low	Crisis intervention; support proceeds to stage 2
2. Has a plan been made?	No	Low	Crisis intervention, support, verbal no-suicide contract
	Yes		Proceed to stage 3
3. Are the means available?	No	Low	Crisis intervention, support, regular monitoring of suicidal thinking and plan, written no-suicide contract
	Yes	Middle	Proceed to stage 4
4. Will the plan be carried out?	No	Middle	Family watch, written no-suicide contract, frequent contact, medication evaluation, removal of the means
	Yes	High	Proceed to stage 5
5. Will hospitalization be voluntary or involuntary?	Yes	High	Assist in finding a placement; ask family or friends to transport client to hospital
	Yes	High	Call appropriate authorities to evaluate for involuntary hospitalization

© Cengage Learning

Digital Download Download at CengageBrain.com

Stage 1: Are There Thoughts of Suicide? The first stage is assessing for suicidal ideation. When clients present with one of the previously mentioned factors or appear to be considering suicide, workers should ask clients directly whether they have had thoughts of harming or killing themselves. Some possible questions are "Have you had thoughts of hurting yourself?" "Have you thought about committing suicide?" or "You mentioned that you are very depressed; sometimes people who are depressed think about suicide and death. Have you?" Workers who are just starting their careers often worry that such questions will make someone want to kill themselves. However, this does not typically happen. If someone has no thoughts about suicide, asking them may help them realize that maybe his or her problem is not so bad after all. He or she will usually respond with an emphatic "no." However, clients who have had such thoughts may feel relieved to talk about them openly.

If a client denies any suicidal ideation, a worker can assess the client's needs and proceed with basic counseling, crisis intervention, or case management, depending on what intervention is appropriate. A client at a low level of risk can usually benefit from a variety of services. A brief description of common interventions follows the section on suicide assessment. If a client reveals ongoing thoughts about suicide, the worker must then proceed to the next stage of assessment.

Stage 2: Is There a Plan? This next stage of assessment determines whether a client has a plan for committing suicide. This refers to the method of suicide a client intends on using. Typical plans include overdosing on pills, hanging, shooting oneself, driving off a cliff, and cutting oneself with a razor. If someone has thoughts of suicide but has no plan, that person may still be assessed as low risk and should be monitored regularly to make sure that he or she still does not have a plan. If a client admits to having a specific plan, the worker must proceed to the next stage of suicide assessment.

Stage 3: Are the Means Available?   The next piece of information needed is whether the client actually possesses the means to carry out the plan. Once a plan is disclosed, workers must find out if a client has a gun, pills, rope, razors, and the like. If a client does not have whatever is needed to carry out the suicide plan, then that person may still be considered at a low risk for suicide. When clients have **suicidal ideation** and a plan, they should be monitored closely to ensure that the means to carry out their plans have not been obtained. A verbal **no-suicide contract** is a good idea. The client is asked to make a verbal contract with the worker, promising not to commit suicide. If a client agrees, it is a good idea to shake hands and solidify the contract. This client should continue in a relationship with one or more human services workers until the ideation subsides completely. A client who has the means moves into the next level of risk—middle risk. Assessment must proceed to the next stage.

Stage 4: What Is the Level of Determination?   It is vital to find out how determined a client is to carry out the plan. Many times a client who has suicidal ideation, a plan, and the means is ambivalent and hasn't carried out the plan because there might be something that offers hope of feeling better. At this stage of assessment, a worker must explore reasons why the client has not attempted suicide, despite having a plan and the means to carry it out. What a client says at this stage helps workers establish their clients' levels of **determination**, which helps establish whether a client is at middle or high risk. The more reasons a client has for living, the better, especially if a specific experience is discussed that would definitely make a difference. For example, if a client says, "I won't want to kill myself if I knew I would find a job in the next six months," a worker has a chance to assist the client in finding a job. Another example might be a client who says, "I haven't killed myself because it would hurt my grandmother. She's always been so loving and kind to me." A worker might encourage this client to focus on this loving relationship and even use the grandmother as part of treatment, perhaps in a family watch.

If something can stop a client from committing suicide, the risk level remains middle risk. Interventions at this stage may include making a written no-suicide contract (see Figure 6.1) with the client, frequent sessions with the client, referral for medication assessment, removal of the means, and involvement of family members. If a client is adamantly determined to commit suicide, making such comments as, "I'm going to leave here and kill myself," then workers must proceed to the next stage of the assessment.

Stage 5: Voluntary or Involuntary Hospitalization?   When a client is determined and has the means to commit suicide, that client is assessed as being at high-level suicide risk. A worker can then offer the client one of two options: **voluntary or involuntary hospitalization**.

If a client agrees to being hospitalized for further assessment and for his or her own safety, the worker proceeds in finding an appropriate placement, usually

> Any human services worker can make a written no-suicide contract with a client. Of course it is not legally binding, but it is psychologically binding and can be effective.
>
> I (client's name) _____
>
> agree that I will not cause any harm to myself or intentionally allow harm to come to me at least until I speak personally with (worker's name) _____
>
> I agree to this contract for the next two weeks.
>
> Date _____ client's signature _____
>
> Date _____ worker's signature _____

FIGURE 6.1 Sample No-Suicide Contract

Digital Download Download at CengageBrain.com

determined by medical insurance and other resources. Some high-risk clients realize that they need protection from themselves and will enter into a facility voluntarily. Other high-risk clients, however, may refuse to voluntarily enter a hospital, and they may need involuntary hospitalization to ensure their safety.

Typically, when a high-risk client refuses hospitalization, specific, usually state-determined, steps need to be taken. In some U.S. states, police are called, along with a member of the psychiatric emergency team (PET). PET workers are trained to assess whether or not high-risk clients need to be held in a protective facility for a brief time period until further psychiatric assessment can be made. It is important to keep in mind that only qualified people can have someone involuntarily hospitalized. In California, for instance, only state-certified PET workers and hospital psychiatrists have the authority to do this. All human services workers must understand how to work collaboratively when conducting suicide assessment and prevention (Kanel, 2015; Wyman, 1982). Figure 6.2 provides an example of a suicide hotline intake form.

Critical Thinking/Self-Reflection Corner

- Do you think human services workers should always prevent suicide?
- Are there any situations in which you think people should be allowed to commit suicide?
- What are your initial feelings about asking clients whether they have been thinking about killing themselves?
- Do you think that other professionals should be responsible for ensuring that people don't commit suicide? Which professionals?

Name (if possible) _____ phone number (if possible) _____

Date and time _____

Are you having suicidal thoughts? Yes _____ No _____

Do you have a plan? Yes _____ No _____

Do you have the means? Yes _____ No _____

Have you ever attempted suicide? Yes _____ No _____

Have you ever been treated for emotional problems? Yes _____ No _____
If so, who were you seeing? _____

Are you still in treatment? Yes _____ No _____

Name of therapist (if different from previously named) _____

Are you taking any medication? Yes _____ No _____ What type? _____

What is stopping you from committing the act? _____

Will you make a commitment with me not to harm yourself? Yes _____ No _____

Will you follow up with a therapist? Yes _____ No _____

Referrals given _____

Follow-up plan _____

FIGURE 6.2 Suicide-Prevention Hotline: Sample Intake Information

Digital Download Download at CengageBrain.com

POSTTRAUMATIC STRESS DISORDER (PTSD)

PTSD is a broad category that applies to people who have been severely traumatized at one or more times in their lives and are not functioning effectively because they have not integrated the trauma. It can be caused by a manmade disaster, a natural disaster, personal victimization, or an unexpected death of a loved one. The *American Psychiatric Association's Diagnostic and Statistical Manual of Mental Disorders*, fourth edition, text revision (DSM-IV-TR) (2000) describes PTSD as being induced after an exposure to a traumatic event in which a person experienced actual or threat of death or serious injury or threat to physical integrity of self or others. The symptoms of PTSD include the following:

- Intense fear and feelings of helplessness
- Recurrent and intrusive recollections, flashbacks, and dreams of the event
- Physiological reactivity when exposed to cues that symbolize the event
- Avoidance of stimuli associated with the event
- Numbing of feelings
- Inability to recall aspects of the event
- Feelings of detachment
- Pessimism about the future
- Sleep difficulties
- Anger and irritability
- Difficulty concentrating
- Hypervigilance and exaggerated startle response.

Gabbard (2000) suggests that "the most common precipitating event reported among persons with PTSD was the sudden, unexpected death of a loved one" (p. 252). He discusses the idea that trauma victims alternate between denying the event and compulsively repeating it through flashbacks or nightmares. This is the mind's attempt to process and organize overwhelming stimuli. He further proposes that most people do not develop PTSD even when faced with horrifying trauma, so there must be certain predisposing factors such as genetic makeup, childhood trauma, personality characteristics, compromised support system, and perceptions that the locus of control is external rather than internal.

One of the unique aspects of PTSD diagnosis is the importance placed upon the causal agent, the traumatic stressor, or as the ABC model of crisis intervention refers to it, the precipitating event. One cannot make a PTSD diagnosis unless this stressor criterion has been met. Because not everyone develops PTSD even when exposed to the same stressor, it has been hypothesized that trauma may be filtered through cognitive processes before it is appraised as an extreme threat, and there are individual differences in this appraisal process. People have different trauma thresholds (Yarvis, 2013, p. 83). Yarvis's supposition corresponds very neatly with the premises of the ABC model of crisis intervention, which focuses on the cognitive aspect of a precipitating event.

Other Interventions for PTSD

In addition to crisis intervention and cognitive restructuring, other methods may be useful in treating PTSD. Eye movement desensitization and reprocessing (**EMDR**) has been shown to be useful. It involves elements of exposure to traumatic stimuli via imaging and cognitive behavioral therapy. It may facilitate the accessing and processing of traumatic material (Shapiro, 2002). Group therapy may also be useful as those with PTSD share their stories and feelings with others who have gone through the same experiences. Medication may also be useful when the anxiety and depression are severe and prevent the person from functioning (Kanel, 2015).

Because a person suffering from PTSD often oscillates between intrusive thoughts of the traumatic event and numbing of and dissociation of the feelings of the event, Gabbard recommends that those working with individuals with PTSD allow for both the withholding of distressing information and gentle encouragement of the memory of the trauma (2000, p. 256). Lindy and colleagues (1984) recommend supporting areas of adequate functioning and reestablishing the individual's personal integrity.

RESPONSE TO TRAUMATIC COMMUNITY DISASTERS

During the past decade, the United States has been hit with a variety of natural and **manmade disasters**. The most recent example of a **natural disaster** was Hurricane Sandy, which caused billions of damage on the East Coast, primarily in New Jersey, a few years ago. Many of us still remember Hurricane Katrina, which occurred in 2005 and devastated most of New Orleans as well as many regions of Mississippi and Alabama. The victims of disasters such as these received services designed to help them get back on their feet. Other natural disasters, such as earthquakes, fires, and tornados, have devastating economic and emotional effects on millions of people. Many communities offer trauma response units to help people manage the consequences of such disasters. When mental health workers talk to survivors of unexpected trauma, it is often referred to as **critical incident debriefing** or **trauma response**. This can be done at community centers, gymnasiums, or even at a bank such as when gunmen enter and rob the bank. The True Stories From Human Services Workers Box relates a real-life incident from one of the authors about her experience of doing critical incident debriefing.

True Stories from Human Service Workers

Critical Incident Debriefing after a Bank Robbery

When I was working as a psychotherapist in private practice, I was contracted with the employee assistance program for a bank. When a gunman robbed this bank, many of the tellers and other employees began suffering from PTSD and were unable to perform their duties at the bank. I was asked to come to the bank and offer critical incident debriefing services to approximately 20 employees. I had them all sit in a big circle and each person was to describe his or her feelings about the robbery. I then had them talk to each other and offer support and share their fears. I explained the nature of PTSD and what they might expect. I urged them to continue to talk about their feelings, write about them, and also to spend some time in enjoyable activities. I listened intently to their fears and concerns and provided empathic responses. I explained that seeking help and talking to others is useful in alleviating anxiety. This session lasted about two hours. Most employees said they felt much better. I gave them my number and offered to provide further counseling as needed. Only one employee called me: the teller who was held at gunpoint. I worked with her for a few weeks.

Manmade Disasters

In 2013, a manmade disaster occurred in Boston during the famous Boston Marathon, when two men detonated bombs that killed and maimed people watching the marathon and those completing it. This was a shock despite the fact that there have been many terrorist attacks in the United States and abroad since the World Trade Center attacks of September 11, 2001. Since 9-11, most of us have been emotionally affected by terrorism even if we don't all develop PTSD. Unfortunately, terrorism isn't the only type of manmade disaster experienced in the United States. Some of the readers will remember the shooting of 20 children and 6 adults at Sandy Hook Elementary School at the end of 2012. Gun violence didn't just begin at Sandy Hook, though. In 2007, 32 people were murdered in a mass shooting at Virginia Tech University. These unexpected shootings reduce feelings of safety and normalcy, often causing PTSD. While the community does pitch in to assist those who are severely affected by both natural and manmade disasters, many still remain deeply affected and have difficulty functioning. This is where human services workers, such as counselors and social workers, are needed to help pick up the pieces that have been torn apart due to these types of disasters.

Additionally, given its nationwide presence, the Veterans Administration (VA) is heavily involved in disaster management, particularly as it affects veterans and their families. Its role is to respond to a range of community emergencies and disasters in part through collaboration with other governmental, nonprofit, and for-profit agencies (Claver, Friedman, Dobalian, Ricci, & Horn Mallers, 2012). For example, the VA was essential in the evacuation and sheltering of nursing home residents during the 2005 hurricanes Katrina and Rita. Current research on these events indicates that physical harm, psychological distress, cognitive decline, and increased social isolation were areas of concern for older adults during evacuation and sheltering. A community-wide response is critical to the safety and well-being of those affected by disasters (Claver, Dobalian, Fickel, Ricci, & Mallers, 2013).

Social scientists have conducted many analyses of the community's response to both natural and manmade disasters of the past decades, and they have shown four phases of community disaster that are the reactions of a community to the psychological and physical consequences of disasters:

- Heroic, or impact, phase
- Honeymoon, or immediate post-disaster, phase
- Disillusionment, or recoil and rescue, phase
- Reconstruction, or recovery, phase

(Mental Health Center of North Iowa, June 2005; National Center for Posttraumatic Stress Disorder, June 2005).

Heroic, or Impact, Phase During the heroic or impact phase, the goal is to get the victims to a safe place where basic needs such as food and water can be met. Once food and water arrive, the victims need to be housed in a safe and sanitary environment. The general goal is to save lives and property. Altruism is prominent while people expend much energy in helping others to survive. Everyone pitches in and is motivated to help.

Honeymoon, or Immediate Post-Disaster, Phase The honeymoon, or immediate post-disaster, phase may last from one week to six months. During this time period, there is a sense by the survivors that the community is available to offer support and resources. They have survived the disaster physically and realize that they are not alone to recover. They feel a profound sense of having shared something very intense with others.

Disillusionment, or Recoil and Rescue, Phase Unfortunately, survivors soon realize that the help and utopia they had envisioned doesn't usually occur. In this disillusionment, or recoil and rescue, phase, survivors start to lose that sense of shared community and must concentrate on resolving their own problems. Often, outside agencies leave the affected area, and community groups may not respond to the ongoing needs of survivors. Some people believe that many Katrina survivors are in this phase as they are yet to completely rebuild their lives, and it seems that the strong community and national support offered during the first six months post-disaster have weakened.

Reconstruction and Recovery Phase In this final stage, survivors assume responsibility for rebuilding their own lives. The reconstruction and recovery phase may last years, depending on the damage and community support available.

Throughout the years, many human services workers have served the victims of these disasters to aid them in overcoming their feelings of powerlessness, grief, and fear. Trauma response models are very similar to crisis intervention, in that the trauma workers must actively listen to the victims, provide them with information, connect them with resources, and ensure that they remain safe. The majority of workers who assist victims of traumas are volunteers. Of course, certain institutions such as the American Red Cross and the United Way provide services related to community disasters by employing permanent administrative employees to ensure continuity of service from the multitude of community agencies providing trauma response. Holding fundraisers, coordinating volunteers, and collaborating with many agencies throughout the nation is a full-time job. Workers who perform these jobs often work long hours for average pay, but the intrinsic satisfaction in knowing that meaningful services are being provided to millions seems to motivate people to continue working and volunteering for these agencies.

MILITARY TRAUMA

Since the terrorist attacks of September 11, 2001, and then when Iraq was invaded due to the fear that it possessed weapons of mass destruction, the United States has been involved in two major wars, Operation Iraqi Freedom (OIF) and

Operation Enduring Freedom (OEF). Over a million men and women have served their country in these two wars and are now returning home. Many of these service personnel bring back with them wounds. Some wounds are physical such as amputated legs; others are invisible such as PTSD, depression, and traumatic brain injury (**TBI**). It is these **invisible wounds** that human services workers are likely to work with in a variety of settings. Although fewer military personnel have died in these wars than in other wars, many are returning with emotional and psychological scars and need help in healing them. Many women have participated in these wars, which has led to an increase in military sexual assaults. The particular nature of military sexual trauma will be discussed in Chapter 9 in the section on rape and sexual assault, so we turn our focus to how serving in these two wars has led to PTSD, depression, and TBI.

PTSD and Military Service

While lifetime PTSD prevalence rates for the general U.S. population are 9.2 percent, the rates for at-risk groups, such as survivors of sexual assault, motor vehicle accidents, and combat, is often substantially higher (APA, 2000). The PTSD rates for veterans of OIF and OEF (the Iraq and Afghanistan wars) are thought to be 12.5 percent (Hoge et al., 2004). Some studies show that two or more deployments could raise the rates of PTSD (Yarvis & Schiess, 2008).

Counselors first became aware of PTSD when they were dealing with war veterans, especially those of the Vietnam War (Kanel, 2015). Vietnam veterans' symptoms have included reexperiencing the sounds of war, suffering from nightmares, and being unable to manage interpersonal relationships effectively. Support groups were set up to allow these veterans an opportunity to discuss their traumas and to find ways to integrate their war experiences into present-day functioning.

The veterans of World War II had similar responses to their combat experiences. Anyone who exhibited signs of trauma was said to have shell shock. Unfortunately, many World War II veterans did not seek or receive mental health treatment when they returned home in the same way that veterans of the Vietnam War and veterans of more recent wars have done. They were encouraged to "buck up" and "be a man." While it is true that veterans of the Iraq and Afghanistan wars have also been told to be strong and deal with PTSD on their own, many have rejected these ideas and have sought treatment despite being told they don't really need it. Recent films such as *Saving Private Ryan* have put a realistic perspective on the extent of the trauma experienced by the men serving in World War II. It is easy to forget that they suffered because, unlike their Vietnam veteran counterparts, World War II veterans received a hero's welcome when they returned home. World War II was a popular war, and most Americans were supportive of the efforts of the military.

When soldiers are engaged in combat and see the trauma of war, some do experience acute stress disorder. They are often treated by doctors and given time to recuperate. However, the military does such a good job of training soldiers to numb themselves to war trauma that the majority are able to deal with combat as it is happening. It is when they return home that they show signs of PTSD. The disorder has been delayed, almost, by training. Once soldiers return home, many have difficulty adjusting to civilian life. They report being preoccupied with the troops that are still fighting. They often feel guilty for leaving the other soldiers and think they should return to help fight.

The recent wars fought in Iraq and the Persian Gulf have also left emotional scars on combat veterans. Some refer to the PTSD experienced by soldiers who fought to free Kuwait in the 1990s as Persian Gulf syndrome. As the soldiers began returning home after deployments in the Iraq and Afghanistan wars, their psychological and emotional reactions have been studied by clinicians treating them in clinics and by other interested social scientists. It has been shown that they too show symptoms of PTSD, acute stress disorder, and depression upon their return and while they are engaged in combat (Kanel, 2015).

A 2008/2009 Research Study of Veterans and PTSD

Kanel (2013) conducted a research project during the period 2008–2009 to study the symptoms of PTSD, acute stress disorder (PTSD symptoms lasting for less than one month after trauma), and depression that the college-enrolled veterans of the Iraq and Afghanistan wars experienced while in combat and after returning home. Additionally, these veterans were asked about interventions that they believed to be helpful to them in overcoming their mental and emotional problems.

Data was tabulated to determine if participants met the DSM's diagnostic criteria for PTSD or acute stress disorder. Twenty-one percent of participants qualified for a diagnosis of PTSD, and 49 percent met the criteria for acute stress disorder.

The symptoms of depression most frequently reported were "depressed mood most of the day, fatigue or loss of energy nearly every day, and insomnia or hypersomnia" with 50 percent, 45 percent, and 50 percent reporting these symptoms, respectively. To meet the DSM criteria for major depression, at least five symptoms must be reported. Twenty-seven percent of respondents answered "yes" to at least five symptoms.

To understand help-seeking behaviors and the types of things participants found helpful in overcoming their symptoms, more questions were asked. Thirty-one percent of participants said they had seen a counselor, and the most commonly reported factor that was said to be helpful was "having someone just listen." A few subjects stated that the following were helpful: expressing how helpless they felt, being in a relationship, being able to talk honestly and face the truth, reassurance, and allowing themselves to explain what they were thinking and going through. A few participants said the following were least helpful: watching the president talk about the troops, reliving the experience, group counseling, and having to explain themselves. Only 5 percent admitted taking psychiatric medication, which they reported as either an antidepressant or a sleep aid.

Of the 59 percent of subjects who had not seen a counselor, 26 percent said at least one of the following helped them overcome negative experiences:

dealing with it, driving on, family, living life without much thought of it, getting involved with a veterans group, family planning, moving life in a forward direction, having a buddy or mate, ignoring negative feelings, having a spouse, and reading the Bible.

From these results, it is clear that this nonclinical sample of Iraq and Afghanistan war veterans have experienced many symptoms indicative of both PTSD and depression. Despite the fact they experienced these symptoms, only 31 percent sought the services of a counselor. This may be due to the military training that teaches soldiers to "deal with it" and "be strong," which were indicated by those who hadn't seen a counselor. Interestingly, even though this was not a clinical sample, 21 percent met the criteria for a formal diagnosis of PTSD, 15 percent met the criteria for major depression, and 49 percent met the criteria for acute stress disorder. The fact that only two participants were taking medication indicates that they may be lacking appropriate intervention. Clearly, these veterans have many symptoms, and this must not be ignored by mental health practitioners or physicians.

Traumatic Brain Injury (TBI)

TBI remains the signature wound of OIF and OEF. Since 2000, an estimated 195,000 service members have been screened for suspected brain injury (Department of Defense, 2009). This disorder ranges in severity from mild to severe and is usually caused from blast exposure both penetrating and nonpenetrating. The improvised explosive devices, rocket-propelled grenades, and mortar rounds so commonly used by enemy combatants in OIF and OEF are the usual cause responsible for moderate to severe TBI and the "invisible wound" of mild TBI (Boyd & Asmussen, 2013).

The symptoms of TBI include loss of consciousness, amnesia, loss of memory, poor concentration, inability to respond to verbal commands, dizziness, pain, fatigue, sleep difficulties, vomiting convulsions, seizures, inability to wake up from sleep, restlessness, confusion, and agitation.

Intervention for TBI includes immediate rehabilitation. Education and support to the family and the person suffering from TBI is useful. Of course, physician involvement is necessary to rule out severe brain injury. Unfortunately, TBI can affect a person's functioning at work and at school. Educating employers and college personnel is useful, and human services workers should advocate for the rights and needs of veterans and their families whenever possible.

Other Interventions for Veterans

It is vital that any human services worker who is working with a veteran be familiar with military culture and issues. While veterans may prefer to be treated by other veterans, civilian counselors and social workers are needed to manage the many cases showing up at agencies across the country.

Many social service agencies have been creating programs within existing county offices that include veterans' services where a veteran may seek assistance regarding rights for services, financial assistance, educational assistance, and disability assistance. Veteran centers are being created in which former military personnel work with veterans and their families individually and in groups to help them deal with PTSD, depression, and TBI-related issues.

Additionally, many colleges and universities have created veterans' centers for enrolled students to go to for support groups, information about their rights, and general counseling.

CHAPTER SUMMARY

Human services workers frequently participate in activities designed to help individuals, families, and communities heal from a variety of traumatic experiences. When people experience natural and manmade disasters, community workers often provide trauma response services. After a disaster, the community usually passes through four phases while people heal: heroic, honeymoon, disillusionment, and reconstruction. Some people develop PTSD and need individual crisis intervention services. Others become suicidal and need a suicide assessment. Those who have served in the military have special issues including TBI, depression, and PTSD, which are often called invisible wounds. Human services workers are needed to help these military personnel return to society and overcome these syndromes so they may function.

Suggested Applied Activities

1. Pair up and have one student role play a client who is either a low-risk, middle-risk, or high-risk suicidal client while the other student role plays some type of human services worker. Using Table 6.1, practice assessing for suicidal ideation, plan, and so forth. Try to develop an intervention based on the assessed risk level. Switch roles and have the new client role play a different risk level. What were some of the difficulties that the human services worker faced in doing this task?

2. Interview a veteran or a family member of a military service member. Inquire about his or her needs and any problems related to military service that he or she had to deal with.

3. Think about a few community disasters that you have experienced personally. What were your reactions and the reactions of others? How did your community respond?

Chapter Review Questions

1. What are the basic steps in conducting a suicide assessment?

2. What are the appropriate interventions for a low-, middle-, and high-risk suicidal client?

3. What types of situations are dealt with when conducting trauma response?

4. What is the purpose of crisis intervention?

5. What are invisible wounds?

6. Name five traumas that might lead to PTSD.

7. Discuss the phases of community disaster.

Glossary of Terms

ABC model of crisis intervention is a three-stage model in which workers first attempt to develop rapport through basic attending skills: (A) identify the problem, (B) offer new ways of thinking about the situation, and (C) offer coping strategies.

Crisis intervention is a type of intervention in which the worker attempts to help a client return to a normal level of functioning by offering adaptive coping strategies to manage a stressful situation and by helping the client perceive the situation in a more manageable way.

Critical incident debriefing or trauma response are forms of intervention that occur after a community disaster or even when an individual or group experiences a serious trauma such as a bank robbery.

Determination is the stage of suicide assessment in which a worker establishes how firmly decided a client is to commit suicide, and if a decision is not firm, what can be done to keep a client from harm.

EMDR refers to eye movement desensitization and reprocessing and is a form of treatment in which a therapist helps a person integrate a trauma cognitively and emotionally.

Invisible wounds refer to the signature wounds of the Iraq and Afghanistan wars and include depression, PTSD, and TBI.

Manmade disasters are occurrences such as bombings and gun violence that affect an entire community.

Means (of suicide) refers to the method a client plans on using to commit suicide, such as a gun, pills, or a razor blade.

Natural disasters are occurrences such as fires, floods, hurricanes, and earthquakes that affect the community and often cost billions of dollars to repair.

No-suicide contract can be either a verbal or written agreement between a client and a worker that has a client promise not to attempt suicide before speaking with the worker.

Plan (to commit suicide) is how a person intends to commit suicide.

PTSD stands for posttraumatic stress disorder and is a result of severe trauma that is perceived as life threatening to oneself or loved ones. Symptoms include hypervigilance, flashback, anxiety, and numbing.

Suicidal ideation refers to thoughts someone has about committing suicide.

Suicide assessment is a structured process of determining how serious a client is about committing suicide.

Suicide risk includes three levels—low, middle, and high risk. Clients at low risk are those who have thought about suicide but have no plans or means to carry out a plan. Clients at middle risk are those who have thought about suicide, have a plan, and the means. Clients at high risk are those who have thoughts of suicide, a plan, the means, and intend on going through with the suicide.

Support groups are typically led by counselors and focus on helping group members increase self-esteem and feelings of empowerment and decrease feelings of social isolation.

TBI stands for traumatic brain injury and is the signature wound of the Iraqi and Afghanistan wars. It usually manifests in people exposed to explosions and can lead to impaired consciousness and concentration.

Voluntary or involuntary hospitalization is recommended for clients who are a danger to themselves or to others. When a client refuses to go voluntarily, the involuntary hospitalization is usually the only option.

Case Presentation and Exit Quiz

General Description and Demographics

Kyle is a 23-year-old male who is returning to college after serving five years in the military. He spent two deployments, a year each in Iraq, and then voluntarily served one year in Afghanistan most recently. He returned to the United States six months ago and has enrolled in a local college to seek a degree in criminal justice. He would like to get a job in law enforcement. He has been finding it very difficult to study and concentrate while in classes. He often gets up and leaves the classroom, feeling very agitated. He doesn't sleep well due to nightmares. He has trouble connecting with his high-school friends and doesn't feel like socializing with his family. He met a girl that he would like to date, but he doesn't know how to approach her.

Kyle has come to see a counselor at the college's veteran center. After explaining his needs and future goals, the counselor discloses that he too served in Iraq. Kyle immediately relaxes and lets the counselor know that he has been feeling suicidal and depressed and that he blows up a lot.

Exit Quiz

1. One of the first things the counselor should do is:
   a. tell Kyle to buck up and be strong
   b. conduct a suicide assessment
   c. encourage Kyle to return to the military for a future career
   d. all of the above

2. Which invisible wound might Kyle be suffering from:
   a. depression
   b. PTSD
   c. TBI
   d. all of the above

3. What type of intervention might be useful for Kyle?
   a. group counseling with other veterans
   b. referral to the veteran's administration office for disability
   c. telling him about a fraternity he could join
   d. all of the above

4. The counselor may be a good match for Kyle because
   a. he is a college student
   b. he understands military culture
   c. he can tell him what to do
   d. all of the above

5. Kyle's difficulties in concentrating might be due to:
   a. lack of desire to learn
   b. low IQ
   c. TBI
   d. none of the above

Exit Quiz Answers

1. b
2. d
3. a
4. b
5. c

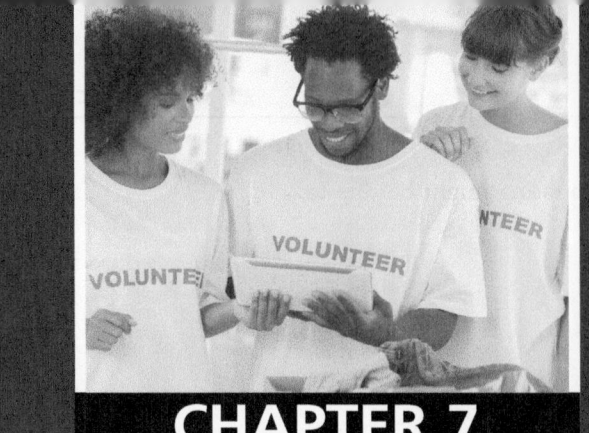

CHAPTER 7

Humans Services Populations

INTRODUCTION

Generalist human services workers are capable of working with and on behalf of many diverse client populations because of their knowledge of people's many needs and issues and of the resources available to enhance quality of life. Chapters 7, 8, and 9 present populations and mental and social issues that constitute common clients or problems addressed in human services delivery.

CHILDREN

Child Maltreatment

From a legal standpoint, children are minors until their 18th birthday. Once children turn 18, they are considered adults and no longer have the protection and assistance they had as children. Unfortunately, while childhood is supposed to be a time to play and grow, many children lack protection and safety. The Child Abuse Prevention and Treatment Act (CAPTA) defines **child abuse and neglect** as, at a minimum:

> *Any recent act or failure to act on the part of a parent or caretaker which results in death, serious physical or emotional harm, sexual abuse or exploitation; or an act or failure to act, which presents an imminent risk of serious harm (Children's Bureau, 2011).*

Physical abuse occurs when children are hit, burned, grabbed, choked, or punished in some way that leaves visible marks such as bruises, scars, welts, or broken bones. These injuries must be sustained by other than accidental means.

Sexual abuse occurs when an adult or a minor who is capable of adult sexual gratification engages in sexual behaviors aimed at sexually gratifying either the child or the adult. This may include sexual intercourse, masturbation, finger penetration, insertion of objects, or exhibition of genitals. General neglect occurs when parents fail to provide for a child's basic needs such as food, shelter, clothing, medical care, and supervision. Emotional abuse occurs when adults repeatedly criticize a child and purposefully tear down the child's self-esteem.

Prevalence

Sadly, child abuse and neglect are one of our nation's most serious problems. In 2011, it was reported that 1,570 children died from abuse and neglect, that is, more than four children every day (National Children's Alliance, 2013). More specifically, there were over 3.4 million referrals of child abuse, estimated to include 6.2 million children, to child protective service agencies. While all children can be victims of abuse, the youngest, under three years of age, are the most vulnerable to maltreatment (Children's Bureau, 2011). Of all children who experienced maltreatment, over 75 percent suffered neglect, more than 15 percent suffered physical abuse, and just under 10 percent suffered sexual abuse (National Children's Alliance, 2013). 2012 data indicate that both males and females are likely victims, with the majority of all cases involving a parent or step-parent or some other relation known to the child. Child abuse occurs at every socioeconomic level, across all ethnic, cultural, education, and religious lines. However, children with a disability, children in foster care, and children of ethnic descent may be particularly vulnerable. Children who are abused may show unexplained injuries, changes in behavior (e.g., in eating, sleeping, or school performance), lack of personal care, risk-taking behaviors (particularly among teens), and inappropriate sexual behaviors. Children who are abused may experience long-term emotional, physical, behavioral, and social problems due to the abuse.

Causality Models

While there is no single cause of child maltreatment, there are several risk factors that increase the chances a child will be abused. From a sociocultural perspective, many people in our society believe that children are to be seen and not heard. Some parents view children as not worthy of adult respect and believe that they have the right to punish or sexually violate them in any way they see fit. Traditional cultural and societal values hold that families have the right to privacy and that children are the property of their parents. It wasn't until 1974 that the federal government stepped in and created laws against child abuse.

Psychological causes of victimization relate to a person's coping skills, such as self-esteem and inner strength. If children are raised to feel badly about themselves and are not equipped with the coping skills to manage life's stresses, they become vulnerable to being victimized. Often, because children are dependent on the abuser for their very survival, many do not tell anyone they are being abused. Sadly, even children who have developed healthy self-esteem may be victimized simply because the adult abusing them is bigger, smarter, and able to manipulate them psychologically. This is particularly true if the parent has poor impulse control, depression, anxiety, or antisocial behavior; if the parent has a history of maltreatment; if the parent drinks; and/or if the parent is young and ill-equipped to parent. Many parents who abuse their children lack appropriate knowledge about child rearing. Research has shown that parents who have misattributions, or negative or incorrect beliefs, about the causes of their children's behavior are more likely to abuse their child. For example, if a mom interprets her three-year-old son's crying as a way to purposefully annoy her she is more likely to react with anger and hit her son. If, though, she interprets his crying as age appropriate and due to his lack of ability to communicate that he is tired, then she will be more likely to respond with empathy and compassion (Twentyman & Plotkin, 1982; Williamson, Bordin, & Howe, 1991).

Sadly, sexual abuse of children may be influenced by the media. Beauty contests, magazine ads, and movies often depict young girls and boys in adult roles and dress. Children are exposed to sexual activities at a younger age than in the past and may appear more sexually sophisticated than they really are. This may make sexual predators feel less guilty about engaging in sex with a child. Additionally, pedophiles are also commonly online, and with the increased use of the Internet by children, child pornography, child sexual abuse, and exploitation are growing problems in society that merit serious attention by human services professionals.

Human Services Delivery in Child Abuse Situations

Emergency Situations and Interventions When a case of child abuse is reported to the police or **child protective services**, an emergency response system takes immediate action. The first step is to assess whether a child is in immediate danger. Such factors as the age and location of a child and the type of abuse determine how soon an emergency worker responds to any given case. Typically, any type of abuse involving infants receives priority status as they are the most helpless of all minors. On the other hand, older adolescents are considered to be more capable of self-care and may be last to receive emergency assessment and intervention.

Any minor who is assessed to be in need of immediate medical care, food, shelter, clothing, or supervision receives emergency services. They are provided with all of these needs by being placed in a government-funded emergency shelter, given treatment in a hospital emergency room, or given food and clothing. If a social worker assesses that a child would be in danger by remaining with a parent or guardian, that child will be removed from the home and put in a temporary emergency shelter run by the government. The child remains under the care of the state until other arrangements are made that can ensure the safe care of the minor. Relatives may be a good resource to turn to in emergency cases.

The same is true if a child is at risk of being physically or sexually abused. If a social worker assesses that another adult in the home cannot protect a child from an abuser, the child will be removed from the home and put in a state-funded emergency shelter. The age of the child and the severity of the abuse increase the likelihood of a child being removed. Children who have been and continue to be at risk of sexual abuse are often provided with special services from social workers, counselors, attorneys, and law enforcement officials who all specialize in dealing with sexual abuse emergency situations. The child is interviewed in the presence of all behind a one-way mirror in an attempt to reduce the trauma of being interviewed. This helps reduce problems when it is time to try the case in court. Also, emergency medical care and psychological intervention are available at these agencies.

The primary goal of emergency care for children who are abused is to ensure that no further abuse will take place and that the child's physical and emotional well-being are taken care of in hopes of preventing deterioration in functioning. Additionally, basic needs for survival must also be provided.

Secondary Intervention Once a child's safety and basic needs are ensured, the focus turns to the psychological trauma. Counseling for children and their parents may be provided to assist in dealing with the possible breakup of the family unit. Safe reunification is the goal in most cases. Even when children are not removed from their homes, family or individual counseling may help families express feelings and fears and learn more appropriate coping and communication skills. Children who are abused often benefit from play therapy, which encourages them to color, paint, play with clay, or use dolls to act out their experiences. Play therapy is effective because it is an easy way for children to express themselves, and they feel most comfortable with play objects in hand while talking about traumatic situations.

Parents who are first-time offenders are often referred to parenting classes in which they learn about normal child development and appropriate expectations, as well as effective disciplinary methods. If drug or alcohol abuse is an issue, parents are referred to drug and alcohol awareness classes or even a 12-step program. Sometimes, parents may attend support groups or even more confrontational groups where they can openly express their feelings about the system and offending or nonoffending parents, and where they can also discuss how their own childhood experiences have affected their parenting abilities. Individual counseling may also be useful for these parents and children.

The goal of the counseling and educational groups is to teach new coping skills, to assist the children and parents to express their feelings and better understand why the abuse occurred, and to prevent any further abuse from occurring. Sometimes children remain in the home while crisis intervention and counseling is provided, while other children live with relatives or in group or foster homes until treatment is completed. The duration of treatment for isolated incidents of abuse may range from six weeks to one year.

Tertiary Intervention Sadly, some parents have treated their children abusively for many years and require longer term services. Whether or not these parents' drug and alcohol addictions or serious emotional problems have caused this abuse, they cannot seem to care for their children properly, despite receiving help from various social services agencies. These cases need ongoing monitoring and case plans, which sometimes last for more than five years. This often means frequent hearings with a judge and many chances to improve in their parenting abilities. Some people just can't seem to pull it together, no matter how many services they receive.

Some need to be involved indefinitely in 12-step groups, such as Alcoholics Anonymous. Others need to participate in support groups, such as Parents United, Parents Anonymous, and other groups designed to help parents stop their abusive behavior. At some point, however, many of these parents lose custody of their children, who are given up for adoption, placed in foster or group homes until they turn 18, or live with relatives while their parents are only permitted supervised visits with them.

Group homes provide counseling services for the children and usually implement a program based on the principles of behavior modification in an attempt to reinforce and teach coping skills and eliminate negative behaviors. Children raised in chronically abusive conditions have many emotional and behavioral disorders and need regular therapy and sometimes medication to manage uncontrollable feelings of rage, fear, and depression. They are at high risk for suicidal behavior, self-mutilation, and drug abuse. Those children placed in foster homes or adopted out must also receive services to help adjust to their new family and resolve feelings they hold toward their own parents. The trauma of being chronically abused as a child often follows the person well into adulthood, and the person often needs ongoing therapy as an adult. Support groups, such as Incest Survivors Anonymous (ISA) and Adult Children of Alcoholics (ACA), offer these people ongoing support throughout their lives. The emotional consequences of chronic abuse can often take 20 years or longer to overcome, even with the help of effective therapy. Because therapy can be costly, it is vital to let clients know about low-cost or no-cost resources available at nonprofit agencies and at 12-step groups.

Primary Prevention On a more optimistic note, many programs are designed to prevent abuse from occurring in the first place. At-risk groups are targeted and provided with assistance in hopes of giving them skills and resources that will increase the chances of successful parenting. At-risk groups such as single mothers, pregnant teens, and low-income families may receive parenting education, financial assistance, and support for housing, child care, and medical care. Hotlines have been developed that allow parents to call and vent frustrations in hopes that this will prevent them from acting out these feelings on their children.

Children also receive services that attempt to prevent abuse from occurring. It might be education at the elementary-school level in which children are taught about appropriate touching, or it might be at the high-school level where teens are taught about proper parenting techniques. Pregnant teens and new teen mothers are also provided with primary prevention services in an effort to reduce the risk of abuse occurring. Many programs teach these teen mothers how to care for a baby before and after birth and how to use resources in their community. Having access to child care and medical care and completing high school are important for these teen mothers. Helping them to become self-sufficient by encouraging them to complete school so they can be competitive in the job market will reduce their stress. Lowered stress reduces the tendency to engage in abusive behaviors with children. Being able to work and support herself and her child will also reduce the likelihood of the child being neglected.

The overall goal of primary prevention is to target at-risk groups and teach them about child abuse, how to prevent it, and how to manage stress effectively.

Other Childhood Considerations

There are many other challenges that human services professionals will address in their work with children. One that warrants critical attention is the issue of childhood custody owing to familial divorce and adjustment to remarriage and blended families. Approximately 40–50 percent of American children witness the breakup of their parents' marriage; of these, many also experience the dissolution of a parent's second marriage. Nearly 40 percent of married couples with children are step-couples, whereby at least one partner had a child from a previous relationship before marriage, and nearly one-third of marriages are remarriages (as cited from Deal, 2013). Also, serial transitions, in and out of marriage, divorce, or cohabitation, are typical for many American children today. What are the consequences of these changes on children? The research on divorce is quite controversial, with many findings indicating that divorce poses negative short-term and long-term outcomes for children; other studies indicate that the outcomes depend on the age and gender of the child, the nature of the divorce, and the level of conflict within the marriage. The result of divorce, structurally, is that many children become part of binuclear or single-parent households, and parents may have sole, joint, or split custody. Upon remarriage, many children will become part of blended or step-families (more positively referred to as reconstituted families). It is not surprising that the United States is witnessing growing family complexity. Each situation poses its own unique challenges; for example, parents with sole custody often experience tremendous financial stressors, burdens, and overload. However, many also report tremendous joy from being able to see their child grow positively as a result of their support and guidance. Split custody, though not as common, can work for many families, but only if arrangements are consistent and children are not being used as a tool to continue the familiar habit of fighting with one's spouse. Joint custody has been shown to have more positive benefits on children as compared to sole custody, including fewer emotional problems, fewer behavioral and academic problems, and higher self-esteem. In reconstituted families, step-parents may have to ensure they do not favor their "own" children over their stepchildren, provide healthy discipline approaches, and make the new children feel welcomed and included in the newly formed family dynamics. This is all easier said than done, and many children and youth struggle greatly with their parents' divorce, their new living arrangements, and their new roles. Human services workers need to be mindful of the living arrangements of the children they work with to gain a better, more comprehensive understanding necessary to meeting their clients' needs, whatever the issue.

Finally, while the scope of this book prevents a thorough or comprehensive discussion of it all, mention should also be made to other prevalent challenges children

Childhood Obesity

Childhood obesity is defined as having a body mass index (BMI) above the 95th percentile. Overweight is defined as having a BMI above the 85th percentile. The average child of every age, family income, nationality, and cultural group is heavier today than in years past. According to the Centers for Disease Control and Prevention (CDC, 2013), childhood obesity has more than doubled in children and tripled in adolescents in the past 30 years, and in 2010, more than one-third of children and adolescents were overweight or obese. Older and poorer children show the greatest increase. These numbers are heavily influenced by the poorer quality of food consumed (e.g., high-calorie, low-nutrition "junk" foods), decrease in exercise, and a co-occurring increase in time spent playing video games and watching television. You may be shocked to learn that the average American child watches 1,680 minutes of television weekly and nearly 1,500 hours in a year! This is sadly in contrast to the 900 hours of time spent in school and the 3.5 minutes per week that parents report spending in meaningful conversation with their children (A.C. Nielson Co. and TV Free America, as cited by CSUN, 2007). Also, obesity may have a strong hereditary component. Additionally, exposure *in utero* (as fetuses in the mother's womb) to maternal obesity or gestational diabetes may also increase the risk for childhood obesity. Unfortunately, being overweight or obese as a child is not a temporary problem; rather, it has long-term consequences, including a risk for diabetes, cardiovascular problems, increased cancer risk, and obesity in adulthood (CDC, 2013), not to mention that obese and overweight children are often teased and are isolated because of the increased risk of being bullied. Prevention and intervention efforts involving schools, families, government agencies, media, and food and entertainment industries are critical.

face. Childhood sex trafficking, obesity, bullying, behavior and academic problems, drug usage, and stress are problems that children, irrespective of age, gender, ethnicity, or social class, currently have to contend with. We urge students though to take the time to learn more about the other salient challenges children face.

Critical Thinking/Self-Reflection Corner

- Do you think you could counsel someone who has abused a child?
- Are you interested in working with children who have suffered abuse? Why or why not?
- How might people's views and behaviors toward children who are obese change when they learn that obesity may not only be a result of poor diet but also have a hereditary component?
- What childhood problem do you think is the most critical to address? Why?
- What would you include in a primary, secondary, and tertiary prevention program for childhood obesity?

ADOLESCENCE

Adolescence is a time of great biological and hormonal changes, brain maturation, moral challenges, increased independence, identity development, and the development of new relationships. In other words, it is a challenging, stressful time (Spear, 2000), and while most teens emerge from adolescence with little turmoil, many teens engage in intense risk-taking and self-destructive behaviors. The issues and needs that underlie gangs and delinquency, pregnancy, runaways, self-mutilation, suicide, depression, and drug use are examples of the many problems that some teenagers face. These particular problems are examined here because they are considered to pose the greatest risk to adolescents' well-being. They are at risk of incarceration, dying prematurely, and developing a dysfunctional lifestyle. If they can be dealt with before they reach adulthood, it is hoped that these dire consequences can be prevented.

Prevalence: At-Risk Behaviors

Gangs and Delinquency While youth involved in **gangs** comprise only a small proportion of the adolescent population overall, these gangs are a significant problem affecting youth safety. 2010 data indicate that about 756,000 U.S. youth, particularly 12- to 15-year-olds, are in over 29,000 gangs (U.S Department of Justice, 2012). Gang activity and its associated violence, including homicides, drug and weapon usage, and turf wars, are a significant component of the U.S. crime problem. While a higher percentage of African American, American Indian, and Hispanic youth join gangs, any race or ethnic group can form a gang, such as the white supremacists known as skinheads. Gang members must swear a loyalty oath that supersedes loyalty to their family of origin and often wear a certain color or style of clothing that indicates affiliation with their gang. Many gang members become **juvenile delinquents**, or law breakers under the age of 18. Sadly, aggression and serious crime are more frequent during adolescence than any other period of the life span.

Pregnancy Not all teens are having sex, but in the United States, 47.4 percent of high-school students reported that they have engaged in sexual intercourse (CDC, 2011). Nearly 40 and 77 percent reported they did not use a condom or birth control, respectively. Over 15 percent reported having sex with four or more partners during their lifetime. There are obviously several negative consequences resulting from teens' involvement in sex, including **sexually transmitted infections** (STIs) and, of course, **unintended pregnancy**. In 2000, nearly half of the 19 million new STIs were among youth, and in 2009, an estimated 8,300 youth had HIV infection. Also in 2009, more than 400,000 teen girls gave birth (see CDC, 2013). Unfortunately, when teenage girls have babies, they often are at risk of dropping out of high school, depending on welfare throughout their lives, abusing drugs and alcohol, becoming victims of domestic violence, abusing their children, and being unemployed (Simpson, Pruitt, Blackwell, & Sweringen, 1997). This does not even address the complications to the baby. If a girl under 15 becomes pregnant, she is at greater risk of almost all possible birthing-related complications, including abortion, **low birth-weight babies**, stillbirth, and even death, as compared with waiting just five or more years to have a baby (Menacker, Martin, MacDorman, & Ventura, 2004).

Runaways Teenagers are considered **runaways** when they leave their legal residence without parental consent. Teens often run away because of a heated argument or to escape abuse. Sometimes, runaways do so to use drugs freely, commit crimes, or to experience what they imagine are the glories of freedom. Others run away due to economic problems faced by their families. Research indicates that one in seven youth will run away and that 75 percent are female (NCSL, 2013), many of whom are pregnant. A high percentage (nearly two-thirds) of runaways are between the ages of 15 and 17 (U.S Department of Justice (2002). Many identify as lesbian, gay, bisexual, transgender (LGBT) or are questioning their sexual identity; many are or were part of the foster care system; and nearly half of all runaways or **homeless youth** report being abused. Sadly, 75 percent have dropped out or will drop out of high school. There are severe consequences that run away youth face, including mental illness and high-risk behaviors such as drug use, unprotected sex, prostitution, and violence (NCSL, 2013).

Self-Mutilation, Suicide, and Depression Adolescence can be a very difficult time for many young people. Pressures from peers, parents, and school may seem overwhelming. In an attempt to cope with this barrage of demands, some teens cut their bodies with razors, knives, or needles to gain a sense of release from these pressures (Whitlock, 2010). This habit often becomes addictive, particularly for girls, and can create a cycle of self-loathing. For other teenagers, these pressures are intolerable, and they see suicide as their only alternative. Many struggle with mental illness such as depression.

Self-mutilation behaviors are seen in about 4 percent of the general adult population, in 12–37 percent in secondary-school populations, 12–20 percent in late adolescent populations (Whitlock), and 40–61 percent of adolescents in psychiatric inpatient settings (Darche, 1990; Diclemente, Ponton, & Hartley, 1991). Often referred to as nonsuicidal self-injury, it is often though associated with suicide.

Youth have the lowest suicide rates compared to any other age group. They are more likely to engage in **suicidal ideation** (thinking about suicide) than actually committing suicide; similarly more teens are likely to engage in **parasuicide** (engaging in a lethal action that does not result in death) and are often relived that they survived. However, this does not imply it is not a problem. It is. Suicide is the second leading cause of death for children aged 10–24 and the third leading cause of death for college-aged youth. Sadly, four out of five teens who attempt suicide have given clear warning signs (Jason Foundation, 2013).

While the general trend among youth is a decrease in confidence from late childhood through adolescence, **clinical depression**—or feelings of hopelessness, lethargy, and worthlessness that last two weeks or more—in adolescents is less common. However, it is still a severe issue that needs to be addressed. Studies estimate that about 8–28 percent of adolescents meet the criteria for major depression and that one in five has experienced depression at some point in their life (National Alliance on Mental Health, 2010). In adolescence, twice as many girls as boys are diagnosed. Psychotherapy, particularly cognitive behavioral therapy (CBT) and interpersonal therapy (IPT), and medications have been shown to be efficacious treatment options.

Drug Usage Most young people have used at least one drug before the age of 18, attempting to enjoy the thrill of what they deem as independence yet denying the risky consequences. According to the National Institute of Drug Abuse (2012), illicit drug use among teens has been on the rise since 2000. Daily usage has also increased. Approximately 17 percent and 22.9 percent of 10th and 12th graders, respectively, reported using marijuana in the past month, with 6.5 percent of 12th graders using it every day. Interestingly, as perceptions of risk deceases, usage increases. Many teens are also using prescription drugs nonmedically (without a prescription or need for a prescription), such as Adderall (a stimulant), Vicodin (pain medication), cough medicines, and sedatives. While alcohol and tobacco usage is on the decline, nearly 14.5 percent and 28.1 percent of 10th and 12th graders, respectively, have reported getting drunk in the past month, and over 17 percent of 12th graders report being current smokers. Hookah water pipes and small cigars are currently raising public health concerns.

Causality Models

It is difficult to pinpoint one single reason explaining why teens would engage in at-risk behaviors. Growth, sexual awakening, emotional intensity, and hormonal rushes may surely contribute. Poor family environments, harsh or chaotic parenting, and stressful childhood experiences are also involved (Repetti, Taylor, & Seeman, 2002). It is also likely, particularly for self-mutilation, depression, and suicide, that there exists a genetic vulnerability that is triggered during puberty.

Researchers and practitioners agree that psychological and social factors also largely contribute to problematic behavior in adolescents. Adolescents are struggling for independence yet still need guidance and emotional support as they venture forward toward **autonomy**. Having a baby may be the only way a teenager believes she can receive the nurturance that her parents were unable to provide. Becoming pregnant may also be a defiant act by some teen girls and their only way to **differentiate** from over-controlling parents. Additionally, a teen girl may believe that having a baby will make her feel better about herself or make her relationship with the baby's father more secure. Teenage girls might also become pregnant because they see no other future for themselves other than having babies and being taken care of by others. Perhaps a girl is unsuccessful in school, and becoming a mother may seem to be a way out of hard work and study.

Peer pressure, absent or rejecting parents, the glamorization of pregnancy, teen drinking, early age at first intercourse, and sexual abuse have been identified as possible factors that put adolescent girls at high risk for becoming pregnant (e.g., Domenico & Jones, 2007). Other factors are living in poverty, being a member of a minority, and being the daughter of a teenage parent. Teen pregnancy can sometimes be thought of as part of the cycle of poverty (NCSL, 2013).

Gang membership is also thought of as being caused by lack of needs being met in the teen's family. Research (National Gang Center, n.d.) has shown that that kids who come from dysfunctional homes where they have been neglected or abandoned are most likely to join a gang. Gang members also tend to have grown up with little verbal communication, lack of structure, and no sense of belonging. In addition, most gang members come from one-parent families in which children and the parent have very little interaction. Poor self-esteem, no sense of personal safety, and little, if any, adult guidance combined with boredom and social alienation also increased the chances of gang involvement. Under such situations, joining a gang that provides loyalty, love, guidance, power, control, and a sense of belonging becomes almost necessary. Other contributing factors include a lack of job opportunities and living in poverty. In many cases, the teen might be raised in an area where his or her parents are part of a gang as well as the majority of people in the neighborhood. Joining a gang may be expected and even necessary for actual survival if one is to live in that neighborhood.

Running away from home is also a way to achieve autonomy and independence. Some feel abandoned by their parents and seek the acceptance of anyone, so they run away to find a sense of belonging elsewhere. Others are seeking independence, but ironically they usually end up being controlled by pimps and other abusive people. The streets are neither safe nor glamorous but are sometimes seen this way by confused and stressed-out teens.

As with all of the above problems, teens who abuse drugs, self-mutilate, or attempt suicide are usually attempting to deal with the tremendous stress of growing up. They either do not feel proper nurturance from their parents and peers or feel too much pressure from both groups.

It is important to note that the teen years are also a time to discover one's identity and try on "new hats." Conflicts at home, along with little maturity, influence teens to rely more on their peers than their parents for guidance. Peer pressure and cliques can become a powerful influence leading vulnerable teens to engage in maladaptive behaviors, with little concern for consequences. Consistent, positive parental support, guidance, and strong, healthy relationships can help even the most vulnerable teen stay on or get on the right track.

Human Services Delivery to At-Risk Adolescents

Emergency Situations and Interventions Adolescents are prone to crises because they have most of the physical and intellectual capabilities of adults, yet lack the emotional maturity, appropriate judgment, and decision-making abilities of adults. They often act before they think, which can get them into emergency situations. For example, they need immediate crisis intervention services after a suicide attempt once medical treatment has been completed. Shelters exist for runaways and offer teens a safe place to stay until they can be reunited with their families. Teens who seek out such shelters receive intensive crisis intervention services, group therapy, and basic needs, such as shelter, food, and medical care.

Teens who discover they are pregnant may also need emergency assistance, particularly if they're having medical problems, such as bleeding or pain. These young girls must be referred to knowledgeable and nonjudgmental medical professionals who can provide treatment for any medical problems, as well as prenatal care and education, and pregnancy termination services, if needed. A teen who is pregnant and wants to end her pregnancy also poses an emergency situation; sadly, many teens will attempt to receive an abortion from unmedically trained personnel or will give birth alone, scared, and in unsanitary environments. Special clinics are available that provide emergency abortions, prenatal services, and adoption services. Trained counselors provide crisis intervention and educational intervention for teens pondering what to do about an unplanned pregnancy. Any female who is pregnant deserves to be informed about her rights to continue with the pregnancy, terminate the pregnancy, or use adoption services. If a teen decides to continue her pregnancy, she will need ongoing services that fall into secondary and tertiary intervention.

Gang involvement may also create a need for emergency intervention. Unfortunately, when teens join gangs, they can put themselves and their families at risk for drive-by shootings and other forms of violence. Additionally, gang involvement increases the chances of being arrested for committing crimes, which creates the need for emergency response by parents. Both medical professionals and law enforcement officials usually handle these types of emergency response interventions.

Teens who self-mutilate or overdose from drugs and/or alcohol also need immediate medical attention or can risk death or serious injury.

Secondary Intervention Many police departments have created gang units that specialize in minimizing the negative effects of gang involvement. They attempt to work with gang members and guide them into other activities. They may even attempt mediation between enemy gangs. Diversion programs are available that provide group educational classes for gang members who have not yet become chronic criminals. The goal is to get the member out of the gang lifestyle as soon as possible. After-school recreational teen centers are available in some communities. Gang members can participate in sports, job training, and other activities.

Interventions for runaway teens at this level include family therapy, group counseling, and individual therapy. The focus is on helping the family make changes that will assist the youth in being able to tolerate living at home. Sometimes, the parents need drug and alcohol counseling. The teen may also need help with drug and alcohol addictions. Teens who run away because they've been abused or because of the violence in their homes need help dealing with these issues as well, often with the aid of child protective services. Many mental health centers are available to provide these types of counseling services. Both community mental and behavioral health centers and nonprofit mental health centers are capable of helping with these problems.

As stated earlier, once a teen decides to continue with a pregnancy, she should participate in ongoing prenatal care with a physician. She may decide to put the baby up for adoption and can receive counseling and legal intervention through public adoption agencies and private and nonprofit agencies. All states have services for these situations at no cost to the pregnant teen. Many communities have homes for the pregnant teen until she gives birth, and sometimes for a period after birth. The goal is to ensure that the teen and her baby are taken care of properly and to provide parenting education. These residential facilities also hope to provide education to prevent future unplanned pregnancies.

Teens who attempt suicide need counseling to help them deal with the situation that led them to such desperate measures. If the situation can be changed, the teen may then return to normal functioning. If the problem is longstanding and the depression is chronic, they may need tertiary intervention.

Counseling is also critical for teens who self-mutilate or abuse drugs and alcohol. Programs, such as Outward Bound, are in place to teach teens who are beginning to demonstrate destructive behaviors. This is often done through wilderness expeditions and efforts to show teens their potential to create healthy, positive environments and life outcomes.

Tertiary Intervention   For any longstanding depression, medication, in conjunction with psychotherapy, is an effective and successful option. Teens, like adults, may need to take antidepressants or antianxiety medications for an indefinite period of time to control severe depression. This may be the only way to inhibit suicidal thinking. In addition to medication, chronically suicidal and self-mutilating adolescents may need ongoing group therapy, individual therapy, or a 12-step group. Mental health clinicians who specialize in these types of adolescent issues should also be contacted when possible.

Chronic runaways may be difficult to treat. They have often had a history of lack of boundaries in the home and don't respond easily to counseling. Because they have often been abused, neglected, or involved in delinquent behavior, such as ditching school regularly, they have developed a lifestyle that doesn't include structure. They may need to be placed in a state-funded group home where supervision is strong. Sometimes they become emancipated if they can work and take care of all their needs on their own. But some teens and their families may need ongoing intervention from family counselors and child protective services to assist in keeping the child safe. Sadly, some families spend years coping with teens who run away, return home, only to run away a few weeks later.

For those teens heavily involved in gang activities, intervention often includes revolving-door incarceration in juvenile hall. Attempts are made to teach these teens how to function outside the gang, how to deal with life stress, and how to express and manage feelings. Group counseling is probably their best chance at being helped during incarceration. It is especially helpful when former gang members visit and share their experiences. In addition to incarceration, programs exist that provide job training for former gang members. They may also have opportunities to earn a high-school diploma through special programs. The focus of tertiary intervention programs is to help the teen stay out of the gang lifestyle and learn how to function as a "civilian." Sometimes, they may need to move to another city or state or spend time in a teen "boot camp." Much of what happens to these gang members depends on the effort exerted by their parents. Some parents simply give up and let their child go his or her own way. Worse yet are the parents who themselves are gang members and encourage their teens to continue involvement in the gang.

For youth who engage in chronic self-mutilation or show dangerous addictions to drug and alcohol usage, long-term therapy, rehabilitation, and harm-reductions models are often useful.

Primary Prevention   Educational programs have been developed that attempt to keep children from joining gangs. These programs usually begin in elementary school and are sometimes presented in junior high school and less frequently offered in high schools.

Former gang members along with law enforcement officials may visit schools and discuss the consequences of gang affiliation. Likewise, high-school programs have been developed that attempt to show adolescents the consequences of pregnancy. Family-life classes often have the teens carry around an egg for a few weeks without letting it drop, crack, or spoil. They have timers that go off indicating when they need to feed the egg, change it, and put it to sleep. Other prevention interventions include educational presentations about the use of birth control, and how abstinence can ensure that unplanned pregnancies won't occur. These usually don't happen until high school, however, and so teens younger than that are missing valuable information.

Drug prevention programs are common in American schools. For example, many schools participated in Red Ribbon Week, where children, beginning in the elementary years, are asked to take a pledge to help create a drug-free America. Primary prevention programs, though, for teen suicide attempts, self-mutilation, and runaways are not always readily available. Society should spend time and money researching the need for these programs.

Other Adolescent Considerations

Similar to working with children, there are many other problems that human services professionals will address in their work with adolescents. This can include, but is not limited to, eating disorders, immigration, vehicular accidents, stress, parental economic stress, Internet and gaming addictions, bullying, and school shootings.

School Violence: Teen School Shootings

- "Teen charged after three students shot near Pittsburgh high school"
- "Oklahoma teen found guilty in school shooting plot"
- "Teen charged as adult in stabbing death of teacher"
- "Teen's school shooting plan included *Call of Duty's* '*No Russian*' Theme"

These are some examples of recent news headlines depicting a teen or teens involved in a school-related shooting. Many of these shootings involved multiple fatalities, followed by homicide. A national Centers for Disease Control and Prevention (CDC) survey indicates that 17 percent of high-school students reported carrying a weapon to school at least once (http://www.teenhelp.com/teen-violence/teen-violence-statistics.html, 2013). Attackers often have in common the following factors: being male, having suffered a loss previous to the attack, having been bullied, having access to a weapon, and showing an interest in violence (Teen Violence Statistics, 2009). Students, administrators, parents, and law enforcement officials all should be part of the prevention process, and even though school shootings make up a small percentage of overall youth violence, they are traumatic events for all involved.

Critical Thinking/Self-Reflection Corner

- Could you provide a pregnant teen with information about prenatal care, adoption services, or abortion services in an objective manner? If not, do you think human services workers should offer unbiased advice?
- What stereotypes do you hold toward gang members? Pregnant teens? Suicidal teens? How might these affect your ability to be empathic with these populations?
- Should government taxes be spent on services designed to help people who seemingly choose to get into trouble, such as teens who get pregnant, join gangs, or use drugs?
- How would you eliminate the problem of unintended teen pregnancy?
- What do you think should be done to completely eliminate gang violence?
- Should a school system be responsible for educating students about birth control and ways to prevent HIV/AIDS? Why or why not?

AGING ADULTS

Most people assume aging is synonymous with disease, *but it is not*. While age is a risk factor for disease, just as are gender, lifestyle, and genetics, it is not causal. Indeed, one's biological age (how fit one's body is) is not the same as one's chronological age. That is why you see 90-year-olds and even older adults running marathons compared to 30-year-olds and younger who can barely walk up a flight of stairs. Not surprisingly, there is so much variability in old age that a single path to growing older does not exist. However, many older adults do suffer, in part due to poor health and lifestyle and also due to poor environmental and social conditions. While it is impossible to provide a full scope of the aging experience in this text, we highlight a few of the more common challenges that many current older adults face. We urge you to take some gerontology courses, particularly because you and your loved ones will also be older one day and because professionally your work in human services will inevitably be for, on behalf of, or inclusive of the aging population.

Prevalence

Demographers estimate that by the year 2050, there will be nearly 87 million adults who are 65 years and older. This is broken down by the **young-old** (65–74 years), which will comprise 38 million people (44 percent of the aging population); the **old-old** (75–84 years), which will comprise nearly 28 million people (32 percent of the aging population); and the **oldest-old** (85 years and older), which will comprise over 19 million people (24 percent of the aging population). By 2025, one in 26 Americans can expect to become a **centenarian** and live to be 100 years or older.

There are many normal changes that occur with aging and impact all people who are fortunate enough to grow old. This is referred to as **senescence** and includes changes in muscle mass, fat tissue, skin, hair, nail, hearing, vision, taste, smell, lung capacity, sleep patterns, and in many other physiological systems of the body. These changes do not typically impact a person's ability to enjoy life and to perform **activities of daily living** (ADLs) and **instrumental activities of daily living** (IADLs) but may require the person to adapt. Most older adults indeed report having good to excellent health, particularly those who have a sense of accomplishment, perceive themselves as having a sense of control in their lives, and experience meaning and life satisfaction.

This is despite the fact that more than 80 percent of adults over the age of 70 have at least one **chronic condition** (as cited in Hooyman & Kiyak, 2011) (**acute conditions** actually decrease with age, although those that do occur are more debilitating, especially for women). The most common chronic conditions, including hypertension, arthritis, heart disease, and diabetes, that occur to older adults are actually preventable. These diseases vary by gender, ethnicity, and socioeconomic status. Unfortunately, there are many older adults who do not have good quality of life and suffer physically, psychologically, and socially, as discussed in the following section.

Elder Mistreatment

"**Elder mistreatment** (i.e., abuse and neglect) is defined as intentional actions that cause harm or create a serious risk of harm (whether or not harm is intended) to a vulnerable elder by a caregiver or other person who stands in a trust relationship to the elder. This includes failure by a caregiver to satisfy the elder's basic needs or to protect the elder from harm" (Bonnie & Wallace, 2003). There exists an increasing trend in the prevalence of elder abuse, with some data indicating that, in the United States alone, over 500,000 older adults are believed to be abused or neglected each year; some estimates indicate, though, that one in four vulnerable elders are at risk of abuse. Sadly, these are likely to be low estimates as most elder abuse goes unreported or undetected (this is known as the **iceberg effect of elder abuse**). Maltreatment includes physical abuse, sexual abuse, emotional abuse, neglect, abandonment, and fiduciary (financial) abuse. This also includes medical abuse (withholding or improperly administering necessary medications) and violation of rights (such as removal from home or placement in a long-term care setting without the elder's consent). While it seems that elder abuse occurs more often to women, it can happen to anyone, particularly to disabled elderly, those with dementia, and those living in institutionalized care. Abuse also occurs in a person's own home, usually by a family member who is financially dependent on the elder. Older adults who experience abuse are at greater risk for death, depression, increased physical health problems, isolation, and loneliness. Despite the existence of the Older Americans Act, the Elder Justice Act, the Administration on Aging's (AoA) Prevention and Elder Abuse, Neglect, and Exploitation Program, and the fact that serious criminal laws are in place to punish perpetrators, elder abuse is still a serious, growing problem that deserves much-needed attention and funding.

Alcohol Abuse

Researchers note that current rates (2.5 million older adults in the United States have problems related to alcohol) are likely gross underestimates and that rates are likely to increase, especially as Americans live longer. Unfortunately, alcohol abuse or alcoholism remains a hidden problem, although it is becoming one of the fastest-growing public health concerns. Heavy drinking among older adults increases the risk of osteoporosis, diabetes, high blood pressure, and ulcers and can cause some older people to be forgetful and confused. Abusive drinking can also exacerbate current medical disorders common in elderly people, including congestive heart failure and hypertension. Alcohol use can also result in falls leading to hip fracture, a leading cause of death for older adults. Alcoholism in older adults is associated with depression, which often goes untreated, overlooked, or misdiagnosed. This is in part due to the fact that there exist stereotypes of drinking that tend not to include images of older adults as drug users (we tend to only associate drinking with youth) and that many health-care professionals are not properly trained to work with older adults.

Poverty

There is a public perception that all older adults are financially better off than all other age groups. However, over 3.4 million seniors age 65 and older live below the poverty line (Center for American Progress, 2013). A large proportion (16.1 percent) of older adults are also near poor (falling just above the poverty line) or are at risk of becoming poor. A strikingly high percentage of ethnic older adults fall within these groups. Older women are among the poorest groups in America, especially those who are frail, over 85, of ethnic descent, living in rural areas, and divorced, widowed, or never married. LGBT seniors are also at risk for poverty due to discrimination and unequal treatment under the law. Challenged retirement benefits, high costs of health care, few opportunities for employment, and housing costs contribute to poverty among older adults. Unfortunately, poverty is highly associated with poorer health, isolation, food insecurity, decreased mobility, unsafe living environments, homelessness, and financial abuse (due to predatory lending).

Frail Elderly

Many elderly also have difficulty meeting their basic needs, especially if they are suffering from illness or physical disabilities. Many elderly, often referred to as the **frail elderly**, require daily assistance with their ADLs (e.g., eating, getting to the bathroom, getting dressed, going to the doctor, or walking). Some elderly do not have enough money to support their needs entirely by themselves, and so they depend on others to supplement their income. Because they can no longer work and bring in new income, they must rely on retirement income, savings, or family financial assistance. Elderly also suffer from more medical illnesses than other segments of the population. They often need assistance simply to get to a doctor or pharmacy because many don't drive.

Alzheimer's Disease

According to the Alzheimer's Association, over 5 million Americans suffer from Alzheimer's disease, a type of dementia that causes problems with memory, thinking, and behavior. It is the most common form of dementia, and it is *not* a normal part of aging. The number of people with this disease is growing, because the longer people are living, the greater the risk is for developing Alzheimer's. One in 10 people over the age of 65 and nearly half of those over the age of 85 are affected. A person with Alzheimer's disease can expect to live an average of eight years and as many as 20 years from the onset of symptoms (Alzheimer's Association, 2013). Currently, there is no cure, but treatments for symptoms are available, and research continues. Elderly people suffering from this debilitating disease usually require a daycare facility or 24-hour family care. This creates much stress on the caregivers, and, in the beginning phases of the illness, on the elderly person as well. The financial burden of caretaking can be as stressful as the emotional burden. Caretakers need to set realistic goals and expectations. They need to make time for activities that bring them joy and satisfaction and to get adequate exercise, nutrition, and rest. They may need to join a support group where they can be honest.

Causality Models

Some mental and health problems that older adults face, such as Alzheimer's disease, may have a genetic component, although most problems are also heavily influenced by poor sociocultural conditions. American culture in particular holds negative attitudes toward the elderly. As has been discussed previously, this is ageism and often leads to poor medical care, manipulation of the elderly person's finances, and outright physical and sexual abuse of the elderly. Some believe that the elderly stop being worthwhile to society and therefore can be treated as less than a real person.

Psychologically, the elderly may experience low self-esteem because they are no longer working or are suffering from poor physical health. Many older adults come from a generation that encouraged remaining silent in their pains. This combination of low self-esteem and society's negative regard of the elderly create situations that are ripe for abusing elderly people. Society and families are also constantly changing (e.g., divorced families and economic challenges), making it more difficult to maintain strong, close family ties with aging loved ones.

Lifestyle is also a contributing factor to many of the health problems older adults experience; most of the diseases that Americans die from are preventable but require changes in behaviors related to smoking, physical activity, and diet, which can be challenging especially for older adults who have spent years engaging in maladaptive habits. Investments in education, food policies, and social support for older adults become even more critical, then, to change the lifestyle. Also, in part due to stereotypes of older adults, even health-care professionals have limited views of aging. Indeed, it is not surprising that there exist deficits in communication between older patients and doctors. Doctors also report that health-care challenges, such as lack of appropriate time, patient competence, and hospital infrastructure, make working with older adults frustrating and limited.

Human Services Delivery to Aging Adults

Emergency Situations and Interventions Because many elderly people need help caring for themselves, many programs provide services that meet immediate needs for protection, shelter, food, and medical care. Not all elderly people are unable to work or provide for themselves, but when aged people have Alzheimer's disease and other forms of **dementia**, are frail, or suddenly become ill, public and nonprofit agencies step in to make sure they are safe and are not being abused or neglected. Many elderly people with Alzheimer's disease may wander outside their homes, putting themselves in unsafe situations. They may need immediate hospitalization or supervision in a daycare center until their behavior can be better managed.

Most government-funded social services agencies include both children's services and **adult protective services**. These adult services provide emergency care for the elderly and disabled adults who cannot take care of themselves and who do not have family to help them. Social workers and nurses often visit elderly people at their homes to ensure their needs are met when it comes to their attention that an elderly person may not be eating, is not managing an illness appropriately, or has basic hygiene and sanitation conditions that are not adequate. Immediate intervention is provided to ensure that the elderly person's basic needs are met. Social workers may transport the person to a hospital, see to it that food is brought to him or her, or hire someone to clean up the home.

Sometimes the elderly are subject to being abused physically, sexually, or financially or neglected in institutions. Adult services serve as a watchdog over such institutions and respond immediately when any abuse is reported. Adult services also respond when an elderly person has been abused by family members or acquaintances as well.

The goal of emergency services for the elderly is to ensure that such basic needs as food, shelter, clothing, medical care, safety, and sanitary living conditions are available.

Secondary Intervention Some elderly people may have their basic needs met but need immediate assistance. These individuals may have fairly good support systems, such as adult children who help care for them. Often, these adult children enter into crisis states themselves because their caretaking responsibilities have become overwhelming. Many programs, such as the Alzheimer Association, have been created to assist caretakers. Counselors at this agency visit a client's home and work with the elderly person on various cognitive and recreational skills, giving the caretaker a much-needed break.

Sometimes the crisis is financial. The elderly person and/or the children often feel overwhelmed with medical expenses or just daily living expenses. People who retire or can no longer work must survive on a limited income. This can be scary. Lifestyles must change, and counseling can help people adjust to these new changes. It can be reframed as a normal transition in the life cycle that everyone goes through, and counselors can assure a person that many resources are available to help. Human services workers often serve as advocates for the elderly, helping them access pension money, social security benefits, and sometimes life insurance benefits after a spouse dies. They may also be assisted in getting federally funded medical insurance, such as Medicare, which pays for most medical care and medications.

Tertiary Intervention Many elderly people can live independently throughout their lives. They are physically and mentally healthy and have sufficient social supports to live on their own. Some elderly, however, cannot manage on their own because they are terminally ill, have cognitive impairments related to Alzheimer's disease or other dementias, or have difficulty getting around and may require a wheelchair. These individuals may need either professional or nonprofessional nursing support indefinitely, which may be provided in their own homes.

More often, however, the needs of elderly people are too extensive and can be met only in a residential facility designed to assist seniors. These facilities range from total care institutions for people who are very ill and disabled to assisted-living apartments for seniors who need help occasionally. The decision to have one's parent live in a facility is often emotionally difficult for adult children who often feel guilty because they feel they should be able to take care of their parents. Unfortunately, most children must work full time and are busy raising their own children and simply cannot take proper care of very ill and needy parents. Social workers and counselors can help these children understand that sometimes their parents are safer in one of these facilities than in their own homes. They can be reassured that their parents may prefer to be around others of the same age.

Primary Prevention Almost every city has a well-established senior center operating on a regular basis. These centers have proven to be very helpful in keeping the elderly physically active, involved in the community, educated about nutrition and good health, socially adept, and emotionally healthier than if they merely stayed at home by themselves. By participating in various groups, such as music appreciation, tai chi, crafts, reminiscent activities, and tax-education classes, these seniors are keeping their minds active, which lessens the likelihood of cognitive impairment. Social interaction can help prevent depression. Being educated about taxes and other financial situations can prevent financial crises.

These centers also provide a place to eat a healthy meal with others, which can help prevent malnutrition. Some of these centers also have programs for seniors who want to volunteer at various agencies. Such programs improve self-esteem and help seniors feel that they are contributing to society.

The overall goal of senior centers is to keep seniors active and healthy for as long as possible. Healthy stimulation and social interaction seem to assist in maintaining good health.

Other Aging-Related Considerations

There are several other areas to consider when thinking about older adults. Many aging adults are at risk for HIV and other sexually transmitted infections, although this topic tends to be overlooked, especially with inaccurate stereotypes that older adults are not sexually active. Depression and suicide are also significant problems affecting many older adults. Discrimination and **ethnic disparity** in health status, health-care access and services, housing, transportation, homelessness, intimate partner violence, and many other issues remain problems facing many older Americans. One of the biggest challenges facing the aging field is that many workers are untrained or unskilled and that there is a shortage of professionals who are motivated to serve older adults.

Human Services Professionals' Interaction with the Aging Population

Research indicates that the growing population of older adults currently outnumbers the amount of trained persons who can provide assistance. Population growth trends are creating a demand for professionals with knowledge and expertise in aging. Additionally, given other demographic shifts among the aging population, many people are working indirectly with older adults (such as childcare providers given the increase of grandparents rearing grandchildren) or in nontraditional ways (such as therapists treating older adults with addictions, which is a growing occurrence). Unfortunately, many direct workers, or those who already work with or on behalf of older adults, have limited knowledge about gerontology and related practices or lack motivation and knowledge regarding how to improve aging-related problems. Many workers also have limited views of aging, assuming inaccurately that all older adults are bedridden or demented and/or are frustrating and boring to work with. Many hold the belief that "little can be done to help elders" (Bial, 2005, p. 51). However, old age is not all about physical health or mental health problems, and a more realistic view of aging, including both positive and negative images, needs to prevail. Unfortunately, most people have a lack of exposure to the aging world or have limited hands-on experience and, thus, do not see the benefits of working with older adults. Indeed, many who work in the aging field report that it is meaningful and fulfilling. Given the growth of the aging population, everyone should be "elder-ready" (Bial, 2005).

Critical Thinking/Self-Reflection Corner

- Would you enjoy working with older adults? Why or why not?
- What do you think it will be like to grow old? What are these images or assumptions based on?
- What experiences have you had with older adults? What stereotypes do you hold of older adults? Are these inaccurate or accurate?
- If you worked in the gerontology field, which area would you want to work in? Similarly, if you were an aging advocate, which topic or problem would be of most interest to you to focus on?

CHAPTER SUMMARY

Many people in society benefit from human services. Children, adolescents, and the aging population may use such services due to a risk of being vulnerable and dependent. It is our job to ensure that all people are safe, protected, treated with dignity, and empowered to improve their quality of life. All people have specific needs, often co-occurring, that must be considered when applying prevention and intervention plans. A better understanding of the causes and risk factors of dysfunctional behavior, abuse, and mental and physical health problems is critical to effective human services delivery.

Suggested Applied Activities

1. Watch a movie or a television show that focuses on one of the populations or problems described in this chapter. Write down the main issues and needs that one of the characters faces.

   _____

   _____

   _____

   _____

   _____

2. Visit one or two agencies. Ask a worker or coordinator of programs to tell you about the different types of services delivered through the agency. Try to categorize each service into primary, secondary, tertiary, or emergency intervention.

3. Browse through your local Rainbow Resources Directory or the web for a list of various human services delivery agencies in your community.

4. Select a population and related challenge or problem. Develop a related primary, secondary, and tertiary prevention program.

Chapter Review Questions

1. What situations might arise for the following clients who require emergency services?

    a. Abused child

b. Pregnant teen

c. Elder being abused

d. Elder living in poverty

2. What are some treatment options for people dependent on alcohol?

3. What are some general principles in delivering human services to those who are abused?

4. Why might a support group be effective for those who have been violated?

5. What should human services workers keep in mind when designing a case management plan for a first-time juvenile gang offender?

6. What primary prevention programs are available for issues related to child abuse, domestic violence, substance abuse, and AIDS?

7. What human services delivery programs are useful for the elderly?

Glossary of Terms

Acute conditions are health problems that are severe and sudden in onset.

Adult protective services are social services provided to abused, neglected, and exploited older adults.

Autonomy refers to one's ability to think, feel, and make decisions on one's own.

Centenarian is a person who lives to 100 years of age and beyond.

Child abuse and neglect is any recent act or failure to act on the part of a parent or caretaker that results in death, serious physical or emotional harm, sexual abuse, or exploitation or is an act or failure to act that presents an imminent risk of serious harm.

Child Protective Services is a governmental agency that responds to reports of child abuse and neglect.

Childhood obesity is defined as having a BMI above the 95th percentile.

Chronic conditions are health problems or diseases that persist or have long-lasting effects.

Clinical depression includes feelings of hopelessness, lethargy, and worthlessness that last two weeks or more.

Daily living activities (ADLs) are self-care activities such as eating, bathing, dressing, toileting, and walking/transferring.

Dementia is a chronic disorder affecting mental processes and characterized by personality changes, memory impairment, and poor reasoning.

Differentiate is the process of becoming autonomous or independent in one's thinking and feeling.

Elder mistreatment is abuse and neglect.

Ethnic disparity in aging refers to the ethnic inequalities that exist in physical and mental health conditions, access to health care, and mortality (death) rates.

Frail elderly are older adults who suffer with a combination of chronic conditions, dementia, or ADL dependencies.

Gangs are self-formed associations of peers that tend to engage in illegal activities.

Homeless youth are those who lack a fixed, regular, and adequate nighttime residence.

Iceberg effect of elder abuse refers to the fact that only a small proportion of elder abuse is ever reported.

Instrumental activities of daily living (IADLs) refer to the more complex activities needed for daily living, including handling personal finances, shopping, meal preparation, and using transportation.

Juvenile delinquents are law breakers under the age of 18.

Low birth-weight babies are those born weighing less than 5 pounds, 8 ounces, which is a risk factor of health problems for some babies.

Old-old are adults between the ages of 75 and 84.

Oldest-old are adults over the age of 85.

Parasuicide is engaging in a lethal action that does not result in death.

Runaways are youth who leave their legal residence without parental consent.

Self-mutilation refers to a complex group of behaviors resulting in the destruction of one's own tissues such as starching, burning, and cutting.

Sexually transmitted infections (STIs) are infections passed from person to person through intimate sexual contact.

Senescence is the condition or process of biological aging.

Suicidal ideation is thinking about suicide.

Unintended pregnancy are those that are mistimed, unplanned, or unwanted at the time of conception.

Young-old are adults between the ages of 65 and 74.

Case Presentation and Exit Quiz

General Description and Demographics

The Paulo family consists of five children, Leona, age 22; Jimmy, age 19; Johnny, age 17; Leticia, age 14; and Maria, age 7. The father, James, age 45, works full time. The mother, Liliana, age 40, does not work outside of the home. James's mother, Maria, age 68, lives with them. James's father died many years ago. Liliana's parents live in a neighboring city, and they all get together often.

Problems within the Family

Johnny has been involved in a local gang since he was 15. There have been drive-by shootings at his house recently. He owns several guns and participates fully in gang warfare. His parents have tried to make him give away his guns and want him to quit the gang. He refuses to move out and is often verbally abusive to his mother and father and physically abusive to his father. Leona has had several arguments with Johnny and has called the police to have him taken away. He frequently steals things from the home to sell. His mother feels sorry for him and allows him back into the house after he has been gone for about one week. She doesn't want to lose his love.

He started using crystal meth about six months ago and becomes more violent when he is high. Before he began using crystal meth, he only smoked pot. His parents do not know what to do. Johnny has been caught stealing money from his grandmother, Maria. She keeps all of her money under her mattress, and one time after she received her social security check, Johnny stole $600.

Liliana has been suffering from *los nervios* episodically. She saw her primary care physician through her husband's HMO medical plan. He prescribed an antidepressant for her. She still suffers from intense bouts of anxiety and rage. This began one month ago, after Johnny stole Maria's money. Liliana's anxiety is so severe that she is afraid to let her daughters leave the house.

In the past week, little Maria has been afraid to go to school. She complains of stomachaches in the morning. The school counselor referred her to a family therapist. Maria tells the therapist that her brother Jimmy sometimes makes her lie in bed with him and touch his private parts, and sometimes he touches hers. Maria doesn't like it and is afraid to tell her mother.

Leticia has a new boyfriend who talked her into having sex at a party last month. She never had sex before, and they didn't use any birth control. Leticia is afraid that she may be pregnant because her period is late. Her boyfriend, who's 22 years old, tells her not to worry about it.

James continues to work daily. He is aware of the problems at home but is passive for the most part. He is satisfied with letting his wife take care of the children. He feels powerless to manage his sons and feels inadequate when communicating with his daughters. James drinks beer every day after work, a habit he's had since he was 15. His drinking rarely prevents him from going to work, but his wife and daughters don't like being around him when he drinks.

On Friday nights, after he gets paid, he goes to a local bar to drink. James is depressed most of the time but accepts that he is not meant to be a happy man.

Exit Quiz

1. Which intervention level should be provided to deal with Johnny's gang involvement problems?
   a. primary prevention
   b. secondary prevention
   c. tertiary prevention
   d. emergency services

2. A factor that might hamper Johnny's ability to stay out of gang life might be
   a. his parents' approval of gang behaviors
   b. his father giving up trying to control Johnny's behaviors
   c. his mother secretly wanting him to steal so she can have some of the money
   d. all of the above

3. An effective intervention for Johnny might be
   a. press charges for robbery and have him go to juvenile hall
   b. have the police come to the house and confiscate the guns
   c. send him to an out-of-state boot camp
   d. all of the above

4. Johnny's substance abuse might be helped by
   a. long-term rehabilitation at a hospital
   b. group counseling and family counseling
   c. residential treatment
   d. medical detoxification

5. When little Maria's family therapist heard about what her 19-year-old brother had been doing, she should
   a. call in the brother immediately and confront him
   b. tell Maria to go home and order him to stop
   c. call child protective services immediately
   d. all of the above

6. Jimmy might benefit from
   a. jail time
   b. personal counseling
   c. mandatory group therapy
   d. all of the above

7. When the family therapist heard that Grandmother Maria had her social security check stolen, she should
   a. help her find a part-time job to earn the money back
   b. report this as financial abuse to adult protective services
   c. tell Maria to open a checking account
   d. none of the above
8. Little Maria might benefit from which level of intervention?
   a. primary prevention
   b. secondary intervention
   c. tertiary intervention
   d. none of the above
9. Liliana's anxiety might best be treated with what level of intervention?
   a. primary prevention
   b. secondary intervention
   c. tertiary intervention
   d. none of the above
10. Who should receive individual counseling?
    a. little Maria
    b. Liliana
    c. James
    d. all of the above
11. Leticia needs which level of intervention?
    a. emergency intervention
    b. secondary intervention
    c. tertiary intervention
    d. none of the above
12. James's drinking problem might best be treated at which level?
    a. primary prevention
    b. secondary intervention
    c. tertiary intervention
    d. none of the above

Exit Quiz Answers

1. c
2. b
3. d
4. b
5. c
6. d
7. b
8. b
9. b
10. d
11. a
12. c

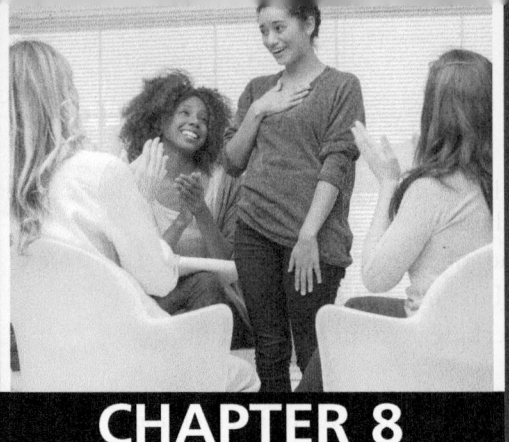

CHAPTER 8

Mental Illness, Poverty, Disabilities, Crime/Violence, and Substance Abuse

MENTAL ILLNESS

Historical Background

As previously discussed in this book, mental illness has been viewed from a variety of perspectives throughout time. Whether mental illness was thought to indicate demonic possession, imbalances of bodily humours, or immorality, mental illness has existed from the beginning of humankind. Scientists today believe they are finally getting a handle on what causes mental disorders and how to regulate symptoms. However, the causes of mental disorders are still in dispute, which leads to disagreements about the best methods of treatment. Additionally, much of mental-health treatment is based on managed care and state-funded programs. Unfortunately, these funding sources control who receives treatment and what kind of treatment is administered. There are laws and professional ethical codes that ensure certain rights for mental health patients. These ethical standards and laws were implemented because of the history of maltreatment of those afflicted with mental disorders.

Definition of Mental Disorders

The term "mental disorder" refers to a variety of syndromes and diagnoses. It has been defined as a clinically significant behavioral or psychological syndrome or pattern that occurs in an individual and that is associated with present distress or disability or with a significantly increased risk of suffering death, pain, disability, or an important loss of freedom. In addition, this syndrome or pattern must not be merely an expectable and culturally sanctioned response to a particular event, for example the death of a loved one. It must currently be considered a manifestation of a behavioral, psychological, or biological dysfunction in the individual. Table 8.1 lists some of the more common mental disorders and the general category under which each falls in the ***Diagnostic and Statistical Manual of Mental Disorders (DSM-V)***.

Prevalence

According to recent data from the National Institute of Mental Health (NIMH, n.d.), mental disorders are common in the United States. Nearly one in four adults (ages 18 and above) suffer from a diagnosable mental disorder in a given year. For example, about 21 million adults suffer from a mood disorder (such as major depression or bipolar disorder), 40 million have an anxiety disorder, 2.4 million have schizophrenia, 7.7 million have posttraumatic stress disorder (PTSD), and over 9 percent have a personality disorder. Mental illness often causes disabilities, and many people suffer from more than one mental condition at a time (**comorbidity**).

Causality Models

Some disorders result from biological factors more than other factors, such as **schizophrenia**, **delirium**, **dementia**, **delusional disorders**, **bipolar disorder**, **major depressive disorder**, **panic disorder**, **obsessive compulsive disorder**, ADHD, and **pervasive developmental disorder**. There is believed to be a strong genetic component to each of these disorders. Scientists believe that neurotransmitters, such as dopamine and serotonin, are not released in sufficient amounts in people who suffer from these disorders.

While it may be true that all disorders have a genetic component to them, some are considered to be more heavily influenced or triggered by psychological and social factors. For example, **personality disorders** are considered to result from early childhood deprivations and deficits in relationship skills. These people didn't receive adequate nurturance, boundaries, or guidance from their parents and therefore do not have the skills necessary to function in society as adults who work and sustain themselves or who can sustain healthy and satisfying relationships.

Many of the other disorders are also considered to be a consequence of exposure to harsh or insecure family environments or the inability to cope with life stressors. **Anxiety disorders**, for example, can be traced to early experiences of serious trauma, such as child abuse, a natural disaster, or war. Also, feelings of

TABLE 8.1 Categories of DSM-V Mental Disorders, Followed by Examples, if Applicable

Neurodevelopmental Disorders	Schizophrenia Spectrum and Other Psychotic Disorders	Bipolar and Related Disorders	Depressive Disorders	Anxiety Disorders
■ Intellectual disability	■ Schizophrenia and subtypes	■ Bipolar disorders	■ Major depressive disorder	■ Agoraphobia
■ Communication disorders	■ Schizoaffective disorder	■ Anxious distress specifier	■ Anxious distress specifier	■ Specific phobia
■ Autism spectrum disorder	■ Delusional disorder	■ Other specified bipolar and related disorder		■ Social anxiety disorder (social phobia)
■ Attention deficit hyperactivity disorder	■ Catatonia			■ Panic attack
■ Specific learning disorder				■ Separation anxiety disorder
■ Motor disorders				■ Selective mutism

Obsessive Compulsive and Related Disorders	Trauma- and Stressor-Related Disorders	Dissociative Disorders	Somatic Symptom and Related Disorders	Feeding and Eating Disorders
■ Body dysmorphic disorder	■ Acute stress disorder	■ Dissociative identity disorder	■ Somatic symptom disorder	■ Pica and rumination disorder
■ Hoarding disorder	■ Adjustment disorders		■ Medically unexplained symptoms	■ Avoidant/restrictive food intake disorder
■ Trichotillomania (hair-pulling disorder)	■ Posttraumatic stress disorder		■ Hypochondriasis and illness anxiety disorder	■ Anorexia nervosa
■ Excoriation (skin-picking) disorder	■ Reactive attachment disorder		■ Pain disorder	■ Bulimia nervosa
■ Other specified and unspecified disorders			■ Conversion disorder	■ Binge-eating disorder
				■ Elimination disorders

Sleep-Wake Disorders	Sexual Dysfunctions	Disruptive, Impulse-Control, and Conduct Disorders	Neurocognitive Disorders	Gender Dysphoria Personality Disorders Paraphilic Disorders
■ Breathing-related sleep disorders	■ Genito-pelvic pain/penetration disorder	■ Oppositional defiant disorder	■ Delirium	
■ Circadian rhythm sleep-wake disorders		■ Conduct disorder	■ Major and mild neurocognitive disorder	
■ Rapid eye movement sleep behavior disorder and restless legs syndrome		■ Intermittent explosive disorder	■ Etiological subtypes (such as Parkinson's disease)	

(Source: *American Psychiatric Association, 2013*). Please note that substance-related and addictive disorder, including gambling disorder, is a main DSM-V category but is not included in Table 8.1.

Digital Download · Download at CengageBrain.com

anxiety and depression can also result from being rejected by peers during childhood. **Phobias** often come after experiencing a scary event (such as being bitten by a dog). **Eating disorders** are believed to be an attempt to be perfect, to compensate for feelings of inadequacy, or to feel in control. Studies have shown associations between family factors, such as **enmeshed** and **disengaged** families, and children with eating disorders. Adjustment disorders, abnormal and excessive reaction to life stressors, usually occur when people do not have the coping skills necessary to deal with an unexpected situation. Although they may try to cope for a while, without help, they can become overwhelmed by feelings of depression, anxiety, conduct problems, risky behaviors, and physical pain, resulting in impaired functioning.

Society and culture may also have some influence on the occurrence or experience of a mental disorder, particularly among those who are vulnerable. For example, the media's depiction of pencil-thin models and the unrealistic emphasis on beauty may contribute to eating disorders. Some cultures consider diseases normal. For example, *ataque de nervios* (discussed earlier in the book) is a culturally defined Latino syndrome caused by acute stress. It can display itself through shouting, crying, and aggressiveness, and although it is considered typical by many Latinos, it is associated with mood and anxiety disorders.

Needs and Issues

Most people with mental disorders need a safe place to talk about their problems. They need to know that help is available and that they are not alone. Privacy is vital, as is trust. Some may need medication and counseling; in most general cases of depression and anxiety, a combination of both is most effective. In more serious cases, hospitalization may also be necessary.

The purpose of counseling is to create a relationship in which clients can be open, honest, and genuine when discussing their life experiences. Sometimes, clients need to discuss childhood traumas. Other clients need to discuss a current situation that they cannot cope with and learn adaptive coping skills. Some people need to learn how to relax and learn stress management skills that include cognitive restructuring and behavioral changes. When problems are due to dysfunctional family rules, clients may need family counseling to help change dysfunctional rules and roles into more adaptive ones. This can be quite challenging particularly when familiarity and maintaining status quo is more comfortable than changing well-established family patterns even when such patterns are unhealthy or damaging.

Human Services Delivery for Mental Illness

Emergency Situations and Interventions Several emergency situations exist in the area of mental illness and emotional disorders. Sometimes depressed people attempt suicide. Psychotic people who have decompensated into a delusional state may be unable to care for themselves. Others may lose control of their anger and attempt to harm others. All of these situations require emergency response from mental health workers. Most communities have facilities and workers designated to evaluate these behaviors and to decide whether involuntary hospitalization is needed to ensure the safety of the individual or of others. These community workers are often members of a **psychiatric emergency team** (PET).

Local law enforcement workers often work closely with these mental health workers to ensure safe transportation of these people to protective environments. After medical issues have been resolved, counselors typically provide crisis intervention to help contain dangerous behaviors. Sometimes, people need medication to help calm them down. Unfortunately, some people need restraints to assist in stabilizing an emergency.

Secondary Intervention If a person has not been assessed to be in immediate danger, crisis intervention is usually provided by mental health professionals and paraprofessionals. If the problem is not a long-standing one, the counselor will identify current life stresses and hopefully be able to assist the client in resolving them. If a counselor cannot personally manage all the problems, then other human services workers may be called in to assist with resolving the problems. People who benefit from secondary intervention are usually suffering from an adjustment disorder or acute stress disorder caused by a severe trauma. People in these situations can access local and national nonprofits for resources, referrals, and support.

Tertiary Intervention Many people suffer from long-standing mental illness and emotional disorders that require more than brief therapy and crisis intervention. Those with personality disorders usually need many years of intensive psychotherapy. They may also need to participate in group therapy and take medication to manage symptoms of depression and anxiety. Likewise, those suffering from eating disorders; obsessive-compulsive disorders; generalized anxiety; dissociative identity disorder; long-standing sexual perversion disorders; and many childhood disorders, such as ADHD, autism, and separation-anxiety disorder, need ongoing therapy and behavior management counseling. They also need medication to assist them in functioning.

People suffering from schizophrenia and bipolar disorders often need medication indefinitely as well as case management services provided by community mental health. When the disorder is very severe, they often live in board-and-care homes. Psychotic people are often hospitalized during severe psychotic breakdowns. They are stabilized and then returned to the board-and-care home. Some can live independently if they comply with medication treatment. They usually see a psychiatrist throughout their lives.

Primary Prevention Unfortunately, few prevention programs are designed to stop people from developing emotional disorders because many of these disorders are either hereditary or result from dysfunctional family dynamics. School systems and government agencies are hesitant to interfere with how parents raise their children. They are even hesitant to talk about self-esteem in schools because this steps on the toes of the parents. As far as genetic counseling, there still isn't a specific test that clearly indicates which genes carry mental illness. Society needs to put more emphasis on preventing mental illness, but this may mean interfering with parental rights to raise children as parents see fit.

Current Efforts to Prevent Depression in Children

Interestingly, alternative medicine and behavioral approaches are being used to prevent depression in children. Yoga is in fact becoming a common tool to improve overall health and prevent mental illness, showing promising benefits. Resilience programs, such as those that teach social problem solving skills and cognitive-behavioral skills (such as identifying negative, irrational thinking) has also been found useful for children. Current research by Froh and Bono (2013) indicate that asking children to reflect on gratitude and what is good in their lives is linked to increased optimism and decreased negative mood.

Critical Thinking/Self-Reflection Corner

- What stereotypes do you hold of persons with mental illness?
- How would you handle a mental illness diagnosis? Specifically, would you share the information with others, discuss it in appropriate settings, or keep it quiet?
- Would you be interested in working with persons with mental illness? Why or why not?
- Does knowing there is likely a genetic basis for most mental disorders influence how you would work with this population?

POVERTY

Historical Background

Meeting the needs of people based on economic status has long been the focus of government as presented in Chapter 1 (Elizabethan Poor Laws). Being poor or living in **poverty** has been viewed in a variety of ways throughout history. At one time, it was thought to be due to immorality. Some people think that poor people are lazy. Others have proposed it is part of a government plan to control the economy.

Definition of Poor/Poverty

Over the years, the economic standard of living as well as government guidelines that determine level of income have changed the definition of poverty. In general, people are considered poor if they can't earn enough money to support themselves and their families. Support includes having a clean, safe place to live; enough food to feed each family member at least twice a day; and clothes that are appropriate for the climate. Support also includes being able to pay for health and dental care and for children's school supplies. Most welfare programs either assist poor people to earn enough money to support themselves or provide money, services, and products to permit a minimal standard of living.

TABLE 8.2	2013 Poverty Guidelines for the 48 Contiguous States and the District of Columbia
Persons in Family/Household	Poverty Guideline
For families or households with more than 8 persons, add $4,020 for each additional person	
1	$11,490
2	$15,510
3	$19,530
4	$23,550
5	$27,570
6	$31,590
7	$35,610
8	$39,630

Retrieved from the U.S Department of Health and Human Services website at http://aspe.hhs.gov/poverty/13poverty.cfm

Digital Download Download at CengageBrain.com

The U.S. government defines and sets poverty thresholds according to income and family size. These definitions are updated annually by the Census Bureau and are used nationwide as a statistical yardstick and to determine government funding for people who fall within the parameters of the thresholds. The first thresholds were based on the U.S. Department of Agriculture's statistics on food budgets for families under economic stress in 1963–1964 and from data on how much money families spend on food. If total family income was less than the threshold appropriate for that family's size, then that family was considered to be living in poverty. As of 2013, federal poverty guidelines define poverty, for a family of four, to be at or below $23,550 (FamiliesUSA, 2013). See Table 8.2 for more examples. Poverty levels vary, though, by state as well as by family size and ages of family members.

Prevalence

Poverty rates have decreased since the 1950s from 22.4 percent of the entire U.S. population to 15.1 percent in 2011, which is nearly 46.2 million Americans. Of this, 16.1 million were children, with a high percentage comprising African American and Hispanic children (ASPE, 2012). Poverty rates tend to be lower for Caucasians and Asian Americans overall. Poverty rates are highest for children living in families headed by single women (47.6 percent) as compared to children in married-couple families (10.9 percent). Many living in poverty are homeless; nearly 3.5 million people are homeless, with 35 percent characterized by families with children. Not all people living in poverty are unemployed. In fact, as of 2011, 28 percent of workers earned poverty-level wages, with a high proportion of such workers being female, black, Hispanic, or between the ages of 18 and 25. Sadly, of those who are able to work themselves out of poverty, 50 percent fall back into it within five years (Oswald, 2005).

Causality Models/Needs and Issues

It would be the rare social scientist who believed that genetics or biochemical imbalances caused poverty. Some people consider poverty to be under a person's control, and others believe that certain people who live in poverty (such as children) have no control over their economic situation. Those who believe that people have control over their situation often feel angry and don't want assistance available for them. Some people think that poor people are merely lazy and are looking for an easy handout. However, it is doubtful that many people would begrudge a small child financial and medical assistance because people usually believe that children cannot control their standard of living. Most people believe that able-bodied adults should work and support themselves without governmental assistance, unlike children or people with disabilities who are physically unable to work and support themselves.

More current thought holds that sociopolitical factors cause poverty. This includes income inequality, racial discrimination, and family structure (single-parent families), as well as decreased economic opportunities (low-paying jobs, sporadic work, etc.), lack of affordable housing and health care, and political factors (such as cuts in human service welfare programs). Government welfare assistance has been based on this philosophy since Queen Elizabeth created her programs in England during the late 1500s and early 1600s.

Individual or psychological factors, such as mental illness, drug addiction, and alcoholism, can exacerbate poverty situations and increase the risk of homelessness. Some people are thought to be unable to work and sustain their own basic needs due to depression or other emotional disorders. It is possible that some of these disorders are due to biochemical imbalances and/or genetic predisposition to mental illness. Indeed, mental illness and poverty are highly associated. In 2010, adults living below the poverty level were three times more likely to have serious psychological distress as compared to adults over twice the poverty level (CDC, 2012).

Learned helplessness is a popular psychological concept used to explain the cause of poverty. Learned helplessness is often caused by depression, low self-esteem, lack of coping skills, ineffective role modeling from parents, and inability to mature and develop emotionally. From a psychoanalytic standpoint, people living in poverty have failed to accept their position as adults in society and are fixated at a primitive, infantile way of functioning. Perhaps their dependency needs were never fully met in childhood, and they are seeking this fulfillment later on in life.

Some believe that some poor people may have chosen poverty as a lifestyle because they are lazy. But what psychological factors lead to such laziness? To consciously decide to live in poverty does not seem enjoyable, so what would make a person lazy enough to desire it? Humanistic theorists might suggest that these people are searching for need fulfillment and have simply not found a safe environment to explore their potential and have just given up trying to succeed.

A behavioral perspective might suggest that people stay poor because they are encouraged to stay dependent on others; that they are part of a culture of poverty that emphasizes "resignation, dependence, present-time orientation, lack of impulse control, weak ego structure…" (as cited in Oswald, 2005). The behavioral model might also suggest that poor people continue to live in poverty because that is what they learned growing up. Acceptance of poverty was role modeled by parents, and children raised in these homes learn to adapt to having very little. Their coping skills might range from stealing to borrowing and begging. Some social scientists refer to the transmission of poverty from one generation to the next as a **cycle of poverty**. These children grow up thinking that this is the only way in which they will ever live and cannot see any other existence as possible. They are raised to adapt to the norms and values often seen in poor families, such as lack of expectations, "make do with what you have," and "life is a struggle so take what you can." Being raised in poverty might also make the children feel deprived, and therefore they grow up believing that financial assistance is normal and expected, especially if they grew up in a home in which welfare was received. The idea of being financially independent might not even occur to these children.

Many times, people's lack of education prevents them from finding jobs that pay enough to support them. Certain cultures may value work more than education, and so people from these cultures are encouraged to quit school and start working as soon as possible. Often, this creates a vicious cycle of poverty.

Different types of people live in poverty and therefore have needs and issues that vary. Whether poverty results from suddenly being unemployed, being raised in a culture of poverty, or being disabled, assistance of some type is usually needed but not always sought.

The so-called **deserving poor**—children, elderly, and the disabled—usually receive government funding directly. This assistance usually does not cover all of a person's expenses, so additional assistance with health care, child care, housing, transportation, and food is critical. Due to physical disabilities and/or age, many deserving poor cannot work and so are given priority for receiving assistance. Children can receive free meals at schools to ensure they're getting proper nutrition.

When a person living in poverty is an able-bodied adult, financial assistance is not as easily obtained. These people are deemed able to work and to take care of themselves, and so only short-term programs, such as homeless shelters and the Salvation Army, are available that focus on helping people find work and improve their job skills. Sometimes these people are eligible for food stamps, but often they look to churches and other charitable organizations to survive. Shelters and other agencies that help the destitute often can provide clothing to those who need it. These individuals often need a boost in self-esteem and supportive counseling while they transition from being homeless to being self-supporting. They may still live in poverty, but at least their dependence on outside assistance has lessened.

> ### True Stories from Human Service Workers
>
> *The Needs of Those Living in Homeless Shelters*
>
> Because of the many needs of individuals and families living in poverty, agencies that serve this population typically offer a multitude of services. As with any human services agency and any population, needs are assessed and then clients are referred to one or more services aimed at meeting those needs.
>
> For example, Cindy Snelling, assistant director of a homeless shelter in southern California, says that "the specific needs of this population are stability, safety, increased self-concept, a job, housing, food, and clothing."
>
> The shelter offers safe and clean housing and food for at least 45 days. This time period creates some stability while its residents look for work. People staying at the shelter are also encouraged to participate in support and educational groups that often improve self-esteem.

Educational programs are also available for single mothers, especially teenage mothers. The intent of these programs is to end the cycle of poverty by encouraging the mothers to be able to secure decent-paying jobs. Often these women and girls need guidance and encouragement regarding their ability to succeed in the work world. They may need education about how to end the cycle of poverty and how to be a role model for their own children.

Many people living in poverty are also addicted to drugs and alcohol and need to be motivated to get into detox and drug-treatment programs. Similarly, people who are depressed or have other emotional disorders need access to counseling services and possibly medication simply to have the motivation and energy to take care of themselves.

Human Services Delivery for Those Living in Poverty

Emergency Situations and Interventions The emergency situations faced by people living in poverty have to do with basic needs, such as food, water, safe shelter, and emergency medical assistance. Social services systems usually offer emergency food stamps and emergency medical care to people who would die or become seriously ill without them. Many hospital emergency rooms will assess a patient's eligibility for **indigent** (services for the poor) medical services. Most hospitals will not turn away critically ill patients because they do not have insurance or money. State and federal taxes fund these programs.

In addition to government-funded programs, many churches provide meals to those in dire need. Other nonprofit agencies provide emergency shelter and food for homeless people. Without these homeless shelters, many poor people would starve to death or die from exposure to harsh weather conditions.

Secondary Intervention These interventions assist people in a temporary crisis, for instance people who suddenly lose their jobs. They may have enough money for food, shelter, and medical care for only 30 days. Although these are not emergency situations, providing assistance to these people as soon as possible can prevent additional problems. They may need supportive counseling that encourages them to "hang in there" and services that provide resources to help find new employment. This approach works best with people who have previously been able to support themselves but are now going through difficulties.

Some homeless shelters are now extending the number of days people can stay because of the difficulties brought about by the current economy. These shelters offer job training and group counseling, as well as food and shelter. Residents are motivated to return to autonomous living in society because they have previously supported themselves and have many coping skills and the confidence to return to that level of functioning.

Tertiary Intervention Some people are **chronically poor** or **cyclically poor**, and their likelihood of ever being able to support themselves financially without assistance is low. While many in this group work, employment is low paying and limited. And for others, dependence on the system to support the family is not considered negative but rather a way of life. The welfare system in the United States is complex and involves many different programs. Unfortunately, many of the poorest Americans are among the least able to navigate the welfare system. Current antipoverty programs include the Supplemental Nutrition Assistance Program (SNAP), a food program for low-income families and individuals; housing assistance; the Supplemental Security Income (SSI) program for low-income adults over the age of 65; the Women, Infant, and Children (WIC) program, which provides healthy food to low-income households and pregnant women; and job training programs offered through the Department of Labor.

The 1996 Welfare Reform Act signed into legislation by the Clinton Administration dramatically reshaped how support is provided to needy families. This law oversees the **Personal Responsibility and Work Opportunity Reconciliation Act (PRWORA)**, which reduced funding for many of the above-stated programs (such as food stamps) and increased funding for child care and for care of children in low-income families. The bill also added a workforce development component, such that welfare recipients are required to begin working after two years of receiving benefits. This Welfare to Work program was an attempt to decrease the cycle of welfare and entitlement and encourage people to support themselves and their families.

Primary Prevention A few programs have been developed that work with children and teens to make sure they feel prepared to enter the job market, manage money, and take care of themselves throughout life. As early as sixth grade, some children are learning how to invest money, how to manage a checking account, why saving money is important, and how to use credit wisely. Many high schools offer courses that focus on family life and independent living.

Perhaps the most common types of programs that aim at preventing poverty are those that focus on encouraging adolescents to complete high school and attend college. Education has a huge impact on income. Primary prevention education with teenagers who are about to become adults can make them realize that finishing high school, getting adequate job skills training, and even going on to higher education can get them out of the trap of poverty that their parents found themselves in. Indeed, the idea of economic mobility in the United States is strongly believed to be based on attaining marketable training and higher education.

Critical Thinking/Self-Reflection Corner

- What images do you hold of persons who live in poverty?
- How would you explain the causes of poverty to a child?
- Would you be interested in working with persons who are poor and/or homeless? Why or why not?
- What can you personally do to help prevent poverty?

DISABILITIES

Historical Background

Persons with disabilities, historically, were viewed as vulnerable and deserving of provisions and protection. Today, while many negative stereotypes and images exist about those with disabilities, and emphasis is still placed on providing services, priority is made to empower and integrate those who have a disability into all areas of life. While modern legislation is in place to protect those with disabilities, the true story of its advocacy began when people "began to challenge societal barriers that excluded them from their communities, and when parents of children with disabilities began to fight against the exclusion and segregation of their children. It began with the establishment of local groups to advocate for the rights of people with disabilities. It began with the establishment of the independent living movement which challenged the notion that people with disabilities needed to be institutionalized, and which fought for and provided services for people with disabilities to live in the community" (Mayerson, 1992, p .1).

Definition of Disabilities

"Disability" is an umbrella term that typically refers to a physical or mental condition or impairment that limit's or restricts a person's ability to engage in one or more major life activities. People described as disabled may have many types of physical and mental challenges, some of which were present at birth. Disabilities that usually receive assistance and protection are typically biologically based, such as mental retardation, blindness, cerebral palsy, and other physical handicaps, but also may include communicative disorders and mental illness. Many disabilities, such as blindness, mental retardation, epilepsy, cerebral palsy, and muscular dystrophy, have a genetic origin. Other disabilities, such as spinal cord injuries, could be the result of accidents causing permanent physiological impairments.

Prevalence

Data from 2011 indicate that 12.1 percent of all Americans have a disability (this is over 37 million people who reported one or more disability). Over 25 million American lives are restricted by the effects of disability. Disabilities tend to be higher among ethnic Americans and women (Cornell University, 2012). A high percentage of those who are disabled are also living in poverty (27.8 percent). One in six children is diagnosed with a developmental disability or delay. Many older adults (1 in 3) report a disability due to arthritis, back pain, heart disease, cancer, and diabetes.

Causality Models/Needs and Issues

Disabilities are caused by several factors including genetics as well as social, environmental, and physical factors, such as brain injury or infection (during or after birth), growth or nutrition problems, child abuse, drug misuse (especially during pregnancy), accidents, bodily wear and tear, poor nutrition, and unhealthy lifestyles. Lack of access to health services and lack of understanding can exacerbate physical health issues that commonly occur with disabilities. Many with developmental disabilities, such as Down syndrome, have poor life expectancy. Many experience depression due to isolation and stigmatization of disabilities, social restriction, and trouble communicating. Many people with disabilities experience abuse and neglect.

Many individuals who have been disabled since birth receive services from **regional centers**, which are federally funded agencies that specialize in developmental disabilities and follow clients from birth to death. The type of needs a disabled person has depends on the type of disability. Some are capable of working and making enough money to support themselves but still need such services as protection from abuse. Some need advocacy services to ensure they aren't discriminated against. Others, however, do require services to take care of all basic living needs, such as food, shelter, clothing, medical care, and daily living care. Some people with disabilities prefer not to be referred to as disabled but rather "differently abled," such as hearing impaired individuals. They usually can work and don't require financial assistance. However, they may be eligible for other forms of assistance due to their disability.

Some persons with disabilities need counseling to deal with depression and anxiety associated with their disability. The families of this population may need counseling to help them deal with feelings of sadness about their family members' disability. Self-esteem and feelings of anger and frustration may present issues for the person who is disabled. Counseling often focuses on the person's strengths, integrating the disability into their lifestyle, and what they can contribute to society.

Human Services Delivery to Persons with Disabilities

Emergency Situations and Interventions People with physical disabilities may be more prone to crisis situations and more likely to need emergency care because various disabilities often make it more difficult to function, create conditions

> **DISABILITY AWARENESS QUIZ**
>
> 1. Just over one in four workers entering the workforce today will become disabled before retiring.
>   ☐ True   ☐ False
>
> 2. Most disabling injuries occur on the job.
>   ☐ True   ☐ False
>
> 3. Working men are more likely to become disabled than working women.
>   ☐ True   ☐ False
>
> 4. Most families in America live paycheck to paycheck.
>   ☐ True   ☐ False
>
> 5. An illness or accident will keep one in five workers out of work for at least a year before the age of 65.
>   ☐ True   ☐ False
>
> 6. Most Americans don't have enough savings to meet short-term emergencies.
>   ☐ True   ☐ False
>
> 7. More mortgage foreclosures are caused by premature death than disability.
>   ☐ True   ☐ False
>
> 8. Most workers receiving social security disability benefits are over 55 years old.
>   ☐ True   ☐ False
>
> 9. Employers may continue to contribute to disabled employees' 401K plans even if they are not earning an income.
>   ☐ True   ☐ False
>
> 10. Most workers today have discussed how they would financially handle a period of disability.
>   ☐ True   ☐ False
>
> Answers: 1. True 2. False 3. False 4. True 5. True
> 6. True 7. False 8. False 9. False 10. False
>
> *Adapted from The Council for Disability Awareness (http://www.disabilitycanhappen.org/docs/Quick_Quiz.pdf)*

more conducive to accidents, and have an unpredictable quality to them. Fortunately, people with recognized disabilities do not have much difficulty receiving medical care. Government funding for such individuals is readily available.

Individuals with disabilities may be vulnerable to abuse and neglect. Government agencies at the county, state, and federal levels have been created to take care of these situations. Many states have in place protocols for reporting abuse and neglect of persons with disabilities. Also in place is the **Americans with Disabilities Act (ADA)** of 1990, which is a civil rights law that prohibits discrimination based on disability. While enacting the ADA, Congress recognized that despite limitations, all person's should have the right to fully participate in all aspects of society, despite the fact that many are precluded from doing so because of prejudice, antiquated attitudes, or the failure to remove societal and institutional barriers. An intensive level of support is also available via special education services and behavior intervention plans.

Secondary Intervention   The goal of secondary intervention with individuals who are disabled is not to cure them of their disability but to manage crises related to the disability. Many of the crisis situations encountered by the disabled population have to do with inadequate knowledge and understanding of a particular individual's disability and failure to establish or keep in place the necessary support systems. As with all crisis intervention, effective treatment of individuals with disabilities is rooted in a system of comprehensive collaboration among various professionals. Additionally, human services workers must be knowledgeable about the many resources available to help them with legal concerns, medical needs, and other needs related to the disability. Societal stigma against this population, discrimination, and embarrassment about dependency are often components of a crisis state for individuals with disabilities and their families. Mental health counselors, both professional and nonprofessional, may serve as a needed support system for a person with a disability. Many people with disabilities are capable of using regular mental health treatment. They deserve meaningful intervention and attention, not to be stigmatized or patronized.

Secondary intervention might include advocacy to receive equal services and treatment at work, school, or at an agency. This requires the human services worker to be knowledgeable about laws and rights. For example, public school systems, on parents' request, must test any child for learning disabilities, and, if a child has a learning disability, the school must provide the intervention that a child with that disability requires. Some parents might seek the assistance of a counselor for this child, not knowing that the school system should be providing services. In such instances, the counselor should act as an advocate for this child to receive the benefits mandated by federal legislation.

Tertiary Intervention Because many disabilities cannot be repaired or significantly changed, much of the intervention for this population is tertiary in nature. That is, the function of intervention is to provide a healthy and as normal a quality of life as possible for the disabled person. Keeping a person functioning in mainstream society as much as possible is the aim. Some students (those suffering from dyslexia or attention deficit hyperactivity disorder [ADHD]) may be able to manage a mainstream class for most of the day, while attending a special resources class for certain subjects. Others may have to attend a special school for students with disabilities, such as the Braille Institute for the Blind or a special school for autistic children. No matter where the child attends school, the goal is to provide as normal an experience comparable to students without disabilities.

Other people with disabilities may have to reside indefinitely in board-and-care homes or residential facilities such as hospitals or group homes. Their disability may be so severe (profound mental retardation, for instance) that it prevents them from meaningful interaction with society. Permanent hospitalization or institutionalization is only considered as a last resort, however. Many previously institutionalized disabled people can now live in board-and-care homes or in private homes with their families and attend special programs in the community for individuals who are disabled, where they go on field trips with trained human services workers. They may even participate regularly in other social activities, such as cooking, singing, dancing, and arts and crafts. These outpatient programs give them a more normal life and a higher quality of existence.

Most people with disabilities receiving tertiary intervention have case managers whose job is to assess the person's needs and connect the person with many community resources. These case managers must know how to use the laws designed to provide a better life for them as well.

Primary Prevention Preventing certain disabilities from occurring may be possible. Some disabilities result from genetic abnormalities. Much research is currently focusing on hereditary disabilities and methods to detect the genes that pass on those traits. Parents who know they may pass on a disability might be able to take medication or get other types of treatment that may slow or even prevent a disability altogether. Some might even opt not to carry the pregnancy to full term.

Other disabilities result from taking certain chemicals, drugs, or alcohol during pregnancy. For example, in the 1940s and 1950s, physicians were treating severe morning sickness with a new drug, thalidomide. This drug created severe birth defects in babies born to mothers who took the medication. So banning the drug for pregnant women prevented further thalidomide-related birth defects. Another preventable birth defect is fetal alcohol syndrome, which is caused by a mother's heavy alcohol use during pregnancy. Prior to the 1970s, pregnant women regularly consumed wine and other alcohol throughout their pregnancies. Studies have since shown that women who drank heavily during pregnancy gave birth to children who were mentally slow and behaviorally challenged. As a result, alcohol consumption during pregnancy is strongly discouraged, which has lessened the incidence of fetal alcohol syndrome.

In general, educating pregnant teenagers early on about the effects that drugs and alcohol can have on their unborn babies is the best preventive way to intervene. Despite all precautions, however, some babies are born with disabilities, the causes of which have yet to be identified. The best that can be done is to detect the disability early in a child's life so that treatment can begin. For example, the sooner a child who is blind learns Braille and how to use a guide dog, the better the quality of life. The same holds true for children who are deaf or autistic. Early intervention can prevent a lifetime of crises and tertiary institutionalization.

Prevention programs related to bullying are also in place. The second author worked with spinal cord injury patients at a regional center in southern California that specialized in the treatment, care, and recovery of those affected by spinal cord injuries. One of their innovative programs also includes education about bullying; their program, Own my Own Power! educates the community about how to prevent bullying of persons who are disabled and how to empower youth to own their strengths.

Critical Thinking/Self-Reflection Corner

- What images do you hold of persons who are disabled?
- What do you think of the statement: There are no disabled people, only disabling environments?
- Why do you think many persons who are disabled are discriminated against?

CRIME/VIOLENCE PERPETRATORS

Historical Background

While human services addresses the needs of victims of crimes, human services workers also often work with people who break the law, which is the focus of this section. Some of these clients behave violently and have harmed others, while others are less violent and aggressive but have still committed crimes. People who commit crimes are often referred to as perpetrators. This term is most often used when discussing those who commit violence against others, such as child abusers. People who fall into this group have also been called criminals, deviants, and sometimes sociopaths. Society has always had to deal with this type of person. As we learned in Chapter 1, corrective action with this group has ranged from humanistic compassion to execution. Our current society still reacts similarly to this population.

Definition of Crime or Violence Perpetrator

Anyone who breaks the law has committed a crime. Crimes range in severity from misdemeanors to felonies. Misdemeanors are not punished as severely as felonies are. Felonious acts are often violent in nature, such as armed robbery, kidnapping, murder, and drug distribution. A misdemeanor might include such first-time offenses as minor drug possession, drunk driving, or passing bad checks. Our system tends to be easier on first-time offenders than on those who have a history of criminal behavior. Individual states often follow their own designated legislation. For example, California's three-strike rule, established in the 1990s, mandates that if someone is convicted of any felony with two or more prior strikes, that person will be prosecuted to the full extent of the law, which could mean receiving a sentence of at least 25 years to life. In 2012, the rule was amended to define the new felony to be serious or violent.

Individual states also vary in how they define crime. For example, states vary in their definitions and considerations of assault and battery, hate crimes, domestic violence, criminal harassment, and even shoplifting. History also influences definitions of crimes, such as spousal abuse, which has only been considered a crime since the 1980s, while murder, has been against the law since the beginning of civilization.

Prevalence

According to the Bureau of Justice Statistics (2013), as of 2011, over 5.6 million U.S adults had ever served in state or federal prison. This includes persons in prison and on parole and those previously incarcerated. Of this population, nearly as many were black as were white (2,166,000 and 2,203,000, respectively), and nearly 100,000 were Hispanic. Among age groups, those between 35 and 39 years of age were most likely to have gone to prison. Also, according to the Federal Bureau of Investigation (2012), there were over 12 million arrests in the United States, which included murder, rape, assault, arson, burglary, property crime, fraud, and vandalism, among many other crimes.

Causality Models

Why do people commit crimes? This question has been studied for the past 100 years by social scientists. Some believe that aggressive behaviors are caused by abnormal biochemistry that causes **bipolar disorder**, ADHD, or personality disorders. Many people argue that those with these sorts of disorders are not in control of their behaviors. For example, psychoanalytic theory suggests that chronic criminality is due to **antisocial personality disorder**. People with this disorder have not developed proper superego capacity and do not feel remorse or guilt for aggressions against others, much like a two-year-old does not feel guilt if he or she hits someone. These people go through life as if the rules don't apply to them. They behave in ways to meet their needs without regard for others' needs. Another personality disorder thought to be associated with certain crimes is referred to as narcissistic. Psychoanalytic theory suggests that this type of person is fixated at an early stage of psychological development (around age 3). His or her behavior is an attempt to satisfy primitive needs for recognition, power, control, and validation. **Pedophiles**, spousal abusers, and child abusers are often thought to be suffering from **narcissistic personality disorders**.

Some perpetrators were abused as children and often attempt to gain some type of restitution by violating another when they become adults. This payback theory is part of the psychoanalytic theory that proposes that people displace anger and aggression onto safer targets because they feel powerless to express their anger on the person who abused them. While being abused may be one cause of becoming a perpetrator, it is not the only cause. Humanistic theory might suggest that these perpetrators were not given enough love or nurturance and are deficit in self-esteem development. They were not raised by parents who were capable of providing a safe or realistic environment.

Social and cultural theories also attempt to explain why people perpetrate crimes. Poverty is thought to lead to crime. When people see others living within a standard of living above theirs, they often engage in behaviors such as theft, robbery, burglary, and drug sales to get what others have. Living in violent neighborhoods may also lead to criminal behaviors. It may be the norm in certain communities to engage in violent acts against others, such as gang violence and partner abuse. If one is raised in an area where guns are prevalent, that person may think it is normal to possess and use guns. Likewise, if someone is raised in an area where drugs are sold and used openly, criminal behavior becomes normative. Some communities have a culture of learned helplessness where people grow up believing that they cannot get out and advance their way of life. They may not even know that there is a different way of life. Using drugs, engaging in criminal activity, and acting out aggression may be seen as exciting. The idea of spending time incarcerated may not even bother this type of person.

Needs and Issues

Because perpetrators range from first-time offenders to chronic offenders, their needs and issues will vary from perpetrator to perpetrator. If someone does suffer from an antisocial personality disorder, that person has been committing crimes since childhood. People with antisocial personality disorders are difficult to treat with counseling and need to face the reality of what they are doing and its consequences. If motivated to change, they can receive help and try to learn that positive results can happen if they can change their behavior. Reality therapy is a type of counseling in which the counselor attempts to create a safe, involved relationship in which the client can feel cared about by a responsible person. The focus is on helping this person meet his or her needs for feeling worthwhile, successful, and loved. It is very difficult to completely cure this type of disorder, but criminal behaviors can be controlled with proper intervention.

Other perpetrators need help gaining access to resources, such as education, employment, and other social welfare assistance. They may need intense guidance on how to become a successful contributor to society as well as intense monitoring on how to maintain a structured lifestyle that does not include involvement with other perpetrators of crime.

Perpetrators of family violence and rape often need intense counseling. They must learn how to empathize with others and learn how to control their own needs. They often have many irrational thoughts and distorted beliefs about their behaviors that have permitted them to engage in violence against those whom they love. These need to be addressed in group, individual, and family counseling. Some of these perpetrators need to spend time incarcerated to keep society safe while they work on these issues. They may also need punishment, such as jail, to help them truly understand that there will be consequences for their criminal behaviors. To be truly helped, perpetrators must deal with their childhood traumas and learn how to successfully meet their needs as adults.

Human Services Delivery for Crime and Violence Perpetrators

Emergency Situations and Interventions When people get arrested, it usually creates a feeling of emergency for the person arrested and significant others. The legal system handles what happens after the arrest. Either the person stays in jail or gets out on bail. The person either hires an attorney or gets one appointed to him or her by the court system. Human services workers are not generally involved in this aspect of intervention.

Secondary Intervention Human services workers, however, do become involved once the preliminary interventions have been completed. Many people who break the law by committing burglary, murder, assault, forgery, and theft go to some type of correctional facility. Human services workers play a larger role in working with first-time offenders and juveniles than with people who have long histories of criminal behavior.

Human services workers are also involved with "family" crimes, such as domestic violence and child abuse. Social workers, therapists, and probation officers, among others, must work collaboratively on these family crimes. These offenders rarely go to prison. The court system and society holds conflicting views on these offenses. It is hard to decide whether these crimes result from emotional disorders, bad choices, or greed—the cause of so many other crimes. These offenders rarely go to prison because society prefers to keep families together when possible. Also, the perpetrator is often the sole bread winner of the family, and so keeping oneself out of prison may help keep a family out of the welfare system.

So if they don't go to prison, what interventions are available? Probation is one common intervention for first-time offenders and juveniles. Probation can be formal or informal. People on formal probation must visit their probation officer about once a month. Probation officers serve as case managers, working with offenders to ensure they are functioning within the law, are attending any required counseling or 12-step groups, and are not associating with the wrong people. As long as offenders comply with the rules of their probation, they do not have to do additional time in a correctional facility. If they break those rules, then incarceration may be inevitable.

Many people involved in crimes related to substance abuse, such as drunken driving, possession of drugs, and public intoxication, may be referred to **diversion programs**. These programs usually consist of drug awareness and drug education groups, individual and family counseling, and community service. The offenders eligible for diversion programs are not usually chronic drug addicts because addicts usually need more intense treatment. However, juveniles and recreational or social drug users may benefit from these programs.

Perpetrators of domestic violence are often sent to mandatory, structured treatment programs for batterers. These programs last between six months and two years and include anger-management groups, individual therapy, drug and alcohol counseling, 12-step programs, and parenting classes. If a perpetrator has a long history of arrests for spousal abuse, he or she may have to be incarcerated.

Perpetrators of child abuse receive intervention plans from child protective services. A social worker assigned to a case serves as its case manager and develops a plan appropriate for the offense. Perpetrators of severe child abuse and neglect go to prison; however, first-time offenders convicted of abuse that was not life threatening may be referred to parenting classes, 12-step groups, individual therapy, and family counseling. The case manager monitors the completion of the case plan and works toward reunifying a family if it is safe for the children.

When a family member sexually abuses a child, intervention is usually geared more toward counseling and reunification than punishment. Strangers who sexually abuse children are more likely to be incarcerated, though not for very long. Perpetrators of incest may be given probation that includes mandatory involvement in group therapy and individual counseling. If, however, these offenders have a long-standing history of child molestation, they may be given significant jail time.

As with all secondary interventions, the goal is to prevent any further offending behaviors. Sometimes crisis intervention is enough, but many problems need more intense psychotherapy and group therapy.

Tertiary Intervention People who commit serious crimes, such as murder, kidnapping, armed robbery, and drug distribution, are usually incarcerated. Sometimes the incarceration is to punish, other times it is to protect society.

Innovative Intervention Efforts for Perpetrators: Prison Pet Partnership

At the Maximum Security Women's Prison in Washington State, the Prison Pet Partnership Program has become a model for the nation in the area of rehabilitation of offenders within the criminal justice system. In the program, inmates learn to train, care for, and board dogs to be used for persons with disabilities. Not only does this provide necessary vocational skills to inmates, it also gives them something meaningful to care for and love, improved self-esteem and coping skills, and responsibility, all of which can improve the chances of successful rehabilitation.

Even some of the family crimes and substance abuse crimes mentioned above receive incarceration sentences from judges. When crimes are not considered to be a crime against another person, such as petty theft, forgery, drug use and possession, offenders may be allowed to serve part of their sentences at a halfway house. These halfway houses provide employment training and counseling, group therapy, 12-step groups, and personal counseling. The offenders learn to function in society as a law-abiding citizen, something they may have never done before. Sometimes, these chronic criminals need daily support to help them avoid involvement with the criminal justice system.

Primary Prevention Sometimes preventing crime is as simple as maintaining strong neighborhoods. Lack of street maintenance, broken windows, abandoned buildings, and broken-down cars are a few examples of a disorganized community that can lead to crime. The implementation of neighborhood crime-prevention programs often assist in primary prevention efforts. Another example of a primary prevention program is the Scared Straight program. Either at-risk juveniles are taken to prison or prisoners visit these juveniles at an agency. The convicts tell the scary truth about incarceration to these youths. A similar program involves having at-risk youth participate for a brief time at a boot camp, a sort of mock prison facility where they must adhere to very strict rules.

Critical Thinking/Self-Reflection Corner

- Can you work with a pedophile?
- Should all people who commit crimes go to prison?
- How should society decide who should go to prison and who should receive counseling and educational courses?
- Do you have empathy for persons who have committed a crime?
- Do you believe criminals deserve a second or third chance? Why or why not?
- Would you enjoy working in the criminal justice system? Why or why not?

SUBSTANCE ABUSE

Historical Background

The use of mind-altering substances has been part of human behavior ever since man first discovered that certain plants induce euphoric states. It is widely known that opium was smoked thousands of years ago by ancient civilizations, such as the Chinese and Egyptians. Wine consumption was discussed in the Bible and was an integral part of ancient Roman ceremonies. Alcohol has been the most used substance in the United States since its creation. At one point, there was an attempt to make alcohol use and distribution illegal. This didn't work, and so alcohol remains one of the most used drugs. The use of other drugs, such as cocaine, opium-based drugs, and marijuana, can be traced back to the 1890s in the United States. At first, they were used medicinally. People then started using these drugs for pleasure and to enhance work performance. These drugs became illegal during the early 1900s under the Harrison Drug Act. Marijuana, the most widely used illicit drug, has of course in recent years become highly controversial regarding its legality. Many argue it should be removed from the criminal justice system and regulated in a way similar to alcohol and tobacco. Others feel that too many misperceptions exist regarding the safety of marijuana and thus its legalization is not a smart move. Synthetic versions of many illicit drugs have been created during the past 100 years and are also illegal. Despite the strict laws prohibiting drug use, many people still abuse drugs. Some are illegal drugs; others are legally prescribed by physicians. We are, in general, a society of alcohol and drug users. Many social events revolve around drinking and using drugs. As such, it can be quite challenging for someone addicted to drugs to recover.

Definition of Substance Abuse

The *Diagnostic and Statistical Manual IV (DSM-V)* (APA, 2013) puts people with **substance abuse** in one of two categories: **substance dependence** or substance abuse. Dependence means that without the drug, users suffer physical withdrawal. This person needs increasingly larger amounts of the substance to feel its effects. The dependent drug user suffers from one or more medical consequences as a result of using the drug. Abuse means that the drug is taken most of the time and creates impaired social, work, academic, or daily functioning. Abusers include both those who drink alcohol and those who take mind-altering drugs. Although nicotine and caffeine are addicting, they will not be addressed in this book.

Alcohol, amphetamines, cannabis, cocaine, hallucinogens, inhalants, opiates, and sedatives are all discussed in this section as they are the most commonly abused substances. Some are more addicting than others. Table 8.3 provides a brief look at the effects of different drugs.

In 2011, nearly 8.7 percent, or 22.5 million Americans, aged 12 and older had used an illicit drug or abused a psychotherapeutic medication (such as a pain

TABLE 8.3 Substance Abuse

Drug	How Taken	Addiction Potential	Pleasurable Effects	Negative Effects
Alcohol	Ingested	Very addictive; may cause convulsions, shakes, hallucinations during withdrawal	Euphoria, disinhibitions, pleasant taste	Slow reaction time; too much causes nausea, blackouts, slurring, falling down, liver damage
Marijuana (cannabis)	Smoked, ingested	Psychologically, not physically, addictive	Euphoria, silliness, laughter, sleepiness, hunger (munchies)	Motivational syndrome, paranoia, depersonalization, brain cell death, tar in lungs
Cocaine, crack, crystal methamphetamine	Snorted, smoked, IV injection	Physically addictive; during withdrawal, feeling sketchy, paranoid, depressed, agitated	High energy, increased confidence, weight loss, diminished need for sleep	Inability to concentrate, poor social interaction, poor sexual performance, heart attack, stroke
Heroin	Snorted, IV injection	Very physically addictive; during withdrawal, feeling sick, vomits, shakes	Euphoria, release from all stress and pain	Nodding out, needle marks, hepatitis, risk of HIV
Sedatives	Ingested	Very physically addictive; during withdrawal, feeling sick, convulsions, hallucinations, seizures	Euphoria, sleepiness, lack of anxiety, relaxation	Feeling out of it, inability to function without the pills, liver damage, emotional vacancy
LSD	Ingested	Not addictive	Euphoria, feelings of unreality, distortions of reality, increased visual and sensual pleasure	Bad trips; paranoia; psychotic feelings of depersonalization, panic, anxiety
Ecstasy	Ingested	Not addictive	Euphoria, heightened sensual pleasures, mind feels open and creative	Heart palpitations, unconsciousness especially when used with other drugs, poor impulse control
Inhalants	Sniffed	Addictive	Euphoria, a rush of excitement	Drowsiness, poor muscle control, suffocation, nausea, vomiting, damage to brain and central nervous system
Analgesics	Ingested	Can become addictive, especially long-term opioid usage	Pain relief	Overdose, sleep apnea, fractures, osteoporosis, infection, sexual dysfunction, depression, anxiety, tooth decay

© 2015 Cengage Learning

Digital Download Download at CengageBrain.com

reliever) (National Institute on Drug Abuse, 2012b). Across a lifetime, 48 percent reported having used any illicit drug (National Institute on Drug Abuse, n.d.), the most common being marijuana, as well as cocaine, heroin, acid (LSD), and ecstasy (MDMA). Other examples of drugs used are inhalants, steroids, and tobacco/nicotine. Interestingly, an emerging public health concern is the increasing use of e-cigarettes, Krokodil (a homemade opiate), N-bomb (synthetic hallucinogens being sold as legal), bath salts (synthetic, amphetamine-like stimulant), and drinking prescription-strength cough syrup. Regarding alcohol abuse, as of 2002, almost 5 million adults were alcohol dependent or alcohol abusing and had at least one child in the home. Other data indicate that the prevalence of lifetime alcohol abuse and alcohol dependence is 17.8 and 12.5 percent, respectively, and these are more common among men than women (Hasin, Stinson, Ogburn, & Grant, 2007). In 2011, 6.8 million adults had a co-occurring substance use disorder and a diagnosable mental illness (SAMHSA, n.d.). Substance abuse among older adults is a growing problem. Some data indicate the percentage of Americans, aged 50–59 years, who reported having abused illicit or prescription drugs during the past year, more than doubled from 2.7 percent to 6.2 percent between 2002 and 2009 (National Institute of Drug Abuse, 2011). Other studies have indicated that community prevalence rates of abuse among those 60 and older range from 2–25 percent for heavy alcohol use and alcohol abuse. For youth, illicit drug use has continued over the years at high rates. For example, in 2012, 6.5 percent of 8th graders, 17.0 percent of 10th graders, and 22.9 percent of 12th graders used marijuana in the past month—an increase among 10th and 12th graders from 14.2 percent and 18.8 percent, respectively, in 2007. Tobacco and alcohol usage among youth, though, has dropped in recent years. Analgesic usage is on the rise. The number of adults with regular use in 2000 were 4.4 million for opioids (including oxycodone, hydrocodone, and morphine), 6.2 million for NSAIDs (nonsteroidal antiinflammatory drugs such as ibuprofen and aspirin), and 6.0 million for acetaminophen. Long-term opioid usage can lead to several adverse effects including respiratory, behavioral, musculoskeletal, and cardiovascular problems (GroupHealth, n.d.). Finally, it has been estimated that the cost to society due to substance abuse and addiction is close to $600 billion a year (National Institute on Drug Abuse, 2011).

Causality Models

There are many reasons that lead to substance abuse. Medical models hold that a family history of substance abuse can make a person more susceptible or vulnerable to becoming an addict. These models argue that addiction is a disease in which substances cause changes to a person's body, mind and behavior, in ways that the addicted person cannot control. From this perspective, addiction is not seen as a sign of moral weakness, overindulgence, or lack of willpower, known as the moral model, but as a genetic, chemical, or brain disease, such as being due to a neurotransmitter imbalance. Those with addiction then would need to engage in lifelong abstinence.

Psychodynamic models of addiction and substance abuse hold that drug abusers are self-medicating due to underlying psychological problems, poor coping skills, and internal struggles. Social models argue that substance abuse is a learned behavior, modeled perhaps from family members, or a result of peer pressure. Interestingly, the media may also influence substance use, particularly when we are bombarded with glamorous images of drinking and smoking. Family models propose that substance abuse regulates family functioning. Having an addict in a family often leads to the creation of roles, such as enabler, hero, scapegoat, and victim, for various members in the family. There does seem to be some truth to this theory because when the abuser stops using, the family often goes into crisis mode until family members learn new ways of relating to one another. People who have difficulty with intimate relationships may use substances to cover up the anxiety they experience being close to others. When the abuser becomes sober, family members must now relate to each other in emotionally intimate ways, which can be felt as emotionally threatening.

Most likely, each person's drug use is a result of the combination of many of the above models. This biopsychosocial perspective holds that addiction and substance abuse is a multifaceted process and that treatment and recovery need to address all aspects of a person's life, such as nutrition, stress, family issues, employment, psychological issues, social support systems, childhood experiences, and more.

Needs and Issues

Many people who abuse substances or are addicted risk several negative outcomes, including impacting their own personal mental and physical health and longevity; their relationships with family; and their ability to function and be productive, as well as facing the risk of increased crime, abuse, and violence. Children of parental substance abuse and addiction face several biological and social consequences.

Recovery and treatment, as well as relapse, are challenging processes that many addicts face. This often includes lifelong therapy, medication usage, and withdrawal, as well as the likelihood of having to develop a new lifestyle with new social connections. Often, addicts' only social ties are with other abusers. They need to learn how to feel pleasure through socially acceptable activities. This process may take years to complete. Some believe it is an ongoing process that is never complete. The philosophy of Alcoholic Anonymous suggests that all addicts are merely recovering and are never cured.

Human Service Delivery for Substance Abuse

Emergency Situations and Interventions Substance abuse emergencies may be either life-threatening or legal emergencies. Life-threatening emergencies, such as suicide attempts, heart attacks, strokes, or overdoses, must be treated in a medical hospital. An illness or injury must be managed and stabilized before any other treatment for substance abuse begins. When substance abusers are arrested for drug possession, driving under the influence of alcohol or an illegal substance, or any other illegal drug-related crime, they need immediate assistance. Once a person has been cleared medically and legal issues have been managed, workers can begin to work with a person on their abuse of drugs or alcohol.

Secondary Intervention Brief intervention for alcohol-related problems may be effective for those who are not alcohol dependent. That is, they report drinking at levels that may be risky but have not yet created serious medical or legal problems in their lives. The goal of this type of brief intervention may be to reduce drinking to moderate levels. If the drinker is alcohol dependent, the goal would be abstinence. Treatment for alcohol dependency is discussed under tertiary intervention.

Common elements of brief intervention include the following:

1. Providing information about health risks associated with heavy drinking
2. Emphasizing that it's the patient's own responsibility and decision to drink
3. Advising on how to reduce or stop drinking and how to engage in "low-risk" drinking
4. Providing strategies to reduce drinking, such as pacing one's drinking, sipping, and so forth
5. Using an empathic counseling style
6. Encouraging patients to rely on their own resources to bring about change and to be optimistic about their ability to change (National Institute on Alcohol Abuse and Alcoholism, 1999)

Short-term counseling and crisis intervention may also be appropriate and effective for some drug users, especially if they have just begun to abuse drugs. In particular, adolescents may benefit from brief intervention if they haven't yet developed a lifestyle in which drug use has become the focal point. These drug users may simply need drug education classes, family therapy, or supportive counseling. The focus of these interventions should be on how to return to their previous level of functioning prior to drug use. The drug user might be encouraged to become involved in productive recreational activities, to rekindle friendships that may have been damaged by drug use, and to increase satisfaction from work or school. Sometimes, the drug use is an attempt to cope with other life problems. Counselors can often help drug users express feelings and talk about problems and learn ways to cope with them without resorting to drug use.

Some people who abuse drugs and alcohol may also benefit from 12-step facilitation. While it may be true that a person who is addicted and physically dependent on drugs or alcohol may need to participate in a 12-step group indefinitely, some might benefit from a 12-step group for a brief time. They may need the support of the group to help them shift their social world into one that doesn't include drug use. A 12-step group for some people can be used as a transitional social world until they have a healthy stable social world developed in their own life.

"**Twelve-step facilitation** (TSF) consists of a brief, structured, and manual-driven approach to facilitating early recovery from alcohol abuse/alcoholism and other drug abuse/addiction. It is intended to be implemented on an individual basis in 12 to 15 sessions and is based on behavioral, spiritual, and cognitive principles that form the core of twelve-step fellowships such as AA. TSF is suitable for problem drinkers and other drug users and for those who are alcohol or drug dependent" (Nowinski, 2000). The goal of TSF is to facilitate the acceptance of the need for abstinence from alcohol and other drugs and the willingness to participate actively in a 12-step fellowship as a means of sustaining sobriety. After a few months of 12-step group participation, some users who are not physically addicted to alcohol or drugs may be able to use alcohol or drugs moderately and still function appropriately in society. However, some people who have had chronic drug and alcohol problems cannot ever drink or use drugs at all and may need to be involved with a 12-step group indefinitely. We turn to those chronic abusers next.

Tertiary Intervention For individuals who drink or use drugs chronically, the goal is complete abstinence. During the TSF process, a counselor attempts to convince these clients that willpower alone is not sufficient to sustain sobriety. Instead, they must surrender to the group conscience of the 12-step group and accept that a higher power is the locus of changing one's life. Clients remain in therapy for a few weeks after joining a 12-step group. This allows clients to discuss with their therapist how they can best use the group, and a therapist can offer encouragement to continue going to the group. A TSF therapist also conducts a few sessions with significant others during this time.

Some individuals with drug and alcohol addictions need treatment beyond TSF and 12-step groups. "No single treatment is appropriate for all individuals. Matching treatment settings, interventions, and services to each individual's particular problems and needs is critical to his or her ultimate success in returning to productive functioning in the family, workplace, and society" (National Institute on Drug Abuse, 2012a).

Intervention for clients who abuse drugs and alcohol chronically may include such medications as methadone, LAAM, and naltrexone, which help those addicted to opiates reduce their dependency on those types of drugs, as well as antidepressants, mood stabilizers, or neuroleptics that help treat mental disorders, such as depression, anxiety, bipolar disorder, or psychosis, that may accompany drug and alcohol addiction. For those with severe physical addictions, detoxification is often necessary. During a detoxification process, an addict may be given medication to ease the symptoms of withdrawal from an opiate, pain pills, alcohol, cocaine, or crystal methamphetamine. This may take three to five days. After a person is stabilized on medication, treatment can begin to focus on the psychological and social aspects of the addiction.

Medical detoxification safely manages the acute physical symptoms of withdrawal associated with stopping drug and alcohol use, but it is rarely sufficient in helping addicts achieve long-term abstinence (National Institute on Drug Abuse, 2012a). Recovery from drug addiction can be a long-term process and frequently requires multiple episodes of treatment. Participation in 12-step groups such as Alcoholics Anonymous (AA), Narcotics Anonymous (NA), or Cocaine Anonymous (CA) is usually considered necessary for long-term abstinence. These are usually attended both during and after formal treatment.

Formal treatment may be on an outpatient basis, such as individual psychotherapy or group therapy at a day-treatment center. Some people are in a long-term residential treatment program, often referred to as a **therapeutic community (TC)**, which could last from six months to a year. The TC model focuses on resocialization of the individual and helping the person develop personal accountability and responsibility to live a socially productive life. This treatment may be highly structured and confrontational and includes cognitive behavioral therapy in which clients learn how to examine damaging beliefs, self-concepts, and patterns of behavior and to adopt new, more harmonious and constructive ways to interact with others. TCs may include employment training and drug testing as well. The residents at the TCs usually have very severe problems with drugs and alcohol as well as involvement with the criminal justice system and mental health problems.

Short-term residential programs follow the 12-step approach and consist of three to six weeks of inpatient treatment, followed by extended outpatient therapy and ongoing participation in a 12-step group. Relapse prevention, supportive expressive therapy, and education are all part of ongoing outpatient therapy models that serve as an adjunct treatment to involvement in a 12-step program.

One widely accepted model of recovery is the developmental model, which identifies six stages an addicted individual must go through for long-term recovery. These include the following:

1. "Transition, the period of time needed for the addicted individual to come to grips with the realization that safe use of alcohol or other drugs for them is not possible;
2. Stabilization, during which the chemically dependent person experiences physical withdrawal and other medical problems and learns how to separate from people, places, and things that promote substance abuse;
3. Early recovery, when an individual faces the need to establish a chemical-free lifestyle and build relationships that support long-term recovery;
4. Middle recovery, seen as time for the development of a balanced lifestyle where repairing past damage is important;
5. Late recovery, during which the individual identifies and changes mistaken beliefs about oneself, others, and the world that caused or promoted irrational thinking; and
6. Maintenance, the lifelong process of continued growth, development, and managing routine life problems" (HHS, 1999).

Because drug and alcohol addictions, as well as recovery, are so complicated, long-term treatment and commitment are essential. The goal is thorough modification of an addict's lifestyle, including social interactions, emotional expression, and ways of connecting with others. Patience and commitment are essential for human services workers who work with this population.

Primary Prevention As with all primary prevention programs, the goal is to educate at-risk people about the negative consequences of drug use and alcohol abuse. Students in elementary school participate in Red Ribbon Week. They sign commitment contracts stating they won't use drugs, smoke cigarettes, or drink alcohol. Nancy Reagan's campaign during the 1980s told children to "just say no." Subsequent to the Just Say No campaign, many local police departments in collaboration with elementary schools implemented the Drug

Awareness and Resistance Education (DARE) program in which the students were educated about drugs and alcohol and given strategies to avoid using drugs. Younger children were targeted because unfortunately by the time children enter junior high school they may have already tried drugs or alcohol. The earlier the onset of using drugs and alcohol can be prevented, the easier it may be to help people avoid becoming addicted or chronic users. One of the oldest and largest drug prevention campaigns in the country is Red Ribbon Week, which "serves as a vehicle for communities and individuals to take a stand for the hopes and dreams of our children through a commitment to drug prevention and education and a personal commitment to live drug free lives with the ultimate goal being the creation of drug free America" (http://www.imdrugfree.com/).

Critical Thinking/Self-Reflection Corner

- If you knew addiction "ran in your family" would you choose to drink or use drugs?
- How have you handled peer pressure to use illegal substances?
- Have you or anyone you know been affected by a loved one's drug use?

CHAPTER SUMMARY

There are many issues and challenges that people face in their lives. Whether it is abuse, addiction, engagement in violence, poverty and homelessness, or a disability, all people deserve to have opportunities to enhance their quality of life and become empowered through the resources available to them. It is in part the job of human services professionals to ensure that all clients are treated with respect, dignity, and fairness, irrespective of their life situation. It is important to be aware that one's personal views and attributions of causes of behavior directly impact treatment and behaviors toward people. For example, believing that addiction is a sign of weakness may cause a human services professional to become angry; if one believes that addiction is caused by a disease, this may increase feelings of empathy. Personal self-awareness, knowledge of the literature and current research, and experience with human services populations will increase the likelihood that one's clients will have better care, well-being, and necessary access to critical resources.

Suggested Applied Activities

1. Interview at least five people who have had experience, either directly or indirectly, with one of the topics discussed in this chapter. What was their experience like? How did it affect them emotionally, financially, and/or physically? How did the experience influence choices and decisions they have made?

2. Watch a movie or a television show in which one or more of the characters are experiencing problems with one of the topics discussed in this chapter. What are their issues and challenges? How do they overcome them? Are the problems and solutions presented in the movie or show realistic and accurate?
3. Read a book about one of the topics presented in this chapter. Discuss with friends or classmates. For example, consider reading *Nickel and Dimed: On (Not) Getting By in America*, by journalist Barbara Ehrenreich, which discusses the impact of welfare on the working poor in the United States.

Chapter Review Questions

1. What services might someone from the following population need?

   a. Mental illness

   _____

   _____

   b. Poverty/homelessness

   _____

   _____

   c. Disabled

   _____

   _____

   d. Crime-related perpetrator

   _____

   _____

   e. Substance abuser or addict

   _____

   _____

2. How might support groups be effective for people who have experienced poverty, mental illness, disabilities, addiction, or imprisonment?

   _____

   _____

3. What might human services workers keep in mind when designing a case management plan for a first-time offender or someone who has relapsed?

4. What primary prevention programs are available for issues related to mental Illness, poverty, disabilities, crime/violence, and substance abuse?

5. What models help to explain addiction?

Glossary of Terms

Americans with Disabilities Act (ADA) protects and preserves the rights of people with disabilities, especially in the workplace and within institutional settings.

Antisocial personality disorder is a pattern of behavior that displays a lack of regard for people and rules. People with this personality disorder lack feelings of guilt, seem to have no conscience, and usually have a history of criminal behavior.

Anxiety disorders are a group of mental disorders in which the primary symptoms are anxiety, fear, worry, and panic.

Attention deficit hyperactivity disorder (ADHD) is found in young children who exhibit restlessness, inability to concentrate, impulsivity, and misbehavior.

Bipolar disorder, previously known as manic depression, is an illness in which sufferers experience extreme mood swings, from feelings of elation to those of deep depression.

Chronically poor include those who are poor over many years, often over their entire lives, and commonly pass poverty on to their children.

Comorbidity is a disease or condition that occurs at the same time as another illness.

Cycle of poverty occurs when living in a state of poverty becomes an accepted way of life that is passed down from parents to children.

Cyclically poor include those who experience intermittent poverty, often due to cycling on and off public assistance, in congruence with economic highs and lows; such are often known as the working poor.

Delirium is a serious disturbance in a person's mental abilities that results in confused thinking and decreased awareness of his or her environment.

Delusional disorders are a type of serious mental illness involving psychosis.

Dementia is a chronic or persistent disorder of the mental processes caused by brain disease or injury and marked by memory disorders, personality changes, and impaired reasoning.

Deserving poor are those that are vulnerable to poor social conditions and outcomes due to environmental and social reasons, not personal control.

Diagnostic and Statistical Manual of Mental Disorders (DSM-V) offers the criteria by which mental disorders are diagnosed in the United States.

Disengaged defines families that are too emotionally distant from one another.

Diversion programs are a form of sentencing designed to enable offenders of criminal law to avoid criminal charges and a criminal record.

Eating disorders are a variety of food-related disorders in which sufferers become obsessively involved with body image and what they are eating and how it will affect their bodies. They usually have unrealistic body images.

Enmeshed defines families whereby emotional boundaries and closeness are lacking.

Indigent people are extremely poor people who have no financial resources whatsoever.

Learned helplessness is the inability to escape poverty or an abusive relationship and instead accepting and living with the situation as if it's the only alternative.

Major depressive disorder is a mental disorder characterized by a pervasive and persistent low mood that is accompanied by low self-esteem and by a loss of interest or pleasure in normally enjoyable activities.

Medical detoxification is a procedure conducted in a hospital by a physician in which medication is used to help a person withdraw from alcohol or drug addiction.

Narcissistic personality disorders are characterized by a constant need for admiration and validation from others to counteract feelings of insecurity and a weak sense of self. People with this personality disorder are usually selfish and incapable of empathy for others.

Obsessive-compulsive disorder is an anxiety disorder characterized by intrusive thoughts that produce uneasiness, apprehension, fear, or worry, by repetitive behaviors aimed at reducing the associated anxiety, or by a combination of such obsessions and compulsions.

Panic disorder is an emotional disorder that involves recurring experiences of shortness of breath, sweating, chest discomfort, nausea, among other things, along with feelings of going crazy and of losing control.

Personality disorders are a group of mental disorders that impair a person's ability to interact and experience the world rationally. They are typically caused from deprivations in early childhood.

Pervasive developmental disorder is used to describe a group of conditions that involve delays in the development of many basic skills, including the inability to socialize with others, to communicate, and to use the imagination.

Pedophilia is a mental disorder characterized by recurrent, intensely sexually arousing fantasies, sexual urges, or behaviors that involve children, nonhuman subjects, or other nonconsenting adults or the suffering or humiliation of oneself or one's partner.

Phobia is an anxiety disorder that causes people to have fearful reactions to an object or a situation that are so extreme that they cause people to avoid the object or situation at all costs.

Poverty is a state of extreme economic distress that results in a substandard quality of life. Poverty, as defined by the government for the purpose of determining the amount of assistance that people need, changes depending on the economic standard of living in society.

Psychiatric emergency team (PET) is a group of mental health professionals who evaluate the mental state of individuals to determine whether they need to be hospitalized involuntarily because they are a danger to themselves or others or just gravely impaired.

Regional centers are government-funded agencies that assist people who are physically and mentally disabled from birth.

Substance abuse occurs when a person uses drugs or alcohol to the extent that they cause impaired social, behavioral, occupational, or academic functioning and whose friends also overuse drugs and alcohol.

Substance dependence occurs when users suffer medical consequences of drug and alcohol abuse and are physically addicted to the substance.

Schizophrenia is a psychotic disorder that causes people to have delusions and hear voices and prevents normal functioning.

Personal Responsibility and Work Opportunity Reconciliation Act (PRWORA) is a federal law addressing poverty and welfare.

Therapeutic community (TC) is a term applied to a participative, group-based approach to long-term mental illness, personality disorders, and drug addiction.

Twelve-step facilitation consists of a brief, structured, and manual-driven approach to facilitating early recovery from alcohol abuse or alcoholism and other drug abuse or addiction.

Case Presentation and Exit Quiz

General Description and Demographics

Samantha, 22 years of age, recently had a baby. She is struggling with postpartum depression; although she had a safe birth, she has limited health-care access and services. Her partner, John, is currently in jail for illegal drug use and possession. Samantha has a high-school education and, prior to having a baby, was working full time at a local clothing store chain. She lives with her grandmother, aged 57, who is disabled but does try to assist Samantha with the baby and bills, although her income too is quite small and limited. Samantha's parents are both drug abusers, and although Samantha did not drink during her pregnancy, she feels overwhelmed by the birth of her new child and desires to drink; she feels it will give her a way to calm her anxiety, feel better, and just escape from reality for a bit.

Specific Problems

Samantha is a multineed client; she is facing severe financial issues, mental health issues, potential drug abuse, and low social support. Although the baby is safe, and grandma is supportive, her disability limits her level of support. Sometimes Samantha worries her grandma will drop the baby due to her poor physical health condition.

Exit Quiz

1. Samantha can get some services for herself and child from through the Supplemental Nutrition Assistance Program (SNAP) and Women, Infant, and Children (WIC) program
    a. True
    b. False

2. Samantha is showing signs of mental illness. She would benefit from
    a. nonprofits' support
    b. local medical clinics
    c. medication
    d. all of the above

3. Samantha's grandma can receive, if not already, additional support through
   a. regional centers
   b. SSI
   c. learning more about the ADA
   d. all of the above
4. When Samantha's boyfriend, and father of her baby, is released from jail, Samantha may benefit from family counseling and leaning more about diversion programs.
   a. True
   b. False

Exit Quiz Answers

1. a
2. d
3. d
4. a

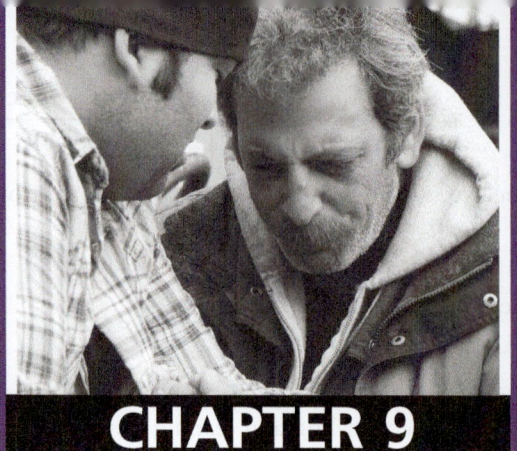

CHAPTER 9

Interpersonal Partner Abuse, Sexual Assault, HIV/AIDS, and LGBT Issues

INTERPERSONAL PARTNER ABUSE

According to research, nearly 29 percent of women and 10 percent of men in the United States have been raped, experienced physical violence, and/or been stalked by an intimate partner (e.g., Black et al., 2011). In fact, two-thirds of rapes are committed by someone known to the victim (U.S. Department of Justice, 2005). Interpersonal partner violence can happen to anyone, irrespective of socioeconomic status, education, race/ethnicity, age, sexual orientation, functional ability, religion, or gender. It happens to opposite-sex and same-sex couples and to couples who are married, cohabitating, and dating. Interpersonal partner violence is recognized as a serious public health concern, although it is most commonly understood to involve male-to-female violence with the female as the victim. Less universally recognized is the occurrence of such violence among teenagers and same-sex partners. This lack of awareness definitely needs to change.

Women and Domestic Violence

Women are at far greater risk of severe, if not fatal, injury from male partner abuse than are male victims. This is due in part to a man's physical size and strength, which make him less physically intimidated by a woman, and to the role of media that often portrays women as sexualized objects (more on this is discussed later in this chapter). Women who are abused by domestic partners live in ongoing relationships in which they are beaten, choked, threatened, stalked, controlled, or raped. This is referred to as domestic violence and may include women who are not married but merely dating or living with someone.

In the past, people often blamed the victim for the assault, speculating that the woman "asked for it." If she was being battered by her husband, she must have done something to provoke him. Women who sought help from clergy or their own mothers were often advised to "just be more loving to him," or "just try to keep the children quiet and have dinner ready," or "pray and hope things get better." Unfortunately, these suggestions do not solve the problems of abuse. While modern-day thought puts more of the responsibility on the abuser, some people still blame the victim.

Prevalence

Some statistical information might give the reader a general idea of how prevalent domestic violence is in the United States. The following box presents some facts and statistics about domestic violence according to Safe Horizon (2013).

Battered Women's Syndrome

Walker (1984) proposed that women stay in domestically violent relationships because they suffer from **battered women's syndrome**, which results from repeated episodes of abuse. The woman comes to believe that the situation is hopeless and that she can't do anything to fix it. She is afraid to leave because her husband may kill her or the children, for fear that she cannot survive on her own, or for fear that family and friends will reject her if she leaves. She may also

Domestic Violence: Statistics and Facts

- One in four women will experience domestic violence in her lifetime.
- Women are more likely than men to be killed by an intimate partner.
- Women ages 20–24 are at greatest risk of becoming victims of domestic violence.
- Every year, one in three women who is a victim of homicide is murdered by her current or former partner.
- Every year, more than 3 million children witness domestic violence in their homes.
- Children who live in homes where there is domestic violence also suffer high rates of abuse or neglect (30–60 percent).
- More than 60 percent of domestic violence incidents happen at home.
- Domestic violence is the third leading cause of homelessness.
- Domestic violence costs more than $37 billion a year in law enforcement involvement, legal work, medical and mental health treatment, and lost productivity at companies.
- Most domestic violence incidents are never reported!

believe that she loves her husband and that the children need their father. Many of these beliefs are irrational and can be altered through cognitive therapy. These feelings of helplessness, hopelessness, and worthlessness cause women to live in a chronic state of emptiness and shock, focusing only on survival rather than escape. This lifestyle is similar to that of a prisoner of war. Both tend to blame themselves and seek their captor's approval without thought of or fear of escape.

Feminist View of Domestic Violence

Many **feminists** believe that women are battered because society permits it. According to this causality model, punishment for domestic violence is not severe enough to deter it. The media portrays women as victims and men as aggressors. Women are taught since childhood that they aren't complete unless they have a man in their life. This often means that a bad relationship is considered to be better than no relationship at all.

Human Services Delivery in Domestic Violence Situations

Emergency Situations and Interventions Domestic violence is the leading cause of injury to women between the ages of 15 and 44 in the United States (Committee on the Judiciary United States Senate, 102nd Congress, 1992). In the United States, more than three women are murdered every day by their husbands or boyfriends (Rennison, 2003). Domestic violence is the leading cause of women's emergency room visits in the United States and one of the leading causes of death. Not only are women at risk for injury, but their children may be in danger as well. Many children who witness violence in their home can experience emotional, behavioral, and learning problems as a result. Sadly, nearly 1 in 10 American children has seen one family member assault another family member, and more than 25 percent have been exposed to family violence during their life (Finkelhor, Turner, Ormrod, Hamby, & Kracke, 2009, as cited by the U.S. Department of Justice, n.d.).

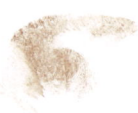

Hospital emergency rooms are well equipped, and the staff is well trained on how to treat women and children who have been battered. Recent legislation made it a requirement for physicians, nurses, chiropractors, and dentists to report suspected cases of spousal abuse to the police because the incidents of domestic violence are so frequent. It was hoped that this would be one way to prevent further abuse from occurring.

Often, domestic violence occurs at night. Many women leave home with their children and nothing but the clothes on their backs to escape a life-threatening situation. **Battered women's shelters** have emergency services available to help these women and children. When an abused woman calls the 24-hour hotline affiliated with a battered women's shelter, an assessment is made to determine if it is an emergency situation; then the woman and her children either drive to a location to meet a worker from the shelter or she is told to go to an emergency room. She may be admitted to the shelter that day or evening, or she may be given vouchers to stay at a local motel until a shelter has a bed for her.

The goal of emergency services for women and children who have been battered is, first, to ensure that injuries are dealt with by medical personnel; second, to ensure that she is no longer at risk of being injured that day or evening; and third, to provide a safe shelter for her and the children where the batterer cannot gain access. All battered women's shelters have confidential locations. In fact, it is a felony to disclose the location of one. This ensures the safety of these women and their children, all of whom are in danger of being killed within the first 72 hours after they leave home.

The True Stories From Human Service Workers box provides an example of work done with victims of domestic violence at a battered women's shelter.

In addition to safe shelter, other emergency services provided at the shelters include food, child care, sanitary sleeping arrangements, and clothing. Legal advice is also provided. The woman who was battered may wish to petition for a **temporary restraining order** as extra protection from her batterer. Most district attorneys' offices connected to local courts have a special department that deals specifically with domestic violence. Trained advocates and counselors provide emergency legal assistance that may include filing for child custody, emergency financial assistance, and filing for divorce.

Secondary Intervention Not all women seeking services related to domestic violence are in emergency situations. They may need assistance from the district attorney's office regarding filing for a restraining order. They may need guidance from a legal aide about how to file for divorce and seek child custody. They may need temporary financial assistance from social services. These women sometimes have access to resources to tide them over until the system kicks in with its help.

Example: A 62-year-old woman visited her physician for a routine medical exam. The doctor noticed bruises on her neck and ribs, as well as a black eye. He found out that she had been battered by her husband. He told her not to go

---

True Stories from Human Service Workers

Working with Battered Women at a Shelter

Battered women's shelters exist throughout the nation. These agencies provide a multitude of services for women and children who leave their homes because the mother has been a victim of physical, sexual, or emotional abuse by boyfriends and husbands. The women and children often stay at the shelters for about 45 days, long enough to develop psychological and emotional coping skills and social resources to be able to live independently.

Example: The director of residential services at a battered women's shelter in southern California says that, "the clients at the shelter have several needs. They have basic needs such as shelter, clothing, and food. They have community resource needs such as county assistance for financial aid and food stamps. They need counseling for post-traumatic stress disorder, suicide prevention, and referrals to mental health workers for serious mental health problems. They may also need help in transitioning to independent housing."

Clearly, these women exemplify the multi-needs client, and the agency appropriately offers a generalist and multidisciplinary team approach.

> ### The Battering Cycle
>
> 1. Honeymoon phase I: In the beginning the couple get along fine and are in love. He is kind and complimentary but may show some signs of possessiveness. He may consider her his girlfriend after just one date.
> 2. Tension phase: Over time, normal tensions and stress arise. Batterers lack communication skills and coping abilities, which creates high levels of tension and makes the woman feel she must "walk on eggshells" in an effort to avoid an argument or a tirade.
> 3. Explosive phase: Unfortunately, for these men, the explosive stage is inevitable and is accompanied by verbal abuse, physical abuse, or sexual abuse. At this stage, the woman is most likely to seek help. She is vulnerable, injured, and scared. During this crisis state, she is usually more receptive to crisis intervention by counselors and law enforcement. If she doesn't get help during this phase, she may easily return to the honeymoon phase, and the cycle continues.
> 4. Honeymoon phase II: The couple return to a peaceful, loving state in which the man apologizes and promises never to be abusive again. She forgives him and hopes for the best, but the cycle usually continues unless he seeks help.

Digital Download   Download at CengageBrain.com

home. He filed a report and recommended she drive to a neighboring county to stay with her grown daughter. This woman had money in her purse, a car, and a place to go. She stayed with her daughter that night, returned to her home court the next day, filed a restraining order, and set up a date to return and deal with money issues. The advocate at the court recommended she schedule an appointment with a therapist to talk about her feelings and develop a plan. She participated in crisis intervention with the therapist. Although she needed immediate services, this situation is not exactly an emergency. She had a place to go, money, food, and access to legal assistance.

Much of the secondary intervention provided for this client was aimed at educating her about the **battering cycle** so she could make choices that would be in her best interest. Many battered women benefit from understanding the cyclical nature of domestic violence.

Over time, the honeymoon phase disappears and the couple live in a cycle of tension and explosion until she leaves him, she gets killed or severely injured, or he goes to jail.

Most battered women's shelters operate on a 45-day model. This is considered sufficient time to help a woman deal with her feelings of rage, fear, and shame; secure employment; apply for financial assistance; file for divorce, a restraining order, and child custody; or enroll in job training courses. If the problem is not a chronic, longstanding one, most women benefit from secondary intervention and function well in society. The hope is that they will neither continue in a relationship with a batterer nor start a new relationship with an abusive person.

Tertiary Intervention   Some women have lived in ongoing abusive relationships for many years. They have participated in treatment and even filed for divorce or restraining orders but return to the abusive partner. Many times these women have developed battered woman's syndrome, which prevents them from leaving because their only focus is on surviving. They may need long-term therapy or case management to assist them in finding relationships that are not abusive. They may live in poverty, be disabled, or have been raised in an abusive home. These factors make it difficult to stay out of abusive situations. They may not have the material, psychological, or social resources to cope with daily stress on their own, and so they tolerate abuse. This type of woman may benefit from support groups, medication, or educational groups.

Human services workers must manage their own frustrations with these women who often return to their batterer or refuse to leave him in the first place. They need emotional support and understanding about why they stay, which is usually because they fear being alone, being killed, taking their children away from their father, and being labeled by society. It might take 5 to 10 years for a woman to finally leave an abusive relationship. She may have needed counseling for 10 years to learn that she can function on her own and that she will have support should she leave.

Primary Prevention As with all the other problems discussed, preventing abuse is by far the most desirable form of intervention. Many programs exist in which human services workers visit high schools and conduct education about domestic violence. Teens are taught about the battering cycle, how to detect a high-risk abusive person, how to assert themselves, and how to communicate and create a healthy relationship. Dating violence is very prevalent, and teens are taught that they don't have to endure it.

SEXUAL ASSAULT

Sexual assault occurs when one person forces any sexual behavior on another. This can include many types of forced physical contact including rape (forced vaginal or anal penetration), forced oral copulation, and other sexual acts that one person is forcing on another.

Most sexual assault victims are women, although men can also be victims of sexual assault, especially in prison. For the lesbian, gay, bisexual, transgender, and queer (LGBTQ) community, little data on national prevalence exists; however, one study indicated that sexual assault rates are likely higher as compared to the general population and that lesbian and bisexual women report greater overall sexual assault (including in childhood) than gay or bisexual men, although the latter are more likely to report sexual assault due to hate crimes (Rothman, Exner, & Baughman, 2011). The remainder of this section addresses only adult female victims of sexual assault.

Prevalence

According to worldwide estimates, at least one in three women has been beaten, coerced into sex, or otherwise abused during her lifetime, with rates of abuse reaching 70 percent in some countries (Heise, Ellsberg, & Gottemoeller, 1999; USAID, 2013).

Rape and Sexual Violence Statistics

According to the U.S. Bureau of Justice (2013):

- From 1995 to 2010, the estimated annual rate of female rape or sexual assault victimizations declined 58 percent from 5.0 victimizations per 1,000 females age 12 or older to 2.1 per 1,000.
- Females 34 years or younger and living in lower income households and in rural areas had the highest rates of sexual violence from 2005 to 2010.
- From 2005 to 2010, the offender was armed with a gun, knife, or other weapon in 11 percent of rape cases.
- From 2005 to 2010, 78 percent of sexual violence involved an offender who was a family member, intimate partner, friend, or acquaintance.
- 57 percent of rapes happen on dates.
- 84 percent of rape victims tried unsuccessfully to reason with the man who raped her or him.
- 55 percent of gang rapes on college campuses are committed by fraternities, 40 percent by sports teams, and 5 percent by others.
- In the 1980s, 5 percent of rape survivors went to the police. In the past 10 years, 30 percent of rape survivors report it to the police. Of those who report it, 5 percent of the time a man who rapes ends up in prison; 95 percent of the time he does not.
- 42 percent of rape survivors had sex again with the rapist.
- 30 percent of rape survivors contemplate suicide after the rape.
- 82 percent of rape survivors say the rape permanently changed them.
- The adult pregnancy rate associated with rape is 4.7 percent.
- 89,000 rape cases are reported annually.
- 16 percent of women experienced an attempted or completed rape.
- 3 percent of men experienced an attempted or completed rape.
- There is a 60 percent decline in rapes since 1993.

Feminist theory suggests that the media, pornography, and overall socialization all contribute to the high rate of sexual assault on women. Some theorists argue that too much exposure to violence against women portrayed via television, music, and advertisements can desensitize people to its real impact as well as perpetuate violence against women as a normative experience; this is especially likely if the woman is depicted as subordinate (Ferguson, 2012). In a classic ad by a famous, worldwide women's clothing designer, four men are standing around a woman lying on the ground with her hands being held down by a fifth man. This ad has been described as "evoking a gang rape and reeking of violence against women." Sadly, such forms of media are not uncommon. While some may still blame the victim for being raped, claiming that she is promiscuous or a scorned lover, or that she was provocative, most social scientists do not hold these views. Instead, the rape victim is viewed as not having anything to do with being raped. She is simply a victim of a rapist who has a need to control and humiliate. Her only role is being female, weak physically, and perhaps too trusting. Some propose that a woman who is raped may not have the psychological resources to protect herself. She may be in shock once attacked and not be able to yell or fight. As date rape is the most common type, a woman may simply not know she is being raped. Some women believe that if they agree to talk with a man, kiss a man, get close physically with a man, or even engage in heavy petting, they are required to "go all the way." Some men believe this too. Some women do not know that they have the right to say "no" at any time. In some states, if a woman does not clearly say "yes" (give verbal consent) to engaging in sexual activity, then the act is legally rape. The point is, a lack of saying "no" does not imply she is saying "yes." Lack of knowledge, then, is another factor that may play a part in sexual assault. This is particularly true for potential male partners. All men need to learn their role in sexual assault and become leaders in the fight against women.

Military Sexual Assault

Military sexual assault is a unique situation due to the sociopolitical aspects of the relationship between the victim and perpetrator. The issues facing victims/survivors of military sexual assault in many ways are similar to acquaintance rape because the victim almost always knows the perpetrator. However, there are many special considerations to keep in mind when working with victims of sexual assault that took place while serving in the military. On October 5, 2005, the Sexual Assault Prevention and Response Office at the Department of Defense created the first agency to monitor and report on sexual assault cases that take place in the military. The goal was to eliminate sexual assaults that take place in the military (U.S. Department of Defense, 2005). The Department of Defense counted about 2,700 victims of sexual assault in 2011, but due to underreporting, it estimates that there were far more, maybe 19,000. The reporting of sexual assault has grown steadily since 2007, from 2,223 in 2007 to 2,723 in 2011 (Kitfield, 2012). Many women describe horrific sexual assault experiences such as being drugged and raped during basic training to being fired for being raped. Others who report being sexually assaulted in the military are diagnosed with a personality disorder for failing to adjust adequately to being raped.

One of the unique aspects of the **Operation Iraqi Freedom (OIF)** and **Operation Enduring Freedom (OEF)** wars was the fact that women veterans will make up nearly 10 percent of the total veteran user population at the Veterans Affairs (VA) by the year 2010. Women occupy more than 80 percent of all military occupational specialties and 90 percent of careers in the military (Pierce, 2006). Currently, women comprise 15 percent of the total active force, and it is expected that this figure will increase (Moore & Kennedy, 2011). Although they don't serve in direct combat, they do serve in combat support roles. Schading (2007) points out that one of the reasons for not allowing women to serve in active fighting is because of the possibility of romance and rape inherent because they are weaker. Unfortunately, because the military has not had zero tolerance of inappropriate sexual behavior, some of this is a reality, not necessarily because the woman is physically weaker but because the rapist is in a position of power. Not only do woman have to struggle with stereotypes if they serve in the military, they also must deal with isolation, and they have few role models and mentors (Moore & Kennedy, 2001).

Military sexual trauma (MST) can be defined as sexual violence occurring while serving in the military and occurs in both men and women, but the prevalence is much higher in women. Women often do not report MST due to fears of revenge, scorn, and negative work repercussions (Pierce, 2006). Katz and colleagues (2007) found that in their sample of 18 women who had served in OIF/OEF that 56 percent reported military sexual assault. All 10 of these assaulted women were sexually harassed (experiencing sexually inappropriate, degrading, or suggestive comments), 6 of the 10 reported unwanted physical advances, and 3 of the 10 reported being raped. They also found that the women who experienced MST reported significantly greater difficulties with readjustment and were rated by clinicians as having more severe symptoms compared to those who were not sexual traumatized. These women are at higher risk for developing PTSD than those who were physically injured or who witnessed others being injured.

Intervention for MST Intervening with this population is still in the early stages as these women are just returning from service and have only begun to open up to mental health workers about their abuse. As with any sexually assaulted individual, a female veteran who has been sexually assaulted needs a sense of community support. Cognitive therapy will be useful in helping her change her thoughts about the assault. Crisis counselors can help her reduce feelings of guilt, shame, and weakness by letting her know that this behavior is unacceptable and was not her fault. She must understand that the perpetrator is the rapist and his motivation was to gain control over her and make her feel humiliated. She can reduce his control over her by holding her head up high, proving to herself she has done nothing wrong, Also, by talking with others, she can feel reassured that she was assaulted. She may need to learn about date and acquaintance rape to better understand what coercion and lack of consent really means. **Eye Movement Desensitization and Reprocessing (EMDR)** might also be useful. Counselors should also be aware of advocacy groups and current laws regarding military sexual assault and encourage the victim to utilize all of the services available.

Crisis workers must also keep in mind that the victim may also be suffering from PTSD due to war-related experiences and depression, suicidal thoughts, anger, and substance misuse in addition to MST. Intervention will include a multifaceted approach.

Human Services Delivery in Sexual Assault Situations

Emergency Situations and Interventions Most communities have created sexual assault victim services either through nonprofit organizations or through existing justice centers. The sexual assault centers provide 24-hour hotline services staffed by trained volunteers and supervised by licensed counselors. They often work collaboratively with law enforcement officials when the victim wishes to press charges against her assailant. The advocates at these sexual assault centers often accompany the sexually assaulted victim to the hospital after the assault and

True Stories from Human Service Workers

Crisis Intervention with Sexual Assault Survivors

At first, many rape survivors are hesitant to attend support groups. Their immediate state of crisis often prevents them from feeling comfortable being around others and talking about their assault.

Example 1: A counselor at a sexual assault center in Orange County, California, says, "Group therapy is vital to the recovery of many victims. Hearing others' stories and sharing their own stories with others helps them realize that they do not have to go through the pain alone. They realize that the heinous crime that was perpetrated against them does not have to be a secret, and they can live full and happy lives despite the awful ordeal."

Example 2: According to the supervisor of client services at a sexual assault center based within the Community Services Program in Santa Ana, California, "We use the crisis intervention model because of its efficiency. It is the only model in which we have been properly trained. Our volunteers respond to hotline and hospital calls 24 hours a day, conduct follow up visits within 72 hours with all clients. Advocates accompany clients to hospitals, law enforcement agencies, district attorneys' offices, court proceedings, and other agencies."

This agency's ability to provide all of these services helps decrease the risk of the victim feeling alone. According to crisis theory and the secondary intervention model, by providing services that meet victims' various and most urgent needs in a timely manner, the agency is helping clients remain functioning in as normal a manner as possible.

---

stay by her side during the rape evidence exam as a support person. Victims often need emergency medical care for injuries sustained during the rape.

In addition to hospital exams, victims of sexual assault need to be in a safe location, such as a friend's or relative's home, a hotel, or a shelter. They may need food and clothing as well, depending on how the assault occurred. During the first 72 hours following the rape, advocates from sexual assault centers conduct follow-up visits as this is when the victim is most vulnerable to psychological shock.

Secondary Intervention After the immediate medical and legal emergencies have been addressed, the victim needs crisis intervention. She usually benefits from treatment that focuses on transitioning her from seeing herself as a victim to seeing herself as a survivor. Both in individual and group counseling, she should be educated about the prevalence of sexual assault and the dynamics of rapists. The goal is to help her see that she is not to blame, nor is she "damaged."

Family members may also benefit from crisis intervention to help them cope with the victim's crisis state. She may be disorganized for a while until she can assimilate the trauma as part of her life.

In addition to counseling, sexual assault victims can benefit from advocates who accompany them to court proceedings and other agencies. After being raped, a victim often feels like she is in a daze and has difficulty communicating with people. It is very helpful to have someone by her side who understands what she has gone through.

Tertiary Intervention Some victims of sexual assault do not seek professional services after the assault. They may not report the rape to law enforcement. In fact, most rapes probably go unreported because date rape is one of the most prevalent forms of rape, and many women simply do not realize that they have been raped when it was done by an acquaintance. Additionally, some victims fail to seek help because of shame, fear, social pressure not to deal with the assault, or lack of knowledge about how to use resources.

After a sexual assault, some victims are able to function at minimally acceptable levels. They do this by using psychological defense mechanisms, such as denial, repression, rationalization, and self-blame. The trauma can sometimes be forgotten for several years. Some victims never tell anyone that they were raped. When a victim waits many years before seeking help, she has usually been suffering from posttraumatic stress disorder (PTSD), as has already been discussed in Chapter 6. Long-term therapy is needed to help her open up about the event that she has spent years trying to forget. The anxiety, nightmares, sleeplessness, numbness, and hypervigilance she experiences are indicative of PTSD. She will most likely need many years of individual, marital, and/or group therapy to work through the trauma and be relieved of these symptoms. The longer a victim waits to seek help, the longer her treatment will be. She has learned coping skills to survive that may have hindered her social relationships, work, and academic functioning and her ability to feel spontaneous joy and comfort in the world.

Primary Prevention Some high schools offer guest speakers to their students who visit campuses and provide educational talks about sexual assault, in particular date rape and drug-induced rape, which can happen when a drug (such as rohypnol, often called "roofies") is slipped into someone's drink. These educational programs aim to encourage young women to assert themselves with men, say no, make a fuss if someone tries to rape them, pay attention to possible clues that someone might be untrustworthy, not put themselves in risky situations, and learn self-defense techniques.

College campuses also provide many opportunities for students to learn about rape prevention through various workshops and support groups in which men and women can address sexual assault issues.

HIV/AIDS ISSUES

Historical Background

Acquired immunodeficiency syndrome (AIDS) was first diagnosed in the United States in the early 1980s. Almost since that time, human services workers have been involved because of the psychological and social impact this disease has on its victims. Stigmas have been attached to those diagnosed with human immunodeficiency virus (HIV) and with AIDS because of the way in which **HIV/AIDS** is usually transmitted. People who have HIV/AIDS may often be ostracized by society, discriminated against at work, and made to feel guilt and shame about having the disease, all of which could prevent people from being diagnosed and treated. To make it easier for those with or who suspect they are ill, special services that specialize in dealing with issues related to HIV/AIDS have become available in most communities. Although HIV/AIDS is not regarded as negatively as it was 30 years ago, the stigma still does exist. The notion that only gay men, drug addicts, prostitutes, and sexually promiscuous people contract HIV is still common among the misinformed who have not bothered to educate themselves about the disease.

Definitions of HIV and AIDS

HIV has been identified as causing AIDS. Someone who is infected with HIV is said to be seropositive or HIV positive, whereas AIDS is the full-blown, active illness.

"AIDS means that the virus has invaded the body and disrupted the immune system so that it can't protect the body from various deadly infections, like cancer or pneumonia. It is a life-threatening disease that sooner or later kills most everyone who has it" (Kanel, 2014, p. 153). An opportunistic infection has invaded the body, or T-cell count is very low, usually under 200.

Prevalence

HIV and AIDS have been decreasing in the United States since testing and medications have been widely used starting in the 1990s. The HIV/AIDS box provides some facts and statistics related to HIV/AIDS according to the U.S. Department of Statistics (2013).

HIV/AIDS Facts and Statistics

- Approximately 1.2 million adults and adolescents were living with HIV infection at the end of 2008, the most recent year for which national prevalence estimates are available.
- One in five living with HIV is unaware of their infection.
- The most severely affected by HIV are young, African American men having sex with men.
- African Americans face the most severe HIV burden.
- Approximately 50,000 Americans become infected with HIV each year.
- More than 17,000 people with AIDS in the United States died in 2009, and over 619,000 have died of AIDS in the United States since the epidemic began.
- Gay, bisexual, and other men who have sex with men represent the majority of persons who have died, accounting for 61 percent of all new HIV infections in the United States in 2009.
- Individuals infected through heterosexual contact accounted for 27 percent of new HIV infection in 2009.
- Women account for 23 percent of new HIV infection in 2009.
- Adults age 50 and older account for 34 percent of those living with AIDS in 2007; postmenopausal women are at particular risk in part due to cultural assumptions that older women are not sexual.
- Injection drug users account for 9 percent of new HIV infections in 2009.
- African Americans account for 46 percent of those living with HIV in the United States in 2008.
- Latinos account for 17 percent of those living with HIV in 2008.

Causality Models

There are five ways that HIV can be transmitted from one person to another: during sexual contact involving the exchange of bodily fluids; by using dirty IV (intravenous) or tattoo needles that had been used by someone who has HIV/AIDS; from an infected mother to her baby during pregnancy, labor, delivery, or by breastfeeding; from a transfusion of infected blood or blood products; and through the bloodstream if contacted with the feces or vomit of an infected person.

What causes someone to engage in behaviors that may lead to HIV/AIDS? Some people are considered innocent victims of HIV because their illness was not the result of promiscuous behavior. Infants who become infected from their mothers and those who have become ill from a blood transfusion are considered innocent, and social attitudes toward them are different from the way HIV-positive IV drug users are regarded. The behavior considered the riskiest for contracting HIV is still unprotected sexual contact between two men. The second riskiest behavior is sharing IV needles. Drug addicts' need for a "fix" is often stronger than the possibility of being infected by a deadly virus. The third riskiest behavior is unprotected sexual contact between a man and a woman (Centers for Disease Control and Prevention, 2002).

Sexual urges, especially when mixed with alcohol or drugs, can also drive people to engage in risky behaviors, such as having unprotected sex with strangers or passing acquaintances. Discussions about sexually transmitted diseases are avoided because such talk may be considered rude in some subcultures. Also, using condoms during sex, which can protect people from infection, is prohibited by some religions. Although for the most part society has opened up the dialogue about sex and HIV, many parents still do not talk to their children about sex, and children remain ignorant about the consequences of unprotected sex.

Until society condones open and frank discussions about sex and disease and makes sexual protection available to teenagers, sexually transmitted diseases will continue to spread. Society also needs to educate people about drug addiction and how it is one of the ways that HIV/AIDS can be spread to the heterosexual population. Although in 1999 gay men made up the largest segment of the U.S. population (42 percent) who were infected with HIV/AIDS, it's important to keep in mind that 33 percent of those with the disease were infected during heterosexual intercourse, and 25 percent became ill as a result of their IV drug use (Centers for Disease Control and Prevention, 2002). Society must let people know that all people are susceptible to contracting HIV/AIDS. For example, as noted earlier, older adults are also at risk. Education about their risk factors, including drug use, unprotected sex, and lack of knowledge about transmission, needs to be shared with all adults irrespective of age.

Needs and Issues

People infected with HIV but who do not yet have full-blown AIDS need to first deal with being diagnosed with a potentially life-threatening disease. They often feel they've been given a death sentence. They need to be fully educated about how to live with HIV rather than die of AIDS. Knowing about available medications and how proper nutrition and exercise can improve their chances of survival can be helpful. They also need to deal with disclosing their diagnosis to any other intimate partners they may have had. This may mean disclosing dishonest behaviors, such as marital infidelities or drug use. Sometimes this may result in relationship break up, and so the person needs a lot of support emotionally and sometimes financially. They also need to deal with their fears about lifestyle changes, such as becoming sober and celibate or using condoms during sex. For some newly infected HIV patients, suicide seems like the only way out, and these feelings must be monitored by counselors and caseworkers.

Once someone has AIDS, he or she has different needs and issues. The infected individual now must deal with the possibilities of death and dying. He or she may need help making out a will and coping with a life of ongoing illness. This will require medical care that may cause a person to be depressed. Being dependent doesn't come easily for some people, and they must learn to adapt to financial dependency and physical dependency. They may have to stop working and have someone take care of them daily. Again, suicide might be an issue and must be monitored (Kanel, 2014).

In general, HIV/AIDS patients need emotional support, social involvement, and normal treatment. They need physical contact with others and to be as productive as possible for as long as possible, which for some may be 20 years or more.

Human Services for AIDS and HIV Clients

Emergency Situations and Interventions Intervention with these clients becomes an emergency when someone contracts an illness that becomes life threatening because of their damaged immune system. Basic medical emergency care will then be necessary.

Another emergency situation related to patients with HIV and AIDS might be suicide attempts. Sometimes, when people discover that they are HIV positive or have contracted a life-threatening disease that may lead to a lot of pain, they try to kill themselves rather than wait for the disease to kill them. Suicide prevention should be immediate and focus on reasons for living. People may need to be educated that HIV/AIDS is not necessarily a death sentence. Medication has done much to prolong the lives of people who have been diagnosed with the disease. They should be encouraged to focus on living as healthy a life as possible. If a person must be hospitalized after a suicide attempt, optimistic support groups should be attended. Here, a person infected with HIV can interact with other HIV-positive people who are living happy lives.

When people with AIDS attempt suicide because they are suffering physically or are worried about financial costs of an illness, they must be helped to see that medication can relieve their pain and also provided with resources that can help cover their medical expenses. Workers can also help people with HIV/AIDS understand that others have overcome opportunistic infections and have continued to live for years. New medical advances have greatly prolonged the lives of those with HIV/AIDS. Many times, family members participate in counseling sessions to share their feelings about the suicide attempt. Patients may decide life is worth living when they hear the sadness and loss their death causes family members to feel.

Secondary Intervention Crisis intervention may be useful for some people dealing with HIV/AIDS issues. For instance, crisis intervention may be helpful for people who are fearful of being tested for HIV. These individuals may have engaged in risky behavior and are now afraid to find out the consequences of this behavior. These clients must be told that knowing whether they are infected may save their lives. If they are infected, they can begin taking antiviral medications, practice healthy nutrition, practice safe sex, and participate in stress management and exercise. These behaviors may prolong their lives. If they aren't infected, they can use their fear as a motivator to ensure they practice safe sex in the future or eliminate possible infection in the future by not sharing needles if they are an IV-drug user.

Another type of person in crisis may be the one who has already tested positive for HIV. They need education about the virus and how to avoid spreading it as well as the differences between being HIV positive and having AIDS. They also need to practice the healthy lifestyle behaviors mentioned previously. These clients may also need assistance in disclosing their HIV status to loved ones. Sometimes they are rejected by family because they may be gay. Other times, they risk losing a loved one because they contracted the virus through infidelity or because they were a secret drug addict. They will need supportive crisis intervention to deal with these emotionally painful consequences. Optimistic support groups are excellent in helping them share common concerns and receive problem-solving advice. They also need to be referred for medical assistance and encouraged to comply with the sometimes burdensome process of taking medication (Magallon, 1987; Price, Omizo, & Hammitt, 1986; Slader, 1992).

The main goal of secondary intervention for those infected with HIV or those worried about getting tested for HIV is to help them realize that HIV is not a death sentence. They need education and emotional support while they learn to adjust to a new lifestyle.

Tertiary Intervention Those who have been HIV positive for several years often require only medication management to keep the virus from duplicating thereby destroying their immune system. However, at some point, they may start developing symptoms related to HIV. When these patients develop illnesses indicative of **AIDS-related complex (ARC)**, they may need medical care beyond antiviral medication. These illnesses include rawness in the mouth (thrush), flu and colds that don't subside, coughs, night sweats, and fever. This may make a person feel dirty and contaminated. They may isolate from others, have to apply for disability and cease employment, and need somebody to help them with daily living. The development of ARC may be seen as the precursor to developing AIDS. They might bounce back after a few weeks and be able to live relatively healthy lives for a while. Unfortunately, another bout of illness may occur in a few months. They need support from groups or case workers while they adjust to not working and relying on others for assistance.

When people develop AIDS, they must grapple with life-threatening diseases and the real possibility of dying. It may not be immediate, but they should get legal counseling to prepare living trusts, wills, and other documents. They may need grief counseling, as will their significant others. They may live in a hospice when the disease becomes terminal. Others live in and out of hospitals, set up nursing care at their own homes, or have significant others care for them. Case workers must provide supportive counseling and guidance for all. They can focus on how this can be a time to become closer as a family. If the person is feeling well enough, support group attendance may be helpful as well. Case managers and counselors should try to encourage AIDS patients to live as long as possible, comply with medication, be optimistic, enjoy life, and create satisfying relationships with others.

Primary Prevention Of course preventing HIV is better than having to treat it. Some high schools offer education about how to prevent sexually transmitted diseases (STDs). However, conservative political philosophy has influenced policies that would require schools to provide such programs and in some cases has limited and even prevented schools from offering this information. In fact, students need a parent's signature to participate in these educational courses, and some parents won't give permission for their children to attend. Additionally, most of these presentations cannot discuss the use of condoms as a means to prevent the spread of STDs. Instead, many simply push abstinence from sex as the only way to prevent pregnancy and STDs. However, some school nurses' offices do offer free condoms to students who ask for them.

Education at the college is more detailed and effective. Condoms are readily available at college health centers. They are also free and available at most public health centers as well. Some attempts have been made to offer drug addicts "bleach kits" so they could clean needles prior to sharing them. These programs, which started in the 1980s and 1990s, did not receive the political support needed for them to continue.

ISSUES FACING THE LESBIAN, GAY, BISEXUAL, AND TRANSGENDER (LGBT) COMMUNITY

Current trends in the United States have shown an increasing tolerance and even an embracing of this population. Television shows such as *Modern Family*, which highlights a gay couple, frequently wins Emmy awards; *Dancing with the Stars* showcased Chaz Bono, a transgender person; Ellen Degeneres's talk show, hosted by an open lesbian, has earned many Emmy awards; and contestants on talent shows are now open about their homosexual orientation. Even the current Pope, Francis, shook up the Roman Catholic world by saying that abortion, contraception, and gay marriage should not be overemphasized at the cost of losing the freshness and fragrance of the gospel (Knickerbocker, 2013).

In the academic community, queer studies programs are on the rise throughout the country. These programs explore how heterosexism, **heteronormativity**, and **transphobia** intersect and collide with national, ethnic, racial, class, and other identifications, fostering a community of learners who grapple with issues of diversity, gender, sexuality, and social justice (California State University, Northridge, 2013). These programs tend to focus on the history and contemporary experiences of lesbians, gay men, bisexuals, transgender people, intersexed people, queer people, and others who occupy nonheterosexist and nonnormative gender positionalities.

While the term "queer" has been used by people for many years, queer theory has only been developing since 1988. It is defined as an approach to literary and cultural study that rejects traditional categories of gender and sexuality (*Merriam Webster Dictionary*, 2013).

There has also been changing attitudes at the federal level, perhaps in response to the changing attitudes in the general population. The U.S. Supreme Court recently joined the tolerance movement by declaring that same-sex marriage would receive the same privileges as traditional marriage when federal laws are involved. Lastly, President Obama signed into law the repeal of the military policy referred to as "Don't Ask Don't Tell." This repeal permits those serving in the military to be openly gay and receive all the benefits of others with no allowance of any negative consequences.

So why then does this population still contend with major psychological and social issues that would necessitate the services of human service workers? Sometimes, individual attitudes don't change as quickly as laws and broader social mores. Think about the abolishment of slavery and the elimination of the Jim Crow laws in the 1960s. While these events outlawed discrimination and slavery, many people's attitudes toward blacks did not change for many years, and there are still many people in the country who continue to have negative racist attitudes toward blacks. Likewise, just because laws have changed related to homosexuality, it doesn't mean that everyone now accepts that lifestyle. Therefore, individuals who are lesbian, gay, bisexual, or transgender still face negative attitudes from others that affect them deeply.

Some Basic Definitions

Here are some definitions of terms often used when discussing this population.

- Lesbian: A woman who feels sexual desire and seeks romantic and emotional relationships with women.
- Gay: A man who is sexually attracted to men and seeks relationships that are romantic and emotional in nature with men.
- Bisexual: A person who experiences social and romantic attraction to both men and women.
- Transgender: A person who has experienced himself or herself socially, emotionally, and psychologically as male if the person was born female, or female if born a male.
- Queer: Any person identifying as any of the persons above or who sees him- or herself as not fitting into normative definitions of what a man or woman should be according to typical societal standards.
- Closet gay: A person who is unaware of his or her homosexuality or is unwilling to publicly acknowledge it: such a person may be thought of as "being in the closet."
- Homophobia: A fear or hatred of a homosexual.

- Heterosexism: The attitude of overt or covert bias against homosexuals based on the belief that heterosexuality is superior (Kanel, 2007, p. 118).

Issues Facing the LGBT Community

LGBT Elders The challenges facing LGBT elders are many. As they age, they often do not access adequate health care, affordable housing, or social services, often due to institutionalized heterosexism (National Gay and Lesbian Task Force, 2013). While some of these issues may be changing, many couples who have been together for over 20 years still do not have rights to hospital visits, tax write-offs, and sharing of financial benefits that heterosexual couples have. Additionally, often, they do not have the family support that other older people have and their needs and issues seem to be understudied by social scientists. In studying people who identify as gay, most samples overrepresent white gay men from urban areas with middle or upper incomes and underrepresent women, people of color, low-income people, and those living in rural areas.

LGBT People of Color Some studies have identified unique challenges facing queer people of color (*Third World Solidarity*, 2013). Often, these people are thought of as doubly oppressed, subjected to disadvantage not only for being black but also for being gay. Within their own black community they may face homophobia. Within the LGBT community, they may face racism. Homophobia in African American communities is one of the factors that make living openly as a gay black person difficult. There is a tradition of high religiosity in the black community, which might lead to lack of tolerance of gays in general. Some have proposed that the LGBT movement has been a "white" movement, thereby disenfranchising blacks in the LGBT circuit.

Older LGBT People LGBT older adults also face significant challenges. Many federal programs that assist aging Americans can be ineffective for LGBT elders. For example, social security, which many older widows and widowers rely on for survivor benefits, does not apply to same-sex life partners. Many tax laws also discriminate against LBGT couples. Perhaps more significantly, many LGBT elders experience increased social isolation and ageism within the LGBT community itself, and many do not receive the same level of social support from family members as compared to heterosexual elders.

General Issues Facing LGBT People Although there is a wider social acceptance of LGBT persons than there was just 10 years ago, prejudice is still prevalent. Coming out to one's family and coming to terms with one's true identity in the face of socialization and peer pressure can lead to high levels of depression and anxiety, including higher suicide rates for teens who are gay or lesbian (Good Therapy.org, 2013).

Of course, gay couples also struggle with the same types of stress that heterosexual couples face, such as money, sex, in-laws, and time, and so a counselor would need to sort out which problems are universal and which are gay-related issues, such as coming out and having a public identity as a gay couple, which a straight couple wouldn't have to face.

Intervention with LGBT Persons

It is important to keep in mind that homosexuality has not been considered a formal mental disorder by the psychiatric community since 1973. However, gender identity disorder remains in the *Diagnostic and Statistical Manual of Mental Disorders* and focuses on the transgender population. This is a current controversy for therapists who may not see this as a disorder, similar to being gay or lesbian.

Crisis intervention, marital counseling, family therapy, and group therapy are all viable forms of intervention for this population. Agencies that focus on this population often have support groups for those coming out, those with HIV/AIDS, and for those who are struggling with suicide and depression. Many help lines have been created for a person who is suicidal or needs a nonjudgmental place to talk. These are often 24-hours-a-day, 7-days-a-week hotlines. Following is a brief list of hotlines available should the reader need help or know of someone who could use this type of help.

- The Trevor Project: 866-488-7386
- SafeHouse Center: 734-995-5444
- EMU Coming Out Support Group: 734-487-4149
- GLBT National Help Center: 1888-843-4564
- Equality Michigan: 866-962-1147
- Ruth Ellis Center: 313-252-1950
- Affirmations: 800-398-4297
- WRAP Resource Center: 734-995-9867
- Gay Men's Domestic Violence Project: 800-832-1901
- Ozone House: 734-662-2222 (Safehouse Center, 2013)

These interventions are useful for secondary intervention needs. Sometimes, the best intervention is advocacy to ensure that discrimination doesn't affect our clients in terms of housing opportunities, economic needs, and other issues such as hospital visits. Even if your duty is primarily that of a counselor, we all need to find the advocate and social injustice worker inside of us in order to eliminate intolerance and institutionalized heterosexism.

CHAPTER SUMMARY

There are a variety of client populations who will seek human services due to having been victimized by perpetrators of violence such as women and some men being abused by intimate partners, and women and men who are sexually assaulted. Some clients seek counseling and social work services due to having contracted HIV or AIDS needing help with emotional and psychological issues related to this sometimes societally rejected disease. Lastly, some clients seek out advocacy, counseling, and social services because they are just trying to live as an openly gay, lesbian, transgender, or bisexual person in a society that often disapproves of it. Human services workers must understand the various issues and challenges in working with these client groups and understand the resources in the community for them.

Suggested Applied Activities

1. Interview at least 10 people. Find out how many know of someone who is HIV positive; is gay, lesbian, bisexual, or transgender; has been involved in an abusive relationship; or has been sexually assaulted. Notice the prevalence of each population and how it compares to the statistics mentioned in this chapter.
2. Watch a movie or television show in which one or more of the client populations discussed in this chapter are part of the plotline. What are their issues and challenges? How do they overcome them?

Chapter Review Questions

1. What is battered women's syndrome?
2. Describe the battering cycle.
3. What are some myths about being raped?
4. What is date rape and how does it differ from other types of sexual assault?
5. What are the special issues facing those suffering from military sexual assault?
6. What is the difference between HIV and AIDS?
7. What are some challenges facing the LGBT community?
8. How can primary prevention assist in reducing HIV and intimate partner abuse?

Glossary of Terms

AIDS-related complex (ARC) is a stage of HIV/AIDS during which a person infected with HIV begins having bouts of fever, vomiting, and other flu-like symptoms but has not yet developed full-blown AIDS.

Battered women's shelter is a residential facility where battered women and their children may live for about 45 days while they manage legal issues, finances, employment, and emotional difficulties.

Battered women's syndrome is seen in women who repeatedly find themselves in abusive relationships. They often begin to lose hope about ever escaping the abuse and focus only on survival within the abusive relationship.

Battering cycle is an ongoing pattern of behavior seen in couples involved in an abusive relationship during which a peaceful period of time, called the honeymoon, is followed by growing tensions that eventually leads to a violent explosion that is followed by another honeymoon period.

EMDR stands for eye movement desensitization and reprocessing. It is a form of exposure therapy in which a trained therapist has the client follow a wand with his or her eyes while the client speaks of a traumatic event and processes emotions and cognitions associated with the trauma.

Feminists are people who focus on equality between both genders and view many issues facing women such as abuse as being due to pervasive sexism in our society.

Heteronormativity refers to the societal value on people coupling with someone of the opposite sex as normal.

HIV/AIDs are often linked together as the virus called HIV may lead to the fatal disease called AIDS because one's immune system become so weak it cannot fight off a series of opportunistic infections.

Military sexual trauma occurs when someone serving in the military is sexually harassed, abused, or raped. It often leads to PTSD.

OEF refers to the recent war in Afghanistan called Operation Enduring Freedom

OIF refers to the recent war in Iraq called Operation Iraqi Freedom.

Temporary restraining orders are provided by the district attorney's office to persons who complain that someone has hurt them or is threatening to hurt them.

Transphobia refers to the feeling of fear when being around transgenders.

Case Presentation and Exit Quiz

Case History and Demographics

Lilly is a 40-year-old Caucasian female who has been married to Jacob for 15 years. They have three daughters, ages 14, 11, and 9, much to the dismay of Jacob, who had always hoped for a son. Jacob works full time at a local factory, and Lilly recently started a part-time job at the local mall when their youngest child started third grade. All of the girls participate in sports and do well in school. They live in a home that they own in a middle-class neighborhood close to school where the girls can walk to school together. The 14-year-old daughter will start high school next year.

Current Problems

Lilly went to her physician complaining of being tired and depressed. Her doctor noticed bruises on her neck and upper arms in differing stages of healing. He asked her how these bruises happened, and Lilly said that she bumps into things a lot. Then she started crying in the office and said that her husband grabs her and chokes her sometimes. The doctor reported this to the police and referred her to the battered women's shelter hotline and walk-in center.

The police visited Lilly and asked about the bruises. She said it was no big deal and that sometimes Jacob just gets frustrated because she doesn't have the house clean and the girls can be loud. She said it was her fault and doesn't want Jacob to get into trouble. The police present the case to the district attorney's office, and they call Lilly. She refuses to press charges, so they drop the case. They refer her to a domestic violence counselor, Shari.

Lilly goes to an appointment with Shari, who is able to identify the marital pattern for the past 15 years. Evidently, Lilly and Jacob go through periods where everything is great and they are very much in love. However, Lilly did tell her that Jacob has a bad temper and gets stressed out all the time. He gets so mad he has punched holes in the wall. Luckily, he never takes it out on the girls, but he does choke Lilly and squeeze Lilly, and has kicked Lilly. Lilly has never thought of leaving him because she believes the girls need a father.

Exit Quiz

1. Which is the most likely reason that Lilly stays with Jacob?
   a. He is very handsome.
   b. He provides for the family financially.
   c. She suffers from battered women's syndrome.
   d. The girls love him so much.

2. When Lilly sees Shari, she should be educated about:
   a. feminism
   b. her duty to stay with a man at all costs
   c. the battering cycle
   d. time management so she can keep her house cleaner

3. The abusive nature of this marriage is most likely to be due to:
   a. Jacob's inability to deal with stress
   b. Lilly's inability to keep the home clean
   c. Jacob's desire to beat up a woman
   d. Lilly's desire to be manhandled

4. Lilly's depression is most likely due to:
   a. a chemical imbalance
   b. menopause
   c. not having a boy
   d. a sense of hopelessness and helplessness, which is part of battered women's syndrome

5. Shari may wish to refer Lilly to:
   a. a psychiatrist for medications
   b. a battered women's shelter
   c. a mental hospital for tertiary treatment
   d. a pastor to ensure she properly understands her role as wife according to the Bible

Exit Quiz Answers

1. c
2. c
3. a
4. d
5. b

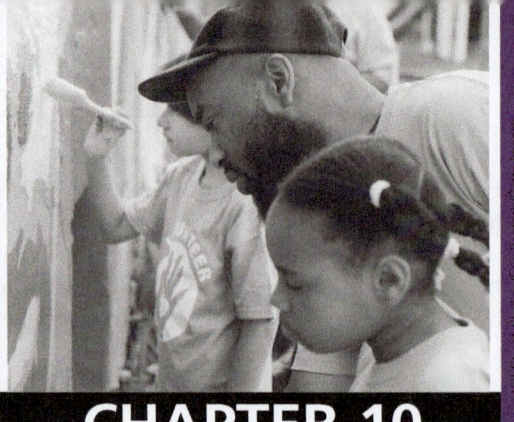

CHAPTER 10

Stress Management

INTRODUCTION

At this point in the semester, the reader may have already taken some exams and may be preparing term papers and other projects, which may have created a certain amount of **stress**. The material presented thus far may have created feelings of anxiety, anger, and sadness. The multitude of problems and needs that people have can be overwhelming and can lead to job **burnout**. It happens to many people in most occupations. Human services workers may be particularly vulnerable to burnout because of emotional stress from trying to assist people who have many emotional and social problems for which they seek help.

Critical Thinking/Self-Reflection Corner

Take a moment now to consider how some of the following questions relate to your own reactions thus far to the course material:

- How long could you continue working happily and peacefully at a shelter where most of your clients are women who come in with black eyes, broken bones, and serious lacerations?
- How would you feel working day after day with children who have been sexually molested?
- How do you think you would be affected by frequently hearing people say that they can't quit using drugs even though it means losing custody of their children?

Don't be discouraged about your career path by the possibility of becoming stressed or angry in those situations. In fact, those reactions are normal responses to a very stressful job.

Before examining **stress management** techniques, a brief discussion of stress and burnout may be helpful. While this discussion focuses on stress at the workplace, it can be universally applicable not only to students stressed out from exams and social pressures but also to clients whose problems are creating stress in their lives.

STRESS AND BURNOUT

What Is Stress?

Stress is the response of individuals to events and experiences (referred to as stressors) in their lives that they have to adapt to or cope with. Anything can be a stressor or trigger of stress, from day-to-day, minor stressors or frustrations, such as getting stuck in traffic, to major life events, such as a death in the family. People often experience stress in situations that require more energy, resources, or experiences than they have. This exerted energy may be physical, psychological, emotional, or intellectual. People also become stressed in potentially threatening situations. Interestingly, daily stressors have been found to have more immediate effects on well-being than major life events, in part because they tend to pile up and accumulate over time that can cause more serious stress reactions (Lazarus, 1999).

Selye (1976) explained that the general process of the stress experience has its foundation in our body's physiological systems; when under stress, the way our body normally functions changes, such that stress disrupts the natural balance, or **homeostasis**, of our bodies. Stress in fact lowers our resistance and can trigger various physiological mechanisms, such as the autonomic and sympathetic nervous systems, which help control and regulate our bodies. If our bodies are always under stress, our resistance is lowered, which can increase our chances of having poor health and disease-related outcomes. In other words, too much stress can lead to wear and tear on the body and, over time, poor physical and mental health problems. This is referred to as **allostatic load** (McEwen, 1998). In fact, this is a lifelong process. For example, it has been shown that children with impaired parent-child attachments or stressful relationships with primary caregivers may have greater vulnerability to stress across their adulthood in part due to impaired physiological reactions that accumulate over time (Horn Mallers, Charles, Neupert, & Almeida, 2010).

However, not all stress is bad; stress indeed can motivate people to grow, discover new abilities, and take new challenges. This sort of "good" stress is referred to as **eustress** and can give a person the feeling of fulfillment and other positive feelings. However, as noted previously, when the experience of stress becomes constant, unrelenting, and too much to handle, known as **distress**, it can have harmful outcomes. When stressful situations persist without hope of resolution, they become overwhelming. People in such situations start to experience anxiety, depression, anger, and frustration. If these feelings continue, impairments in daily functioning can occur. As discussed in Chapter 6, an inability to cope with impaired functioning can bring about a crisis situation. People in a state of crisis often seek professional help. Not getting the appropriate help can lead to serious consequences such as suicide, drug and alcohol abuse, or emotional withdrawal from life.

The truth is that stress is a natural part of life. For example, Chang (2005) suggested that stress is an inevitable consequence of pressure-laden jobs. The good news is that most people can cope with a certain amount of stress on a daily basis; some even seek out stressful situations. Also, while some stressors are objectively more stressful than others (compare a death to being late), our perceptions and experiences also influence our reactions to stressors. This will be discussed in greater detail later in this chapter. No matter what, it is important to remember that stress is a normal and inevitable part of everyday life. As noted at the beginning of this chapter, human services professionals therefore need to be aware of their stressors and learn to cope in healthy ways.

What Is Burnout?

Simply put, burnout is job-related anxiety and dissatisfaction that hampers people's abilities at work and in other areas of their lives. Physical illness, a short temper, impatience, and frustration are typical signs of burnout (Russo, 1980). Maslach and Jackson (1986) identified three symptoms of burnout:

- Lack of personal accomplishment
- Emotional exhaustion and depersonalization
- De-individuation of clients

They proposed that burnout is a reaction to chronic stress on the job. Vettor and Kosinski (2000) suggested that when human services workers have these symptoms, their attitude toward clients may become negative and cynical, and workers may be unable to provide clients with the support they need. Pines and Maslach (1978, p. 224) have defined burnout as "a syndrome of physical and emotional exhaustion involving the development of negative self-concept, negative job attitudes, and a loss of concern and feelings for clients."

The causes of burnout are many and varied. Working in human services may increase the likelihood of burnout because workers often experience conflicts between the ideal and the real. Human services workers enter the field to help others, but when resources are unavailable, the agencies for which they work are unsupportive, and clients are unmotivated to receive help, workers experience a sense of "what's the use?" Burnout may be a defense against feelings of helplessness.

Human services workers may find it emotionally taxing to deal with populations that resent them, with limited capabilities to help themselves, and with performing tedious bureaucratic tasks daily with little positive feedback from authority figures (Gomez & Michaelis, 1995). It may also be emotionally taxing for human services workers to be faced with ongoing conflicts between their personal values and knowledge of the right thing to do and the norms of the organization (Russo, 1980).

Norms are the unwritten rules and guidelines that are understood and followed by the members of an organization. It may be difficult to believe, but some organizational norms may include behaviors that many consider to be morally wrong or at least incompetent. An easy example to illustrate this is the norms in prisons that allow guards to be physically brutal with inmates. Most people think this is wrong, and in the beginning, the guards probably thought it was bad. As time goes on, however, many workers slip into previously unacceptable behaviors because the norms of the institution encourage them. Another example might be the norm of arriving to work on time. In some agencies, there is an understanding that workers may arrive 30 minutes late with no repercussions. To a new worker, this feels unfair. One can understand that a typical response would be to simply start coming in late so as not to experience feelings of resentment toward those who seem to "get away" with it.

Other conflicts may occur while working for human services agencies as well. Personality conflicts with supervisors and coworkers can be a precipitator of burnout and stress, especially if a worker receives no support from anyone. Cliques and factions are natural when groups of people interact regularly, and of course most people tend to gravitate toward those who are most like them. When there is no one around with whom a worker can relate, burnout may occur. In addition to personality conflicts, outright competition and professional jealousy may occur. It's bad enough to have to deal with clients who have a multitude of personal needs, but having to deal with coworkers and supervisors with emotional problems creates added stress on the job. When coworkers are insecure, paranoid, and feel threatened, the risk of becoming burned out is high. In a job where the undercurrent is anxiety and diminished loyalty and commitment to workers, morale is eroded. Chaotic and dysfunctional work environments where individuals are devalued and discounted lead to physical and mental exhaustion in employees (Anonymous, 2005).

In addition to stress from organizational demands and coworker behaviors, human services workers may be at risk for burnout because many times they are not able to help in the way they want to help. It is difficult to accept that some clients may not get better, change, and live happy, productive lives. They may die, get killed, or remain nonfunctional despite the best efforts of human services workers. Burnout may occur when the helping professional evaluates him- or herself negatively when assessing work done with clients (Vettor & Kosinski, 2000).

THE IMPACT OF STRESS AND BURNOUT

Just as the causes of burnout and stress are many and varied, so too are the symptoms and behaviors manifested as a result of burnout and stress. Burnout usually manifests in physical symptoms, cognitive and emotional impairments, social deterioration, behavioral impairments, and impairments on the job.

Physical Symptoms

Humans are hardwired to react to stressful situations with a fight-or-flight response in which the two hormones adrenalin and cortisol are produced. Overproduction of these two hormones can cause long-term damage to health (Anonymous, 2005). Many workers suffering from burnout complain of physical problems such as dizziness, nausea, headaches, fatigue, heart palpitations, shortness of breath, or ulcers, high blood pressure, and other psychosomatic illnesses (Sparks, Simon, Katon, Altman, Ayars, & Johnson, 1990). Stress is increasingly appearing as a diagnosis on medical certificates as physicians now think that overall health will be improved by the reduction of stress levels. The Health and Safety Executive in the United Kingdom (Goldman & Lewis, 2005) commissioned a study on the effect work stress had on the development of musculoskeletal disorders and found that individuals under stress at work are prone to illness.

Cognitive and Emotional Symptoms

An inability to concentrate and memory loss are both cognitive symptoms of burnout. Two common emotional symptoms are depression and panic disorders (Sparks et al., 1990). Many see no hope for things getting better, and others perceive themselves as inadequate and incompetent. People who have had traumatic experiences on the job may show signs of posttraumatic stress disorder.

Example: A woman worked for AAA, a well-known road assistance agency. One day her supervisor yelled at her and berated her in front of a customer. This was typical of her supervisor's management style. The woman broke down and sobbed for a few minutes. Then she became unable to speak. She was so traumatized that she sought the help of a therapist. The woman experienced nightmares, was hypervigilant, and reexperienced the trauma in her mind repeatedly. An interesting symptom was her inability to speak English after the trauma. She began thinking and speaking Swedish, which was her first language. She had apparently regressed to a childlike state to cope with the work trauma.

Social Deterioration

Social withdrawal and poor family relationships are also reported to exist when someone has experienced burnout (Freudenberger, 1975; Maslach & Jackson, 1986). A normally pleasant person may become tense and impatient with people including the public and loved ones. Individuals may not feel like interacting with their children, spouses, or friends. They may interact in a numb state with very little emotional connection. All of these behaviors are signs of social deterioration.

Behavioral Deterioration

Some people who experience burnout may increase their drug and alcohol consumption. This increase in substance use may be a form of self-medication to relieve feelings of anxiety and depression. Others have difficulty in sleeping, eating, and performing other normal activities of daily living. When the behavioral deterioration of daily living is severe, individuals may apply for worker's compensation or disability to compensate them financially during the time when they cannot work.

Impairments in Work Performance

All of the previously mentioned symptoms and behaviors affect an individual's ability to perform his or her job adequately. Human services workers are particularly susceptible to having their work performance affected because of the human-to-human contact usually required on the job. When a worker merely sits behind a desk and does paperwork, it may be easier to hide burnout symptoms than when a worker must listen patiently to other people's problems.

Absenteeism, tardiness, and lowered productivity often occur when workers are burned out. One company reported that 44 percent of those surveyed said that they lose at least an hour of productivity a day because of stress, whereas 47 percent estimated that in the course of a year, they had been at work anywhere from one to four days when they were too stressed out to be effective (Chang, 2005). In a 2001 study of community crisis workers (Kanel, 2014), 45 percent stated feeling angry at the system when working with someone in crisis, and 52 percent said they think of quitting their job between one and five times a month! Table 10.1 provides a summary of the types, causes, and symptoms of burnout.

TABLE 10.1 The Various Types, Causes, and Symptoms of Burnout

Definitions	Causes	Symptoms
Anxiety and unhappiness at work that affects job performance and other areas of life	Conflicts between ideals and reality	Physical: diseases and physical problems such as dizziness, heart palpitations, fatigue, and high blood pressure
Lack of personal accomplishment	Lack of resources available to help clients	Cognitive impairments: poor concentration and memory
Emotional exhaustion	Lack of company support and very little positive feedback from authority figures	Emotional impairments: feelings of helplessness, depression, panic, low self-esteem
Depersonalization	Lack of client motivation and limited capabilities to receive help and help themselves	Social deterioration: impairments with coworkers, clients, family, and friends
De-individuation of clients	Dealing with resentful clients	Behavioral deterioration: changes in activities of daily living such as sleeping, eating; increased substance abuse
Negative self-concept	Dealing with tedious bureaucratic tasks	Impairments in work performance: absenteeism, tardiness, lower productivity
Negative job attitudes	Conflicts between personal values and organizational norms	
Loss of concern and feelings for clients	Competitions and jealousy among coworkers	
Physical exhaustion	Negative self-evaluation of work done with clients	

Digital Download — Download at CengageBrain.com

Critical Thinking/Self-Reflection Corner

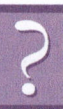

Before moving on to the next section, examine your responses to the following questions to assess your own levels of burnout and stress.

- Have you ever felt like you didn't want to go to work? Why? Are you tired, bored, scared, or preoccupied with something else?
- Have you felt like you didn't want to go to class? (Don't worry, about answering honestly. Even professors sometimes don't want to go to class and teach!) Why? Is the teacher boring? Is the material irrelevant? Do you have something else on your mind?
- How is your functioning with your friends and family just before a midterm or final exam?
- Do you often feel worried before an exam?
- Do you worry when a paper or project is due?
- Do you believe you study enough? If not, why not?
- Do you blame your feelings on others, like the teacher, the boss, or your parents?
- What do you think are some effective ways to manage stress?
- What have you done to try to feel differently in some of these situations?

Now that you have had a chance to think about your own burnout and stress, let's take a look at how to manage these situations. These suggestions may come in very handy at this point in the semester and at your job. Share these ideas with coworkers, supervisors, family, friends, and clients as well.

MANAGING STRESS AND BURNOUT

Learning to manage stress and burnout requires that we understand more about the stress process. Several factors, including individual differences in stress, can influence how we cope. For example, individuals have different levels of resilience and vulnerability to stress due to socioeconomic factors, educational level, gender, personality (for a review see Almeida, 2005), and even age (Almeida & Horn, 2004). For example, older adults, compared with young and midlife adults, report their stressors as less severe. Overall, our individual upbringing, previous and current life circumstances, and type of stressors experienced previously all influence how we cope.

There are several ways to cope. Our cognitive attributions or perceptions can be important, especially as it relates to one's sense of personal control. People who have an internal locus of control, or believe they have choice in their lives, including how they handle external events, cope better with stress. This is compared to people who have an external locus of control and believe they are at the mercy of external events.

In the context of work settings, talking about stressful experiences is also cathartic. For example, a 2001 study of community workers who regularly assist people in crisis suggests that talking with coworkers about one's stress helps relieve its emotional consequences (Kanel, 2007). Of the 67 workers surveyed, 80 percent stated that they talk with coworkers when feeling emotionally stressed after working with people in crisis. This is a great solution for work stress if there are supportive coworkers at the workplace. It may not be a practical solution if coworkers are competitive and when conflict is high among coworkers. In fact, the work environment itself may be the very source of stress. Stress may result from coworker conflict as well as unsupportive supervisors and conflicts with organizational norms. Of course, if a work environment is extremely dysfunctional and oppressive, people might consider quitting as a way to reduce work stress. Unfortunately, not everyone has that luxury. People usually need their jobs to pay bills, eat, and take care of family needs. So, while it would be great if we could all just leave when the work environment, coworkers, or supervisors became unbearable, quitting isn't necessarily the most practical solution. At some point, learning the coping skills necessary to manage the normal, daily stresses in almost all work settings is essential.

The best solution for work stress is to teach managers how to create stress-free work environments and how to interact with staff members in ways that make them feel supported and appreciated. Then all employees could be instructed and coached on how to communicate with one another so that no one feels hurt or inadequate. If everyone learned to cooperate and get along, work would be wonderful. Does this sound realistic to you? Of course not. That doesn't mean that some of these things can't be increased. In fact, many companies offer in-service training, staff retreats, and workshops to improve employee morale and increase competence among those who supervise.

While individual counseling for employees who are stressed may be temporarily helpful, if the company doesn't deal with the root causes of the stress, counseling is "like cleaning up the fish in a pond but then putting them back in the dirty water" (Mendoza, 2005, p. 2). Not every organization offers stress-management training or even effective managerial training about how to help employees who are stressed. Managers may be aware that employees are stressed but may feel incapable of implementing strategies to deal with workplace stress. Some may even view workplace stress and stress management as simply a current trend that need not be taken seriously (Mendoza, 2005).

A Four-Pronged Approach to Managing Stress

- Recognize your own problem areas
- Work on your own problem areas
- Improve interpersonal communication
- Maintain a sense of humor

After reviewing the details of the four stress-management strategies that follow, take a look at the worksheet in the Suggested Applied Activities section, which may be useful during times of stress.

Recognize Your Own Problem Areas

Before deciding to quit a stressful job, individuals should examine their own part in any problems at work. (Students can do the same for stressful situations at school.) Most stress-management strategies focus on perceptions of the problems and ways to change those perceptions. This approach is helpful because it gives people control of their own thoughts, whereas it is much harder to be in control of others' behaviors. Cognitive-behavioral therapy approaches have been instrumental in helping people learn how to rethink their situations so they can deal with them more easily. The basic philosophy behind these approaches is that the situations themselves do not make us feel bad, rather it is our perceptions of them that lead to negative feelings such as anger, depression, and anxiety. In the first century A.D., the Greek philosopher Epictetus said, "people are disturbed not by things, but by the view which they take of them" (cited in Ellis, 2001, p. 16). Since then, cognitive theory has become a major force in counseling and stress management.

Ellis's rational emotive behavioral therapy model (briefly presented in Chapter 5) is simple and easy to implement: When trying to change personal perceptions and reduce stress, consider using the following five steps:

1. Identify irrational, ineffective thinking.
2. Examine whether these thoughts have been beneficial in the past.
3. Identify alternate thoughts that are more realistic, more rational, and based on facts.
4. Make an effort to say these more rational thoughts when feeling badly.
5. Evaluate whether these new thoughts have improved stress levels (Ellis, 1962).

What follows are some common types of **irrational and self-defeating thoughts**. These thoughts may be self-imposed or may come from others. Regardless of their source, it's important to eliminate them and to start thinking more realistically.

Self-Critical Thoughts People in stressful situations often resort to **self-critical thoughts**, such as calling themselves stupid, ugly, fat, worthless, inadequate, and so forth. It's bad enough to deal with stress without adding labels like these. If people can just stop calling themselves bad names, they might be able to focus on resolving the stressful situation. When people calls themselves one of those names they're going to feel horrible, which makes it more difficult to cope with the demands of daily life. Over time, stress builds, and people become burned out. The trick is to stop that inner, name-calling voice and realize that no one is perfect. Once people accept that mistakes are inevitable and don't make them horrible people, they can join real life. Mistakes, instead, might be thought of as a way to learn about what to avoid and what to improve on next time.

That can be hard to do if people view their mistakes as just additional evidence of their stupidity. Likewise, losing weight can be made more difficult when people think of themselves as being a "fat pig," "ugly," or "disgusting." These words make people feel bad about themselves, which can sabotage their positive intentions, such as eating sensibly and exercising.

Critical Thoughts About Others Self-criticism is as self-defeating as criticizing others is. Just as some people tend to blame themselves when things go wrong, other people look for others to blame when something goes wrong. Blaming leads to feelings of anger and resentment. These feelings are not conducive to solving problems and feeling happy. Ellis (1962) proposed that no human being should ever be blamed for anything he or she does and that it is the therapist's job to help rid people of thoughts in which they blame themselves, others, or fate and the universe.

Irrational Thoughts Frequently, people tell themselves that they just can't stand it if things don't go the way they want them to go. They tend to exaggerate the gravity of certain situations and blow them out of proportion. Doing this tends to make people feel anxious or enraged. A typical example might be when a driver cuts someone off on the road. He or she may be telling him- or herself, "How dare he do this to me! I will not let this rest! I cannot stand it when people are rude to me!" The rational counterpart would be, "I sure don't like it when people drive dangerously, and accidents are likely when people take chances. I would prefer that people consider me when they drive."

Another example might be when someone doesn't get hired for a job or a student scores poorly on an exam. Thoughts such as, "This is not fair, I shouldn't have to take such hard exams," and "How dare they not hire me, it's not fair!" make people feel angry. This anger often prevents the person from learning from the situation and improving the next time. In general, when people turn their preferences into demands, they are thinking irrationally, and they will feel bad. The reality is, "You can't always get what you want" and "People don't behave the way they should or the way you want them to behave."

Critical Thinking/Self-Reflection Corner

- How often have you thought or said to someone, "It's not my fault. You are to blame"?
- Has anyone ever told you, "It's your fault"?
- How do these statements make you feel?
- Can anything productive come of these statements of blame?

Reality shows us over and over that people are fallible. They make mistakes, and so do you! You will be a chronically angry person if you expect that all people will be competent, nice, fair, and respectful at all times.

Work on Your Own Problem Areas

When people experience painful or negative feelings, a few steps can be taken toward eliminating or reducing these unwanted feelings. The first step is to identify the **precipitating event** that has activated a negative feeling or behavior. Next, identify the irrational beliefs about this event. Once the triggers of the emotional distress and the unrealistic beliefs and thoughts about it have been identified, the next step is to begin disputing the irrational beliefs and substituting more realistic and rational thoughts. Last, an assessment should be made to decide whether changing those thoughts was helpful in changing the negative feelings and behaviors. If not, then there may be other irrational thoughts that are maintaining the negative feelings. The following examples of two common situations illustrate how to implement Ellis's approach.

Example 1: Negative feelings of anger and bitterness

Precipitating event: Receiving a "C" on an exam

Irrational beliefs: "It's the teacher's fault; he didn't give us a study guide. He didn't tell us the right things to study. The material was too confusing. I should get a 'B' because I always get 'Bs' and 'As'. It's not fair. It's horrible to get a 'C' because now I can't get into graduate school."

Disputation and substitution of realistic beliefs for irrational beliefs: "Where is it written that teachers must provide study guides? They don't all do this. It's really up to me to study and take responsibility for studying. Unfortunately, some teachers don't focus on assisting students in passing exams, and some teachers don't present material clearly. I'd certainly rather earn a 'B' or an 'A' on all exams. Many people get into graduate school even if they get a few 'Cs.' It's always possible to retake a course if need be. Unfortunately, life is not always fair, and things don't always go the way we want."

Evaluation of effect of disputation and substitutions: "I'm feeling less angry and more empowered to take charge of my own studying and grades. Although I'm not exactly happy that life is not fair or that I can't always get what I want, I realize that this is reality and I can't fight reality."

Example 2: Negative feelings of depression and thoughts of suicide

Precipitating event: Breakup of a romantic relationship

Irrational beliefs: "No one will ever love me again. I can't go on living without him or her. I'm not worthy of love. Something is wrong with me, or else why would this happen to me? I'm ugly and fat. I'm stupid, and I shouldn't have put so much trust in one person."

Disputations and substitutions: "It is sad and difficult to experience a loss. But where is the proof that no one will ever love me again? As an adult, I can live without another person, although I may feel sad and lonely sometimes while I grieve. But loss is a normal part of life. We all risk the chance of experiencing loss when we become close to someone, because, as sad and disappointing as it is, people change their feelings, they grow in different directions, and it often has nothing to do with anyone but themselves. Just because someone doesn't want me now, it doesn't mean that was always true. People change, and at least I know the truth now. The extent of my grief indicates the attachment and love we both shared. Loss can be a time for both celebrating what I had experienced as well as a time to feel sad at not having that anymore. It is an opportunity to grow and seek new experiences."

Evaluation: "I am still sad but am beginning to believe that I might be able to make it through this breakup. I sure don't like it, but it isn't the end of the world."

Reframing Critical and Irrational Thoughts Cognitive-restructuring approaches are similar to what strategic therapists call "reframing" and using "positive connotations" (Haley, 1976; Palazzoli, Cecchin, Prata, & Boscolo, 1978). These approaches help people view their problems as possible opportunities for growth and can reshape perceptions of negative events into more positive, more acceptable experiences. Therapists who use reframing techniques first need to understand a client's—and often the entire family's—frame of reference before being able to put the problems in a solvable light. The following examples illustrate how reframing and positive connotations can be used.

Example 1: A 54-year-old woman tells her therapist that she wants to kill herself because she is a burden to her family. Since her back surgery, her children must drive her to doctor appointments and help her clean her house. If she kills herself, she believes, she'll be a good mother by unburdening her children from having to care for her.

Client's frame of reference: She's a good mother, and committing suicide is a sign of being a good mother.

Therapist's reframe: Client would be a bigger burden to her children if she were to kill herself because they will forever feel guilty and sad that she killed herself because she didn't want to be a burden to them. A good self-sacrificing mother would just put up with being taken care of by her children so that they can still feel her love and her presence.

Example 2: A new intern at a battered women's shelter answers a hotline call. The person on the phone is a female who wants to know where the shelter is. The intern figures that since the caller is a woman it would be alright to tell her the address. When the intern tells her supervisor what she did, the supervisor says that it is a felony to give out the address of a battered women's shelter.

Intern's frame of reference: She feels she is horrible and stupid for giving out the address.

Supervisor's reframe: It's a good thing this time that she gave the address to a safe person and that she told me about it right away. Mistakes like these are helpful because they remind all of us about this most important issue. The trainer at the orientation failed to mention this legal issue, and it would have been overlooked if the intern had not brought it to my attention. It would have just been assumed that everyone knew about the policy.

Notice that the reframes and positive-connotation method allow both people to save face and leave the situation with their self-esteem intact.

The main thread that all of these approaches have in common is that individuals can examine their own thoughts that lead to stress and can change them. The change in perception leads to reduction in negative and painful emotions. Not only is cognitive restructuring used in American workplaces and private counseling offices, but it is being used effectively in other countries as well. The following two examples explain how it is being used in Wisconsin and in China.

Example 1: Using cognitive-restructuring theory at the Ho-Chunk Casino

The management of this casino designed a stress-management program called Rethinking Stress, which teaches employees how to accept responsibility for their own reactions to stress. It does not allow employees to blame their stress on outside forces, but it motivates them to change their own behaviors rather than expecting others to change. Participants in the program reported saving an average of 6.25 hours per week and using an average of 2.92 fewer sick days for stress-related issues (Lee, Dolezalek, & Johnson, 2005).

Example 2: Targeting work-related stress at a company in China

A company in China has begun a training program in managing emotional intelligence, a twist on conventional stress management. The focus is on helping employees manage their emotions in the face of crisis or change and even transform negative emotions into positive ones (Caplan, 2005).

Maintaining a Healthy Lifestyle While much stress and burnout come from an individual's thoughts and beliefs, a person's lifestyle and behaviors can also create stress. Eating habits, exercise, and recreational activities play a big part in both controlling and reducing stress. A person's home life and social interests may provide clues to why some people have more difficulties coping with stress and burnout than others do. While feeling productive and fulfilled at work is healthy, using a job as a substitute for living is not. When human services workers' personal lives and needs take a backseat to those of their clients, no one benefits. It does feel good to be needed and respected by clients, but when workers' own needs of being needed and liked are motivations for helping others, the support and help workers provide become confused with the support and help that they need. Such confusion can lead to unwise choices as well as mixed messages (Russo, 1980).

Human services workers must develop and maintain healthy personal lives outside of their jobs. They must eat healthy food and exercise regularly. It is vital to take time to relax and to get involved in activities and interests that are not related to work. When a human services worker (or student) begins feeling stressed or burned out, it may be time to focus on outside interests. If the stress seems unmanageable and overwhelming, seeking the services of a professional counselor is advised. By using these stress-management tactics, workers can make sure that clients receive the most effective and ethical interventions.

The mental health of human services workers is probably the most important resource that a worker gives to clients and the agency.

Just as problematic, however, are human services workers who begin to care too little about clients and their jobs. They disengage from their own personal feelings for clients and coworkers and become bureaucratic technicians. They carry out institutional procedures and rely solely on the rules and regulations to make decisions without letting their personal values and feelings get in the way (Russo, 1980). While this may prevent their personal needs from interfering with their work with clients, it may lead to feelings of emptiness and lack of satisfaction at work. Obviously, the trick is to allow oneself to care about clients and the organizational goals while at the same time allowing oneself to be involved in an outside life that fulfills one's needs socially and recreationally.

Improving Interpersonal Communication

While much work-related stress and burnout comes from an individual's cognitions and behaviors, at other times conflicts with coworkers, difficulties with work-related responsibilities, and other real job-related problems are to blame. Many of these problems can be eliminated by talking assertively with supervisors. The Health and Safety Executive in the United Kingdom (Goldman & Lewis, 2005, p. 13) recently identified six key areas that may affect work stress and burnout. When workers have problems in any of these areas, they should speak with a manager or supervisor to attempt to resolve the problems.

1. *The demands of the job*: Both employee and supervisor must ensure that the employee can cope and handle the job requirements, and if not, training and guidance should be provided.
2. *The degree of employee control over his or her work*: Employees should communicate with supervisors if this is a problem, and supervisors should allow employees to have a say in how they should go about their work.
3. *The level of management and colleague support provided*: Supervisors should provide information and support through accessible policies and procedures and give regular and constructive feedback. If employees do not feel this is occurring, they should speak up and ask for more training and positive reinforcement when work activity is productive.
4. *The quality of work relationships*: Employees must speak up if they experience intimidation, bullying, or other unacceptable and unprofessional behaviors from others. Sometimes this can be done in staff meetings, retreats, or through union representatives. As the study of community workers discovered, talking with coworkers is invaluable in dealing with work stress. Getting along with coworkers is worth fighting for, and to survive at an agency, employees must feel an alliance with at least several other workers. Sometimes open warfare must precede a more cooperative spirit among coworkers. Effective managers must be competent in creating a work environment in which coworkers can get along. At times, an outside mediator may be called upon to manage serious employee conflicts.

5. *Employee role within the organization and how it is managed:* An employee's roles and responsibilities should be clearly defined. It can be stressful to not know what is expected. It is very stressful to receive negative evaluations for duties that the employee didn't even know were his or hers. It is the manager or supervisor's job to ensure that each employee knows his or her duties clearly.
6. *The management of change:* When an agency makes changes, employees should be involved and allowed opportunities to communicate with management about their feelings and thoughts. Change is scary for employees and management because there is always a risk that new rules and ideas won't work as well as old ones. Employees may worry about being replaced or fired (Goldman & Lewis, 2005).

The key to all of these problems is open communication between employees and management. Of course, that is the ideal solution, not necessarily the way things work out in reality. Some managers and supervisors are incompetent and insecure. They may behave in less than professional ways. If a worker wishes to continue in the agency with this type of management style, then the worker must take responsibility to speak up and attempt assertive resolution. Sometimes it is possible to go above one's immediate supervisor and complain. This is referred to as breaking chain of command and is not usually greeted with open arms. Status quo is threatened when you go around your immediate superiors, and you may pay a price for doing so (Russo, 1980). Some problems must be addressed by upper management, such as in cases of sexual harassment. For the most part, though, most organizations prefer that immediate supervisors and their staff resolve complaints and problems.

Developing mentoring relationships can be helpful in managing job-related stress, especially for beginning human services workers. A mentor is someone that an employee or intern can trust, respect, and communicate with openly. The mentor must be someone who has time to spend answering questions and listening to fears, struggles, and other issues. Usually, a mentor is an experienced human services worker who is available to offer ideas about how to perform job duties and how to get along with coworkers and survive in the system.

Aggressive, Passive, and Assertive Behaviors Many people confuse being **assertive** with being **aggressive**, and so they behave passively to avoid aggressive behavior. Passive, aggressive, and assertive behaviors are three very different styles of interpersonal communication. When people communicate assertively, stress levels are typically reduced, while aggressive and **passive** styles of communicating often increase stress. Learning how to communicate assertively is helpful to everyone, no matter what they choose to do with their lives. By learning these few assertive tactics, the reader has the opportunity to improve his or her own relationships and reduce stress as well as pass the information on to future recipients of human services. Assertive behaviors make it likely that the people get what they want when possible. They allow people to negotiate and express themselves appropriately and respectfully. Before introducing specific assertive techniques, a brief discussion about aggressive and passive communication will be presented.

Aggressive communication usually leaves both parties feeling bad. While someone may get his or her needs and wants met, the other feels disrespected, unheard, and manipulated. This type of interacting only concerns itself with one person's needs without any regard as to how the interaction affects the other. The person on the receiving end often feels angry, resentful, scared, and bad about him- or herself. The aggressive person may temporarily feel powerful and in control, but over time he or she may destroy relationships with others. The aggressive person often appears to have a "chip on his shoulder" and may unwittingly turn others away from him or her. While he or she may get what he or she wants at the moment, he or she is losing the love and respect of others in the long term. Aggressive people intimidate others in order to succeed. How content would you be to have relationships with others based on fear?

Passive people often complement aggressive ones. They keep their feelings and needs inside for fear of creating conflict. They don't speak up but rather let others walk all over them. The price people pay for avoiding conflict is often to be viewed and treated like a doormat. At first, others may think it is positive that someone is so easygoing. Over time, though, passive people may lose the respect of others because they don't command respect. Another consequence of being passive is a buildup of resentment. Instead of expressing disagreement and anger directly, passive people often let their angry feelings out indirectly. This is referred to as being passive-aggressive and leads to relationship dissatisfaction. For example, instead of telling her spouse that she is tired of his coming home late for dinner, a wife might simply burn his food and leave it on the table cold.

Simply put, assertive behavior allows people to express their own needs and wants in a way that does not harm others. Assertive people respect themselves and respect anyone else with whom he or she is interacting. While it may not always be possible for everyone to get whatever they want and need all the time, there is frequently room for compromises and negotiations when people relate to one another with respect and empathy. The key to assertive communication is to avoid blaming others or placing responsibility on others for one's own feelings and behaviors. The assertive person expresses needs and wants by making "I" statements instead of "you" and other attacking or blaming statements. In general, when people interact with respect for others as well as for themselves, everyone has a good chance of feeling good about themselves. When people feel good and respected, problems can be solved more readily and conflict can be resolved. The following lists provide examples of aggressive, passive, and assertive statements.

Examples of Aggressive, Ineffective Statements

- "You make me so mad!"
- "You shouldn't talk that way to me."
- "You really have issues, don't you?"
- "You made the wrong choice, and now I have to suffer."
- "You never have enough time to spend supervising me."
- "Why does Janice get to leave early? She doesn't even do as much work as everyone else."

Examples of Passive Statements

- "I guess it's alright if you borrow my book, although I do need it to study tonight."
- "Sure, I don't mind skipping lunch today."
- "You need me to work this weekend? I suppose I can always watch the video of my nephew's graduation."

Examples of Assertive Statements

- "I feel angry when you ignore me because your attention and respect is important to me."
- "When we disagree, I would appreciate it if you could lower your voice and not use curse words."
- "I don't understand why you are upset with me right now."
- "I'm upset that what you've done affects me."
- "I feel that I need more supervision time with you. Can that be arranged?"
- "Although it may not be any of my business, I feel confused as to why Janice leaves earlier than the rest of us. Another thing that's bothering me is when she often refuses to pitch in and help the rest of us. Are you aware of this?"

Assertive interaction includes calm, realistic attempts to solve problems without blaming anyone. People think more clearly when they don't feel attacked and are more likely to come up with viable solutions than when they feel blamed. The assertive person must accept that sometimes the best one can achieve is a compromise.

Suppose you loaned your textbook to a classmate who lost it. You need it to study for the final exam. You don't have enough money to buy a new one and neither does the other student. Because you really need the book immediately, you may have to arrange a plan in which you pay for half of the book along with the other student to ensure you get the book soon. Although it isn't exactly fair, you will get what you need. You can always set up a plan for the classmate to reimburse you with small payments over the next few months. The focus should be on how to get the book you need, not on whose fault it is that you don't have it. You are likely to get reimbursed if you handle it assertively instead of passively or aggressively. If you were to yell and scream and blame your classmate, she might just tell you "tough, you're out of luck." If you don't speak up at all, she may just let you pay for a whole new book on your own.

Human services workers may be especially vulnerable to stress, given the nature of their work with clients and their other duties. Of course, handling criticism can be difficult for everyone, but responding assertively may reduce stress. Instead of fighting the criticism, an effective technique to manage the negative feelings associated with being criticized is to simply agree with the criticism or try to more clearly understand it. This gives the person a chance to learn from any mistakes to make improvements. When someone criticizes another person, there is often the tendency to defend or explain oneself. This is not necessary. The best thing to say to a supervisor, coworker, or a client who's being critical of others is, "What you say may be accurate. What exactly is it about my behavior that you find objectionable? What do you think would be a better way to handle things?" Even if they were wrong to make a comment, by saying these things, they are forced into taking responsibility for their criticism. Assertive people don't allow negative remarks to go by easily. They respectfully ask others to communicate without attacking or blaming. The following lists provide some examples of how to handle criticism assertively.

Examples of Handling Criticism From a Supervisor
- Criticism: "You didn't write these case notes very legibly."
- Assertive response: "I guess you're right, they are a bit messy. What would be the best way to fix it?"
- Aggressive response: "So what? Everyone else writes messy too."
- Passive response: "I'm sorry. I was in a hurry and didn't concentrate. I'll do them over."

Examples of Handling Criticism From a Coworker
- Criticism: "You were rude to those clients."
- Assertive response: "Wow, if that is the case, I sure didn't mean to be. What exactly did I do that seemed rude to you?"
- Aggressive response: "They were rude to me first. Whose side are you going to take anyway?"
- Passive response: I'm horrible. I guess I should quit.

Handling Criticism From a Member of a Substance-Abuse Group
- Criticism: "You're too young to be a group counselor. How can you know anything?"
- Assertive response: "Yes, I am young. What is it exactly about my age that bothers you? What would make you feel better?"
- Aggressive response: "Well, at least I went to college. How about you?"
- Passive response: "Yeah, I know. Maybe I'll wait until I get older to run groups."

Maintaining a Sense of Humor

Using humor appropriately to manage stress on the job, even when working with clients, can relieve tension and create a bond between people. True, one should not laugh at client's problems, but humor can be useful in a variety of ways. Psychologists often use humor in promoting healing in their clients (Fry, 1993; McGuire, 1999). If it is a healing process for clients, then it is probably beneficial for anyone experiencing stress. Studies have demonstrated that laughter boosts the immune system and lowers blood pressure (McGuire, 1999). That alone is extremely beneficial for someone who feels stress. Humor also allows people to think about a situation in new ways, and it effectively reduces feelings of anxiety and depression.

Some tips for adding humor into one's life include interacting with funny, playful people; taking time to play every day; observing children and animals; searching for things to laugh about; and posting cartoons where they can be seen. It's important to avoid sarcasm and abusive humor, as well as to avoid discounting serious emotions by laughing them off. Humor should facilitate, not interrupt, the healing process (McGuire, 1999).

CHAPTER SUMMARY

Stress occurs daily. It is not abnormal but must be managed effectively if we are to function at our best. Human services workers may be prone to stress on the job because of ongoing contact with people in crisis and suffering. It is vital that human services workers practice stress management to perform their duties appropriately. Clients deserve to receive services from workers who are not burned out. Cognitive restructuring, assertive communication, talking to coworkers, and recreation are all helpful in managing stress.

Suggested Applied Activities

1. Using the worksheet below, think of a current situation in which you find yourself feeling negative emotions or engaging in destructive behaviors. Fill in the blanks and try to reduce your irrational thoughts and negative feelings.

Worksheet to Help Reduce Irrational Thoughts and Feelings

Negative feelings: _____

Precipitating event: _____

Irrational beliefs: _____

_____

Disputations and substitutions: _____

_____

_____

_____

Evaluation: _____

2. The next time someone criticizes you, try to handle the criticism by asking the person what it is about your behavior that bothers them so much. Perhaps you might even agree with the criticism and ask for suggestions on how to improve. Don't explain yourself or defend yourself. Evaluate how this type of response makes you feel.

_____

_____

3. Keep track of your daily activities. Make sure you incorporate a fun, playful activity every day. How often do you laugh during a day? Try to engage in activities that make you smile and laugh.

_____

_____

_____

_____

Chapter Review Questions

1. What are five symptoms of burnout?

_____

_____

2. What are five causes of burnout?

_____

_____

3. Name three ways to manage stress on the job?

_____

_____

4. What is the difference between assertiveness and aggressiveness?

_____

_____

5. How might cognitive therapy help reduce stress?

_____

_____

Glossary of Terms

Aggressive is a type of interacting in which a person takes care of his or her own needs without regard for others.

Allostatic load is the wear and tear on the body due to too much stress and adaptation.

Assertive is a type of interacting in which a person demonstrates self-respect as well as respect for others.

Burnout refers to job-related anxiety and dissatisfaction that adversely affects job performance and other areas of a person's life.

Cognitive restructuring involves changing the way people think about their experiences.

Disputation is an internal dialogue that helps people think rationally about a situation that was previously thought of as negative and that led to irrational beliefs.

Distress is the negative outcome of too much stress.

Eustress is the positive experience of stress.

Homeostasis is the natural, physiological balance of one's body.

Irrational and self-defeating thoughts are not based on facts but are habitual ways that people think which often make them feel bad.

Passive is a type of interacting in which people do not command respect for themselves and their needs but instead take care of others' needs in order to avoid conflict.

Precipitating event is a situation that causes a reaction in an individual.

Self-critical thoughts are negative thoughts that people use to label themselves bad in some way. Rather than thinking through a situation rationally, people simply think badly of themselves and feel terrible.

Stress is a state of being physically, psychologically, emotionally, and intellectually overwhelmed. It can manifest itself in physical symptoms as well as negative emotions and thoughts about a situation.

Stress management is a group of behaviors used to reduce stress. This includes cognitive restructuring, maintaining a healthy lifestyle, and assertive communication.

Case Presentation and Exit Quiz

General Description and Demographics

Kara is an undergraduate in the human services department of a local university. This is her second semester in the human services program, and she's beginning her first internship, which is at a group home. Kara is an excellent student, and her grade point average has been 4.0. She has a keen understanding of various theories and counseling techniques, has knowledge about case management, and has excelled in her course dealing with cultural issues. Currently, in addition to her internship class, she's taking courses on crisis intervention, child development, self-awareness, and abnormal psychology. Kara's career goal is to be either a social worker or a family counselor. Kara is 20 years old.

The group home where she is interning is an approved agency site for the human services department. It is a nonprofit agency that contracts with the county department of social services for funding. The agency also holds yearly fundraisers to increase its budget. Kara's supervisor, Emma, is a 38-year-old pediatric counselor who has a bachelor's degree in child development. Kara's stated responsibilities include monitoring the children while they do homework, helping children resolve conflicts with one another, supervising children on the playground, and escorting children on field trips. Kara, Emma, and Kara's fieldwork instructor all agreed on these responsibilities.

The children who live at the group home have all been placed there by the courts because they have been physically, sexually, or emotionally abused or severely neglected by their parents. Many of their parents are in jail, in mental hospitals, or are substance abusers. The parents have failed to follow through with case plans. Many of the children suffer from behavioral and emotional problems. They often act out their anger and frustration at their situation by lying, stealing, hitting, yelling, and swearing. The group home operates under a behavior-modification model. Children receive rewards when they follow the rules and suffer consequences when they break them. Each child is assigned to a personal therapist, either a licensed clinical social worker or a licensed marriage and family therapist. Some children with extremely severe problems receive treatment from psychologists, and some are on medication prescribed by a psychiatrist. Older children often participate in group counseling. They all go to school at the group home and are only allowed to leave the home when accompanied by a staff member.

Kara's Stress

Kara has always wanted to work with abused children. She was abused physically as a child and wants to help abused children feel better about themselves. When she was first accepted to intern at the group home, she felt excited and couldn't wait to start. After interning there for only three weeks, she finds herself dreading the days she works at the agency. She has begun to oversleep on those days she is supposed to go to the agency, and on weekends, she's been going to a lot of parties and getting drunk. She feels guilty about disliking the agency because she tells herself that she should want to help those poor kids. Kara believes that if she doesn't help them, they will grow up to be losers and she would be partially to blame.

When Kara is at the agency, she handles the children very competently. She usually knows the right things to say and is able to help the children manage their conflicts and aggressive feelings very effectively. In fact, she is so competent that her supervisor has left her alone at the agency while the paid staff all go to lunch. At other times, Kara is left alone because several staff members called in sick. Kara doesn't feel comfortable being there by herself and has told Emma that she feels a little nervous. Emma told Kara not to worry because Kara is more competent than half of the paid staff.

Another of Kara's concerns is that she has been asked to drive some children to dental and medical appointments. She never agreed to do this when she signed her contract. Kara knows she isn't supposed to drive them in her own car because the university doesn't allow it. One day a child became violent when Kara was at the home alone. Kara phoned Emma, but Emma didn't answer her cell phone. Kara called the on-call licensed supervisor, who told her to call the police and she'd be right in.

Kara is afraid to tell her class instructor about what is going on because she thinks that the instructor will be angry or that she will get in trouble for performing duties not on her contract. Kara can't handle another day at the agency. Thank goodness she gets to go to her internship class tomorrow.

Kara finally opens up to her instructor and to the rest of her classmates. She learns that other students have had similar experiences at their internship sites. The students and instructor offer some ideas to Kara about how to manage her stress.

Kara takes their advice, and over the next few weeks she slowly starts to feel better about going to the group home.

Exit Quiz

1. Kara shows which signs of burnout?
    a. Physical energy
    b. Overly positive self-concept
    c. Negative job attitudes
    d. All of the above

2. All but one of the following is probably a cause of Kara's burnout:
    a. conflict between the ideal and the real
    b. dealing with tedious bureaucratic tasks
    c. lack of client motivation and limited capabilities to receive help and help themselves
    d. conflicts between personal values and organizational norms

3. Kara's drinking is
    a. an attempt to manage her stress
    b. evidence that she is an alcoholic
    c. a sign that she shouldn't be a social worker
    d. cause for dismissal

4. Kara's instructor asked her what she was thinking that made her feel guilty about not wanting to go to the group home. Kara replied:
    a. "The children don't really want me there."
    b. "If I don't help them, they may grow up to be losers."
    c. "I really am not qualified to help."
    d. None of the above

5. The instructor tells Kara that working with abused children is difficult for even the most experienced counselor and that most of them go through a period of anxiety and depression when working with this population. This is an example of
   a. assertion training
   b. changing the agency structure
   c. cognitive restructuring
   d. all of the above

6. The instructor has Kara role-play a conversation between Kara and her supervisor Emma. Kara is told to tell Emma what she wants in an assertive manner. Which of the following statements is not an example of assertive communication?
   a. "I feel very uncomfortable being alone at the group home and believe it is inappropriate for an intern to be alone with so many abused children."
   b. "You are so unethical leaving me alone. I should report you to the better business bureau."
   c. "I can no longer drive the children in my personal car to doctor appointments. It is against my university's policy for interns."
   d. "I would like to continue working at the group home, but some things need to change for me to be able to continue."

7. What can Kara do to help relieve some of her stress while interning at the group home?
   a. Talk to coworkers about her feelings when she's at the agency
   b. Engage in recreational activities such as swimming
   c. Watch a funny movie
   d. All of the above

Exit Quiz Answers

1. c
2. b
3. a
4. b
5. c
6. b
7. d

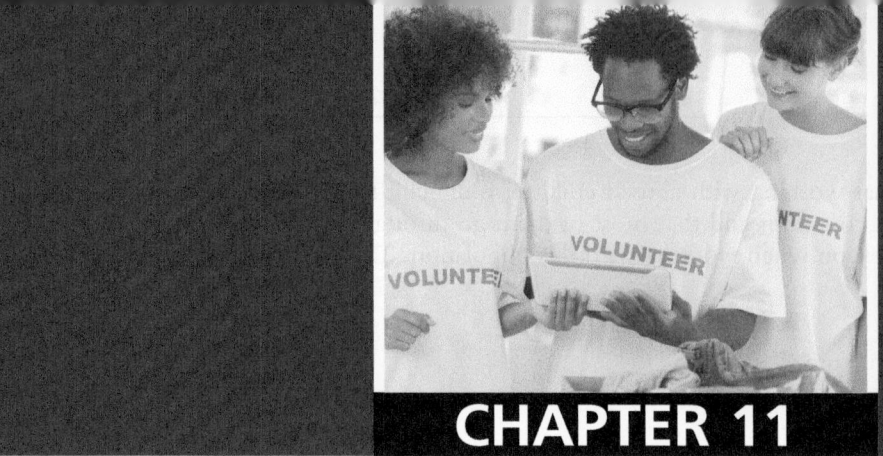

CHAPTER 11

Case Management

INTRODUCTION

Case management as a duty of human services workers has been steadily increasing over the past 30 years. It epitomizes the generalist perspective discussed in Chapter 1. Case managers must be familiar with a multitude of services that recipients of human services frequently need. In addition to serving as brokers of community services, they must be able to provide direct services such as crisis intervention, guidance counseling, giving testimony in court, writing reports, and maintaining case notes, just to name a few job responsibilities. Case management is done in many types of human services agencies including mental health, social services, probation, gerontology, and substance abuse programs. Although it may feel a bit dehumanizing to refer to clients as cases, this is the typical term used in public, nonprofit, and profit agencies.

WHAT IS CASE MANAGEMENT?

In the human services field, a case may be thought of as an individual client or a family with whom a worker is involved over a period of time to achieve resolution of a problem. The case file involves a collection of client communications, forms, process documents, and reports needed to manage any compliance or audit issues and to help the case manager keep track of the progress of the case (Global Community of Information Professionals, 2013). According to the State of New Jersey Department of Human Services, Division of Developmental Disabilities (2013), case management services help individuals learn about and gain access to any services that can help address their needs including medical, social, education, county, and municipal services.

The primary function of case management is to increase the quality of life of clients. Case managers assess the needs of the client and connect them with appropriate services depending on need. It is practiced in a variety of social service settings including hospitals, nursing homes, mental health facilities, and drug and alcohol rehabilitation centers. It is a broad category that involves coordination of care, advocacy, and discharge planning as well as counseling and therapeutic support. It aims to assist clients in navigating social service systems (Renata, 2013).

Some universities offer degrees in case management. For example, the University of California, Davis, offers a certificate program in human services case management in which the focus is on enhancing skills to address the complex needs of individuals and families such as coordinating and providing direct services and assisting clients to manage their abilities and resources in ways that lead to self-sufficiency (UC Davis Extension Center for Human Services, 2013). The department in which the two authors are housed is in the process of developing a master's degree in human services leadership, which entails case management development. Many gerontology programs also offer courses in case management.

TYPES OF TREATMENT FREQUENTLY SUGGESTED FOR RECIPIENTS OF HUMAN SERVICES

Even though most case managers do not provide direct treatment for their cases, they often work collaboratively with other human services workers who do provide the treatment. It is vital that case managers understand these types of treatments and how clients may or may not benefit from them.

As discussed in earlier chapters, services can be broken down into **micro level** (working with an individual), **mezzo level** (working with families and groups), and **macro level** (working with communities and broader statewide and nationwide areas). Case managers focus on referring clients to micro- and mezzo-level services but must still be aware of policies that affect clients at broader levels as well.

Micro Level

Typical micro-level services include individual counseling, psychotherapy, or one-on-one medication evaluations. These services are usually done at an agency or at a private office. Sometimes, clients receive individual services at hospital settings as well as group counseling. Some clients receive individual therapy while they also participate in family counseling.

Individual Counseling or Therapy The various approaches to counseling and psychotherapy have been discussed at length in Chapter 5. This type of service is provided at hospitals, offices, agencies, schools, and correctional facilities by licensed therapists, nurses, case managers, psychiatrists, volunteers, and interns. The focus is on helping an individual work through problems presenting in the here and now or deeper, long-standing issues.

Medications Many clients' behaviors and coping abilities improve by taking medication (sometimes referred to as chemotherapy). Although **medication** may be the best option for certain clients, most clients on medication are also encouraged to participate in other services. Medication may be prescribed by a client's primary care physician or psychiatrist.

Example 1: A 27-year-old man, diagnosed with bipolar disorder, recently suffered an intense manic episode during which he assaulted someone at a local bar. When he went to court, the judge put him on probation and ordered him to see a psychiatrist and stay on his medication. He went to a court-appointed psychiatrist and began taking Depacote (an anticonvulsant drug). After three weeks, he was stabilized and no longer had drastic mood swings.

Example 2: A woman suffering from severe panic attacks went to a therapist who thought she should see a psychiatrist, who could evaluate her need for medication to treat her panic attacks. The therapist continued with counseling, and the psychiatrist will continue with medication management.

Mezzo Level

Twelve-Step Programs These groups are run by group members, not professional human services workers. They have proven to be successful for people struggling with addiction and are a great referral resource for clients because attendance is free (although voluntary donations are asked at each meeting), and clients can attend daily meetings if they choose. In 1935, Bill Wilson founded Alcoholics Anonymous (AA), which was the first of many **twelve-step programs** that followed. The AA program of recovery suggests using 12 steps (listed below), which can be used in any way members find helpful.

1. We admitted we were powerless over alcohol—that our lives had become unmanageable.
2. Came to believe that a Power greater than themselves could restore us to sanity.
3. Made a decision to turn our will and our lives over to the care of God as we understood Him.
4. Made a searching and fearless moral inventory of ourselves.
5. Admitted to God, to ourselves, and to another human being the exact nature of our wrongs.
6. Were entirely ready to have God remove all these defects of character.
7. Humbly asked God to remove our shortcomings.
8. Made a list of those persons we had harmed and became willing to make amends to them all.
9. Made direct amends to such people wherever possible, except when to do so would injure them or others.

10. Continued to take personal inventory and when we were wrong, promptly admitted it.
11. Sought through prayer and meditation to improve our conscious contact with God, as *we understood Him*, praying only for knowledge of His will for us and the power to carry that out.
12. Having had a spiritual awakening as the result of these steps, we tried to carry this message to alcoholics, and to practice these principles in all our affairs. (www.alcoholics-anonymous.org/)

Since its founding, many other twelve-step programs have used AA's principles to treat other kinds of problems. These programs are for people with other types of addictive behavior, such as eating disorders (Overeaters Anonymous), sexual promiscuity (Sex Addicts Anonymous), and gambling (Gamblers Anonymous). In addition, there is Alanon, which is for spouses and families of addicts, Co-Dependents Anonymous (Co-DA) for people who find themselves in codependent relationships, and Incest Survivors Anonymous (ISA) for people who have survived incest.

Support Groups **Support groups** comprise people who all share common problems and issues. Sometimes these groups are led by counselors who facilitate group discussions. The focus is usually on current daily living problems that are often the result of deeper problems. Some support groups are led by volunteers, paraprofessionals, or members who take turns leading the discussions, such as with Compassionate Friends, a group for parents who have lost a child to death, or Breast Friends, for breast cancer survivors.

Example 1: A 20-year-old woman is raped by a friend of her brother. She is scared to press charges but wants to talk about the rape with people that she doesn't know. The rape crisis hotline refers her to a local support group. A volunteer counselor runs the group for women who have been raped by an acquaintance.

Example 2: A counselor has about four women in their late 70s who are all depressed and feeling lonely since their husbands died. She decides to start a support group where they would all come to see her at the same time instead of individually so they could share their common feelings with each other. One of the positive outcomes of this support group was that some of the women decided to start a bridge club. Some began to meet at the local mall to walk in the mornings.

HMOs **Health maintenance organizations** (HMOs) are a special breed of assessment and intervention model. Originally, their main focus was on keeping families healthy and providing early intervention when a family member became ill to prevent the need for long-term care. HMOs have existed since the early 1900s but have received more impetus for growth since the passage of the Health Maintenance Organization Act of 1973, which was considered a building block in a national system for maintaining health rather than a system for treating illnesses (DeLeon, Uyeda, & Welch, 1985). Recent estimates put the number of Americans enrolled in HMOs at well over 50 million. HMOs provide specific health services to enrollees for a prepaid, fixed payment. If the HMOs can find ways to keep enrollees healthy rather than providing them the various health services to which their payments entitle them, the HMOs stand to profit considerably. Keeping enrollees healthy sounds like an admirable goal; however, many therapists and physicians complain that their decisions about who needs services and for how long are being micromanaged by HMOs. The policies mandated by an HMO often reduce the autonomy by which many mental health workers typically practice. Because people pay less for HMO mental health services, private practice clinicians may feel in competition with HMOs. Some HMOs are located in a particular building as is often the case with the HMO called Kaiser Permanente. Patients, whether they're being treated for medical or psychiatric problems or receiving preventive educational services, all go to the same building for services. Other HMOs contract with individual providers who service patients at their own offices. Although clients are seen at various locations, all providers must follow the policies and practices of the HMO. This includes filling out specific forms, obtaining authorization to treat people, and providing justification for treatment.

Despite some of the complaints by providers about losing autonomy, HMO involvement has increased knowledge about how mental health practitioners other than physicians play a vital role in the overall care of many multineed clients. HMOs tend to operate within the multidisciplinary team model because of the variety of providers contracted with an HMO. Providers have access to the names of specialists and may refer their own clients to those who have contracted with the HMO. Not only is it easier for physicians to call on mental health clinicians to aid in treating various medical conditions, but mental health clinicians also may have easier access to physicians to aid in the biological components of emotional conditions (Tulkin & Frank, 1985).

The line separating patients' physical health from their emotional health has grown thinner since medical doctors began working closely with psychotherapists within HMO systems. The role of the psychotherapist within that system may be seen as that of a behavioral medicine specialist rather than merely a psychotherapist as mental health providers do so much more than simply provide psychotherapy. This phenomenon is a function of the growing evidence that 60 percent of visits to physicians are really to treat emotional problems (DeLeon, Uyeda, & Welch, 1985). Including mental health providers in the traditional physicians' world has reduced medical costs because mental health clinicians are trained to treat emotional problems more successfully than general physicians are (Herr & Cramer, 1987). HMOs also allow a variety of clinicians to collaborate on the needs of an entire family and not exclusively on an individual's needs.

HMO policies have encouraged mental health practitioners to create treatment models that are brief and cost effective. Clinicians who have been trained in long-term models, such as psychoanalysis, often object to limits being put on them by insurance policy makers. HMO policy has dramatically affected how mental health providers work with clients. Crisis intervention skills, family therapy models, and cognitive behavioral models have come in handy for providers contracting with HMOs because they are usually short-term models that effectively help clients within 20 weeks. Some mental health providers still object to cost effectiveness being the ruler of mental health treatment, but it is, for now, a huge reality in the provision of mental health services.

HMOs usually have services available for many complaints. They have educational groups, support groups, individual therapy, family therapy, and medication services. Additionally, most HMO plans are contracted with psychiatric hospitals and partial hospitalization services. Most of the human services workers employed by HMOs are licensed therapists, such as licensed clinical social workers (LCSWs), licensed marital and family therapists, psychologists, and psychiatrists. Some interns may also be employed. HMO hospitals often employ medical social workers to assist with patient discharge plans and other social issues.

Macro Level

Macro level focuses on creating new community-based programs and new legislation and policy. This will be discussed in Chapter 12.

Specific Types of Treatment

Both micro- and mezzo-level services are provided in a variety of locations by a variety of human services workers. Case managers should understand these services in order to be better able to conduct an effective **assessment** of the client's needs and offer referrals and support to clients. These services may be aimed to help people going through an emergency or a crisis (**secondary intervention**) or to help people manage long-standing problems (**tertiary intervention**).

In all cases of assessment and decisions regarding treatment plans, human services workers must assess all the needs of an individual or of a group, decide which type of intervention is most appropriate, and then assist them in accessing services to meet the needs or to personally provide services to meet the needs. Knowledge of various interventions is vital when assessing a client's needs as it guides the human services worker through the assessment and subsequent referral process. Also, human services workers often work collaboratively with others to best meet the needs of clients, and so the assessment process includes considering which community agencies and which types of human services workers should be involved in the case. Assessment includes determining the needs of a client and the appropriate services to meet those needs.

Assessing needs can be quite tricky, especially when needs are comprehensive, multifaceted, and personal. As noted by Maslow's Hierarchy of Needs, people need to have their most basic needs (physiological needs like air, food, water, and sleep) met before they can begin to obtain higher order needs, including safety (e.g., safe living conditions and financial opportunities), social (e.g., community connection), esteem (e.g., self-respect and reputation), and self-actualization (e.g., truth and sense of wisdom). It is critical for a human services worker to ensure the appropriate need is being met first. The second author recalls working with a therapist while struggling with postpartum depression and being asked what her relationship was like with her mother—a higher order need. In retrospect, what should have been ascertained first was whether or not she was getting sleep following the birth of her baby—a key factor in the cause of the depression. Additionally, sometimes it is difficult for clients to verbalize or assert their needs. Sometimes the clients' needs range from extreme to minimal. While human services workers cannot ever assume what is needed, strong communication skills and research-based knowledge can assist the worker to navigate through the assessment process.

Outpatient Treatment Outpatient treatment usually refers to private or group counseling held at an agency or a therapist's office. Sessions usually take place once a week for about one or two hours at a time. The client continues to work and live at home during this treatment.

Example 1: A 28-year-old man begins seeing a psychologist because he's been very depressed and having trouble concentrating at work after his girlfriend of two years broke up with him. His therapy focuses on his loss and how to deal with being alone. He participates in therapy for the next eight weeks and begins to socialize more, concentrate better at work, and feels less depressed. He spent most of the time expressing his feelings and talking about what went wrong in his last relationship.

Example 2: An 18-year-old woman sets up an appointment to attend educational and support groups at a nonprofit agency that helps women who are recovering from substance abuse. Groups are run by marriage and family therapy (MFT) interns who are supervised by licensed MFTs. She attends weekly, hour-long educational and support groups. Because she is unemployed, she can only pay the minimum of $8 for each group. After 16 weeks of group counseling, she gets a job and terminates her participation in the groups. Of course, she continues going to AA meetings, which she intends to do for many years to come (tertiary prevention).

Partial Hospitalization, Day Treatment, and Daycare Some recipients of human services need treatment more frequently than once a week. Instead, they need daily programs in which they participate in various groups and receive services, such as lunch and medical exams. These clients usually live at home under the care or supervision of their family when they're not at their day-treatment facilities. Clients who participate in **partial hospitalization, daycare, or day-treatment** services have various difficulties, such as people with Alzheimer's disease who have become dangerous to themselves when home alone and those who are severely depressed and need supervision because they are suicidal. If the setting of service is a hospital, the intervention is referred to as partial hospitalization because the patient sleeps at home and doesn't attend on weekends. Day-treatment programs may occur at hospitals or other centers and clinics, but basically include a full day of group activities and lunch.

Example 1: A 58-year-old woman has been at high risk for suicide. She was recently released from a psychiatric hospital after a three-day involuntary hospitalization following a suicide attempt. Because she still has suicidal ideations, she and her psychiatrist believe she needs intensive treatment but feel comfortable with her sleeping and eating dinner at home with her husband who is willing to monitor her for suicidal behaviors. The client attends various educational and support groups at a hospital from 8 a.m. until 5 p.m. She eats lunch at the hospital but goes home before dinner. She attends these groups Monday through Saturday for the next six weeks until her suicidal ideation disappears.

Example 2: A group of people diagnosed with schizophrenia attend a variety of groups run by mental health workers at a local community mental health agency from 9 in the morning until 5 in the evening, after which they return to their board-and-care homes to eat dinner and sleep.

Example 3: A 78-year-old man suffering from Alzheimer's disease has begun to wander when left alone at home. Both of his grown children must work all day but can afford to have him go to a daycare program where he participates in various social and occupational groups from 7 a.m. until 6 p.m. His daughter and son take turns picking him up at the daycare center. He eats dinner and sleeps at one of his children's homes at night. The children alternate taking care of him so neither gets too burnt out from caretaking responsibilities.

Inpatient Treatment This type of treatment involves a client being admitted to a hospital or other **residential facility**. An aim of **inpatient treatment** is to protect clients from harming themselves and others and to ensure clients' basic needs, such as eating and medical care, are provided. They receive intensive group and individual therapy, medications, and often participate in a therapeutic milieu model in which the entire hospital program is aimed at changing behaviors. Some clients function at such low levels that they remain hospitalized permanently, although this approach is not considered fiscally sound. Others are released from inpatient care and referred to board-and-care homes, to their families, or to partial hospitalization or daycare programs after a two- to four-week stay at the hospital.

Example: A 45-year-old woman has been excessively self-mutilating and recently told her therapist that she was going to kill herself. Because she refused to be hospitalized, she was involuntarily admitted to a psychiatric hospital. She stayed in the hospital for the next six weeks, attending group and individual therapy and taking new medications. Because her suicidal ideation was not subsiding, she stayed longer than the usual length of treatment.

Residential Treatment Facilities, Halfway Houses, and Board-and-Care Homes Certain facilities provide housing and therapeutic care for a variety of clients who have serious problems and are at risk for severe deterioration in functioning if they do not have daily monitoring and care. They may live in the halfway house for six months to two years. During their stay at residential facilities and halfway houses, clients are usually required to participate in group and individual counseling. They often receive job-skills training as well as social-skills training by human services workers who do not live at the facility but rather work in three different shifts to provide 24-hour supervision.

Board-and-care homes are privately owned homes that usually house up to six residents who are provided with food and shelter. The board-and-care owners monitor the taking of medications and contact professionals if clients appear to be deteriorating. Some clients live in board-and-care homes for the rest of their lives. Others, such as abused children, might live in a foster home for one to two years while their parents complete a rehabilitation program. Although the owners of the board-and-care homes and foster homes do not provide counseling services, they often work with counselors to ensure continuity of care for clients. For older adults, board-and-care homes also provide support with instrumental activities of daily living (IADLs) such as grocery shopping and preparing meals, as well as activities of daily living (ADLs) such as bathing and eating.

Example 1: A 32-year-old man was recently released from prison after serving three years for first-offense drug trafficking. Because he had been a model prisoner, he was let out on good behavior two years before his sentence was up. The judge ordered him to live in a halfway house for those two years so he might have a stable environment to learn job skills, learn new social skills, and receive counseling for his substance abuse problems.

Example 2: A 39-year-old woman recovering from methamphetamine addiction applied to live at Phoenix House, a well-known residential facility for recovering addicts. This environment allowed her to stay sober, learn job skills, learn basic independent living skills, and participate in counseling. She stayed for one year until she got a job and had more confidence in her ability to stay sober.

Example 3: A 70-year-old woman with Alzheimer's disease receives necessary supportive and health care services in her home-like board-and-care facility where she lives with five other residents who also suffer from dementia.

Take a few moments now to reflect on a few questions listed below:

Critical Thinking/Self-Reflection Corner

- What are your feelings about a career as a case manager?
- Do you believe that most mental health providers could treat clients appropriately and effectively without administrative watchdogs?
- What are your own experiences in being a patient at an HMO?

SPECIFIC TASKS OF CASE MANAGERS

The Intake Process

An initial assessment is often referred to as an **intake**. The initial assessment is typically recorded on an intake form provided by the agency. The information gathered on an intake form varies from agency to agency and from profession to profession. In general, an intake interview may be conducted by phone, or it may be conducted in person. An intake interview may be conducted by a worker who will continue to provide ongoing services to the client, or a designated intake worker may conduct nothing but intake interviews. The purpose of an intake interview is to get a brief idea of the reasons the client is seeking services. Demographic information, nature of the problem, and history of similar problems is typically assessed during an intake interview and recorded on an intake form. A few examples from different types of agencies are presented here. Corresponding figures provide sample forms that are commonly used at agencies during intakes.

Examples of Intake Assessments at Various Agencies

Intake Assessments Example 1: Suicide Hotlines Workers who answer hotline calls usually make their intake assessments by phone. Hotline workers may use a specific form for gathering intake information and ask the client questions to record on the form. Of course, not every caller is willing to provide all the information asked for, but a counselor can at least try to get the information. Figure 11.1 provides an example of an intake form from a suicide hotline.

Intake Assessments Example 2: Child-Protective Services Most communities have standard child-abuse reporting forms that are completed prior to calling the information in to a child-protective services worker. Social workers receiving the call complete their own version of an intake form that includes the information in the child-abuse report that the caller will eventually send to the department of social welfare (see Figure 11.2).

FIGURE 11.1 A suicide-prevention hotline's sample intake information

Name (if possible) _____   phone number (if possible) _____

Date and time _____

Are you having suicidal thoughts? Yes _____   No _____

Do you have a plan? Yes _____   No _____

Do you have the means? Yes _____   No _____

Have you ever attempted suicide? Yes _____   No _____

Have you ever been treated for emotional problems? Yes _____   No _____
If so, who were you seeing? _____

Are you still in treatment? Yes _____   No _____

Name of therapist (if different from previously named) _____

Are you taking any medication? Yes _____   No _____   What type? _____

What is stopping you from committing the act? _____

Will you make a commitment with me not to harm yourself? Yes _____   No _____

Will you follow up with a therapist? Yes _____   No _____

Referrals given _____

Follow-up plan _____

© Cengage Learning

FIGURE 11.2 Child protective services' sample intake information

Party making the report: Name/title _____

Address _____

Phone _____ Date of report _____

Party receiving the report: police department, sheriff's office, county welfare, or county probation

Address of receiving party: _____

Official contacted: _____

Phone number: _____

Date and time of report: _____

Victim(s): Name, address, birth date, sex, race, present location of child, phone number

_____

_____

Siblings of victim: Name, birth date, sex, race

_____

_____

Parents of victims: Names, birthdates, sex, race, address, phone numbers

_____

_____

Date/time of incident: _____

Place of incident: _____

Type of abuse: _____

Narrative description/summary of what the abused child or person accompanying the child said happened: _____

Known history of similar incidents for this child: _____

Digital Download — Download at CengageBrain.com

Intake Assessments Example 3: Battered Women's Shelters   An initial intake that comes in through a shelter's hotline is answered by an advocate worker who asks callers a variety of questions to ascertain whether they are eligible for acceptance into the shelter or to provide referral information when they are not. Figure 11.3 is an example of the questions on a typical intake form.

Intake Assessments Example 4: Outpatient Mental Health Clinic   If clients have HMO insurance, they will probably phone the HMO plan and speak with an intake worker who will gather brief information to properly refer the client to the best counselor. If clients seek mental health services from nonprofit agencies, community mental health services, or from private practitioners, they will most likely be asked to complete a brief intake form before their first appointment (see Figure 11.4).

FIGURE 11.3   A battered women's shelter's sample intake information

Name: _____

Location: _____

Number of children and ages: _____

Are you currently in danger? _____

When was the last abusive episode? _____

What happened? _____

Have you ever been to a shelter to escape abuse? _____

When and where? _____

Are you being treated by a psychiatrist or therapist? Yes _____   No _____

Name of therapist _____   For how long? _____

What medications are you taking? _____

Do you use drugs or alcohol? _____   How much? _____   For how long? _____

Are you employed? _____

Do you have access to any money? _____

Do you need to leave now? _____

Tentative Plan _____

> **FIGURE 11.4** An outpatient mental-health clinic's sample intake information
>
> Name: _____
>
> Date of Birth: _____
>
> Social security #: _____
>
> Address: _____ Phone: _____
>
> Insurance: _____
>
> Physician name and address: _____
>
> Previous mental-health treatment? _____
>
> By whom? _____ When? _____
>
> Presenting problems: _____
>
> History of similar problems: _____
>
> Informed Consent: (this part explains to clients their rights to voluntary treatment, voluntary termination, any risks involved in treatment, fees, cancellation policy, and confidentiality rights. This section should explain that a counselor is mandated to report abusive behavior to children, elders, disabled-adults, and dangerous behavior to others. Clients should also be made aware that the counselor may breach confidentiality if a client becomes suicidal).

Digital Download Download at CengageBrain.com

Once an intake session is conducted, workers begin the process of developing a plan for intervention.

Treatment Planning

Most human services agencies require workers to complete formal treatment plans. These plans may be written on a form provided by the agency, or in some cases, workers may merely write up their version of the treatment plan. Some agencies might refer to these treatment plans as **case plans**. An effective treatment plan includes clear and specific needs and problems to be worked with, goals and objectives, interventions, and timelines for completion of the plan. Human services workers should include as many interventions as are available in the plan. In this way, the clients have a better chance of achieving their goals. Figures 11.5 and 11.6 provide sample treatment plans for a mental health agency and child protective services, respectively.

FIGURE 11.5   A mental health treatment plan

Name of client: Jane Doe

Intake Date: 03/27/2006

Symptoms/Complaints	Goals	Interventions	Proposed timeline
Uncontrollable crying daily	Reduce crying	Refer to psychiatrist	4 weeks to once a week
Suicidal ideation	Eliminate S.I.	Crisis intervention Verbal no suicide contract	2 weeks
Feels hopeless and worthless	Increase feelings of hope and self-esteem	Cognitive therapy	4 weeks
Conflicts with husband and children	Learn more productive communication	Family therapy	4 weeks

<u>Multiaxial Diagnosis per DSM IV–R</u>
AXIS I: Major Depression, recurrent, moderate
AXIS II: No personality disorder noted
AXIS III: No physical illness related
AXIS IV: Occupational stress, conflicts with husband and children
AXIS V: Current GAS- 55 Highest in past year- 75

Progress Notes

In addition to treatment and case plans, human services workers must also maintain ongoing **progress notes** for every client. These notes not only help workers remember each case and each session with clients but also serve as a form of protection for workers. Proper documentation should include information that demonstrates ethical and competent practice. Notes should be written in an organized manner as well as clearly and objectively. These notes provide continuity in the care of clients. Continuity of care is essential because many times new workers take over the case from a previous worker, or clients transfer to different areas. Having detailed information about a client's treatment with one worker is helpful for another worker who may be called upon to provide services to the client for different problems as well. The progress notes also help the client and worker see when a client has completed the plan and no longer needs services. Finally, many funding agencies, such as Medicare, require certain information in a client's chart to provide proof that appropriate services are being

FIGURE 11.6 Child protective services case plan

Mother's Name: Jane Doe

Minor's names: Johnny Doe, 5/13/95; Chelsea Doe, 8/6/98; Heather Doe, 10/23/2002

Date of alleged abuse/neglect: 04/05/2005-04/05/2006

Name of alleged perpetrator: James Doe

Description of abuse: Chelsea Doe claims that from approximately April 2005 until April of 2006 her father, James fondled her genital area every day after school. She claims that her mother was working during these abusive episodes and that he would take her into his room and abuse her on her parent's bed. Johnny denies that he was ever molested. After a careful examination of Heather, it does not appear that she was victimized either.

Case plan: James Doe must move out of the family home and lose all custody and visitation rights with all three minors until such time that all case plan requirements are fulfilled. James must participate in group therapy at Parent's United for a minimum of 1 year before any visitations are allowed. James must participate in individual therapy once per week for one year. James will enroll in a 16-week parenting class. James may not talk with the children by phone until such time that the children's counselors state that it would be appropriate.

   Jane Doe may maintain custody of all three minors if she fulfills all conditions of this case plan. Jane may not allow James to enter the family home. Jane must attend an educational and support group for non-perpetrating parents approved by CPS. Jane must participate in family counseling with her children. Jane must ensure her children attend individual therapy as recommended by their counselors.

   Chelsea Doe must participate in individual therapy as long as recommended by her counselor. She must see a therapist who specializes in the treatment of child sexual abuse. Chelsea will participate in family counseling as recommended by the counselor.

   Johnny Doe will be seen by a therapist for an evaluation to ascertain whether he needs individual therapy. He will participate in family therapy as needed.

   Heather Doe will participate in counseling if she begins to show any signs of having been molested or exhibits any other emotional problems.

   This case plan will remain in effect for the next year at which time it will be reviewed and revised.

FIGURE 11.7 An example of a progress note

Clinician: Dr. Kristi Kanel, MFT

Client: John Doe

Date of service: 05/16/06

Type of Service: Individual therapy

S: Client complains of feeling very sad this week. He is having difficulty letting go of his wife. He can't think about anything else but her leaving him. He says he alternates between being sad and enraged. He calls her everyday, but she doesn't wish to talk with him. He says his work performance is affected. He speaks exclusively about his wife and his feelings of loneliness without her. He denies feelings suicidal and has no plan to do anything self-destructive. He is devoted to his children.

O: Client is teary while he speaks. His eyes look very tired and he speaks slowly. His affect is congruent with the content of his verbalizations.

A: Client continues to grieve the loss of his wife. His denial about the loss is lifting, and so he is more in touch with sadness and anger.

P: Client should continue taking the antidepressant medication prescribed by his physician. Client will continue with weekly counseling focusing on leaning how to adjust to life without his wife and how to put his energy into being a father. Will consider referral to a support group.

Digital Download — Download at CengageBrain.com

provided for appropriate problems. Figure 11.7 is an example of a widely accepted form of progress notes referred to as **SOAP**.

The SOAP Method of Progress Reports

- S=subjective: This refers to the subjective view of the client. The workers documents what the client says during an interview.
- O=objective: This refers to the worker's objective view of the client's state. The human services worker often describes emotions observed, interpersonal behaviors, hygiene, and other information seen from the worker's point of view.
- A=assessment: Human services workers document their own analysis of the client's needs and progress at this point. The worker may describe a theoretical analysis as well.

- P=plan: Specific interventions are presented here along with the reason for the plan. This may include referrals, medications, and other interventions described earlier in this chapter.

Keep in mind that many agencies provide their own forms for documentation. Human services workers are typically trained on how to complete required paperwork.

Report Writing

Writing formal **reports** is an important skill for human services workers in all agencies. Some reports will be written for reviews by judges. Others will be written to collaborating human services workers to enhance multidisciplinary team work. Written reports should be organized under specific headings and be written in neutral and succinct language. Many human services students have been trained to write formal essays in college. This essay format is not how reports are typically written, however. While there is much variance in how a report should be written, there are some general rules about how to proceed. Hollis and Donn (1980) have developed a framework for a variety of reports that human services workers generally write. Of course, there is not just one way to write a report. How and what is written will depend on the purpose of the report from the writer's point of view as well as the purpose from the recipient of the report's point of view. According to Hollis and Donn, some of the purposes for writing reports include:

1. Requesting assistance from another person
2. Receiving a request from another person
3. Making referrals
4. Developing conjoint and consultative reports
5. Adding information to existing records
6. Obtaining objective data
7. Obtaining objective data plus interpretations
8. Obtaining diagnostic information
9. Obtaining recommendations
10. Obtaining progress report
11. Obtaining preliminary report
12. Recording baseline information
13. Summarizing psychological support information
14. Reporting research studies
15. Reporting for legal purposes
16. Periodic summary reports
17. Agency reports associated with professional activities
18. Special reports (may be associated with grant writing or funding issues) (Hollis & Dunn, 1980, pp. 6–15).

> **FIGURE 11.8** Topics included in recommendation reports
>
> **Identifying Data:**
>   Identification of person to whom report is sent
>   Identification of person about whom report is written
>   Identification of person writing report
>   Report Title
>   Date of examination(s)
>
> **Behavioral Symptoms and Characteristics:**
>   Symptoms observed directly by the therapist
>   Symptoms reported by others
>   Symptoms reported directly by client
>   Client's relationship to the environment
>
> **Other Characteristics:**
>   Physical characteristics of the client
>   Organic concomitants of the disorder
>
> **Summary**
>
> **Diagnosis**
>
> **Recommendations:**
>   Environmental changes
>   Treatment Procedures
>
> **Anticipated length of treatment**
>
> **Prognosis**
>   With the recommendations followed as given in the report
>   Without treatment

Digital Download — Download at CengageBrain.com

The format for a report varies, but it should generally be written in an objective manner with little embellishment. In other words, reports should not look like literary works. They are correspondences constructed to provide specific information. Many reports are written with the purpose of providing the receiver a recommendation about the client. At times a psychologist may write a report to recommend that a parent maintain or lose custody of a child. Sometimes, mental health clinicians write reports to probation officers and the court to recommend that a client remain on probation, go to prison, or be released. Some reports are written to help school officials develop a treatment plan for a learning-disabled child. Figure 11.8 provides some typical topics for consideration in making a recommendation report.

Think about some of the questions in the Critical Thinking/Self-reflection Corner.

> ### Critical Thinking/Self-Reflection Corner
> - Why are detailed progress notes and treatment or case plans vital to the provision of human services?
> - What are your initial reactions to the idea of report writing?
> - How is a report written by a human services worker similar to and different from a typical book report?

CHAPTER SUMMARY

Case management is a process in which a case manager coordinates a case. This may include referrals to other professionals, collaborating on treatment, writing reports and case notes, or providing direct service such as counseling. Case managers should be familiar with macro-, mezzo-, and micro-level interventions for a variety of populations and in a variety of locations. Micro level focuses on individual services, mezzo level focuses on groups and families, and macro level focuses on community intervention and policies. Interventions occur in outpatient offices and agencies and in inpatient facilities such as hospitals and residential agencies and may be offered throughout the day, evening, or both.

Suggested Applied Activities

1. Watch a movie or television show. Select a character who might seek the assistance of a human services worker due to emotional problems, poverty, child abuse, domestic violence, criminality, substance abuse, etc. Write out a mock treatment plan or case plan for the character.

Chapter Review Questions

1. What does HMO stand for?

   _____

   _____

2. What is the nature of a twelve-step program?

   _____

   _____

3. Who might live in a halfway house?

4. What type of clients might benefit from hospitalization?

5. What is the difference between micro-, mezzo-, and macro-level interventions?

6. What are the typical duties of a case manager?

Glossary of Terms

Assessment is a process in which human services workers interview a client or the client's family to gather information about the needs of the client. The purpose of an assessment is to determine what intervention strategies should be implemented.

Board-and-care homes are private homes that usually house about six residents who are disabled physically or mentally. The operators of the homes receive money from each resident. Residents typically receive government support because of their disability. The homes distribute medications, provide food and supervision, and assist with transportation needs.

Case plan is a written document that specifies the problems assessed which need addressing and intervention plans.

Health maintenance organization (HMO) is a privately funded agency in which medical, psychological, optical, and even dental needs may be serviced through a family's insurance plan.

Inpatient treatment usually refers to a hospital setting where clients reside and receive various treatments, such as group therapy, medication monitoring, and individual therapy. Because of the high cost of a hospital stay, this type of treatment is usually reserved only for people who are a danger to others or to themselves.

Intake is a first-assessment interview that establishes what the client's needs are and possible interventions.

Macro level refers to the focus on community organizations and creating new policies.

Medication refers to any psychotropic drug prescribed to stabilize a client's mood, reduce anxiety, manage impulsive behaviors, or lessen psychotic symptoms.

Mezzo level is a level of intervention that focuses on working with groups and families.

Micro level is a level of intervention that deals with individuals.

Outpatient is a type of intervention in which clients receive treatment at an agency or in an office. This is most suited for people who can function in society appropriately.

Partial hospitalization, daycare, and day treatment are programs for clients who don't need to live in a hospital but who benefit from group therapy and individual therapy for several hours a day at a hospital.

Prognosis refers to the potential outcome of a problem—the chances of a problem being resolved satisfactorily or unsatisfactorily.

Progress notes are the written summary of a session in which a worker officially documents the services provided.

Reports are written for various purposes by human services workers to communicate a variety of aspects of a client's situation.

Residential facilities usually house about 8 to 20 people, all of whom are dealing with a common issue or problem, such as parolees, drug addicts, or battered women. Counselors, caseworkers, psychiatrists, and employment advocates usually work with these clients to help them transition back into society.

Secondary intervention is a type of intervention that attempts to treat emergency situations and problems that are not chronic. The aim is to prevent a client's problem from becoming chronic.

SOAP is a method of writing progress notes in which a worker documents the subjective statements of the client, the objective observations of the worker, the worker's assessment of the client's needs, and the plan of action.

Support groups are typically led by counselors and focus on helping group members increase self-esteem and feelings of empowerment and decrease feelings of social isolation.

Tertiary interventions are aimed at helping people adapt to their long-standing problems. People with chronic problems often need some form of intervention throughout their lives.

Twelve-step programs are groups that use the twelve-step approach to recovery, of which Alcoholics Anonymous was the first. These groups seem to be one of the most effective methods for people with addictions to maintain their sobriety. They are considered mutual self-help groups and are not led by professional counselors.

Case Presentation and Exit Quiz

General Description and Demographics

Jim is an 18-year-old male who is single and living with his parents. Jim has never held a job but has graduated from high school. During the summer after graduation, he began having feelings of overwhelming anxiety and depression. He told his parents that he felt people were out to hurt him and were always talking about him. Jim stopped leaving the house and mostly stayed in his room watching television. When he did come out to eat, he would usually talk about a buzzing sound in his room and that his television was broadcasting special messages to him. Jim told his mother that he sometimes wants to kill himself because he can't stand being so depressed.

Jim's mother arranges for Jim to talk to their longtime family physician, Dr. Rogers. Jim and his mother tell Dr. Rogers about Jim's complaints, which he's had for the past three months. Dr. Rogers refers Jim to a colleague of his, Dr. Jones, who is a psychiatrist.

Dr. Jones meets with Jim and his mother. Dr. Jones inquires about Jim's feelings of wanting to kill himself. Jim says that he has a plan to do it but does not have the means. Jim says that he hears a voice telling him that he would feel better if he could just shoot himself with a silver bullet because that would get rid of the demons inside him. Jim, however, doesn't have a gun or access to one. Jim tells the doctor that if he could just feel better, he wouldn't want to kill himself.

Jim denies using any drugs or alcohol. He has no friends and no hobbies. He is beginning to argue with his father over just about everything. Jim yells sometimes but doesn't remember the fights. Jim is afraid that something is wrong with him, but he doesn't know what it could be. Dr. Jones discovers that Jim began hearing voices two years ago, but Jim never told anyone.

Dr. Jones's Treatment Plan

Dr. Jones prescribes Haldol, an antipsychotic medication, and suggests that Jim start taking it immediately. He also refers Jim to a social worker who works at the same HMO as Dr. Jones. The social worker will consult with Dr. Jones about how to proceed.

Assessment by the Social Worker

John Madison, a licensed clinical social worker, meets with Jim and his mother. John discusses Jim's history with them. John also asks about Jim's social relationships, school performance, suicidal feelings and history of suicidal ideation, and symptoms and complaints. John writes up his session as follows.

Social Worker's Progress Notes

Jim is an 18-year-old male who complains of depression, anxiety, and loneliness. For the past two years, he has been hearing voices, which have gotten stronger the summer after he graduated from high school. He says the voices tell him that to feel better he should shoot himself with a silver bullet to rid himself of the demon inside. Jim denies having access to a gun and seems motivated to feel better. He reports various delusions, such as feeling like the television is talking directly to him. He also experiences delusions of reference, such as believing that everyone is talking about him when he goes out in public. Jim has been unable to work because of his anxiety and depression. He has begun to fight frequently with his father but doesn't remember doing so.

Jim was cooperative during the interview but lacked emotional expression or humor. He was anxious and at times expressed himself in a confused, disorganized manner.

Jim is showing symptoms of paranoid schizophrenia. Although Jim has some stress in his life, such as graduating from school and having no job or money for himself, these stresses do not appear to be causing his symptoms.

Jim will continue taking the Haldol prescribed by Dr. Jones. I will refer Jim to the day-treatment center at St. Joseph's Hospital, which is covered by his medical insurance. I will oversee his treatment there and serve as case manager while he attends various support groups, educational groups, employment training groups, and socialization groups.

Symptoms	Treatment Plan	Duration
Hearing voices, delusional	Medication prescribed by Dr. Jones	Indefinitely
Depression	Case management, medication, socialization groups at day treatment	Indefinitely 6 months to 1 year
Suicidal ideation	Case management, medication, crisis intervention	Indefinitely 6 months to 1 year
Bored, inactive	Various groups at day treatment	As needed

John Madison's Treatment Plan

Symptoms	Treatment Plan	Duration
Hearing voices, delusional	Medication prescribed by Dr. Jones	Indefinitely
Depression	Case management, medication	Indefinitely
	Socialization groups at day treatment	6 months to 1 year
Suicidal ideation	Case management, medication	Indefinitely
	Crisis intervention, case management	As needed
Bored, inactive	Various groups at day treatment	6 months to 1 year

Exit Quiz

1. At this stage in Jim's life, his schizophrenic symptoms can be considered
    a. chronic
    b. severe
    c. unmanageable
    d. all of the above

2. The treatment plans designed by all of the workers fall into which category?
    a. Primary prevention
    b. Secondary prevention
    c. Tertiary prevention
    d. None of the above

3. Jim's suicidal risk is most likely
    a. low
    b. high
    c. middle
    d. no risk at all

4. When John Madison writes that Jim was cooperative during the interview but lacked emotional expression or humor, which part of the SOAP method of writing notes was this?
   a. Subjective
   b. Objective
   c. Assessment
   d. Plan

5. When John writes that Jim's symptoms of schizophrenia are probably not related to stress, John was addressing which part of the SOAP model?
   a. Subjective
   b. Objective
   c. Assessment
   d. Plan

6. When John describes Jim as saying that the voices tell him that to feel better, he should shoot himself with a silver bullet, which part of the SOAP model is he addressing?
   a. Subjective
   b. Objective
   c. Assessment
   d. Plan

7. According to John's treatment plan, which statement is most accurate?
   a. Jim will live in the day-treatment center for 1 year.
   b. Jim will attend outpatient psychotherapy.
   c. Jim will live with his parents while attending groups during the day.
   d. None of the above.

Exit Quiz Answers

1. b
2. c
3. b
4. b
5. c
6. a
7. c

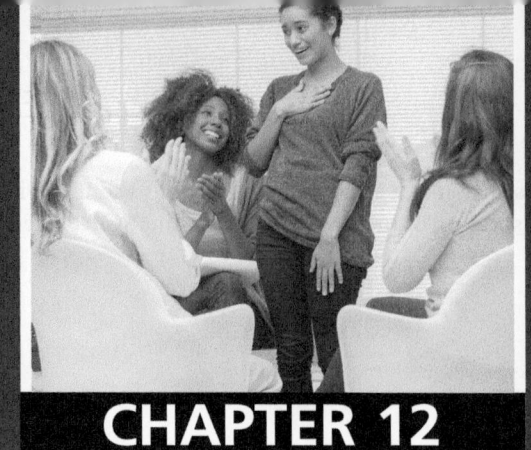

CHAPTER 12

Macro-Level Practice

INTRODUCTION

Macro-level practice is a broad term, but it tends to incorporate several activities, including working with communities and organizations, such as nonprofit agencies and public agencies; engaging in social welfare administration and research; and working with groups for social reform. This can include examining major social issues, policies, and organizational structures. According to Brueggemann (1966), macro-level practitioners "try to correct social conditions that cause human suffering and misery ... They work to develop new programs and changes in policies" (p. 3). Kirst-Ashman and Hull (1993) describe macro-level practice as a process that focuses on changing or improving policies or procedures that regulate distribution of resources to clients, developing new resources when clients' needs cannot be met with available ones, and helping clients to obtain their due rights. Overall, macro-level practice is about intervening with organizations, communities, and groups of people (Meenaghan & Gibbons, 2000); it is not just, the "betterment of individuals and families," but also the "betterment of the mass" (Richmond, 1917, p. 25).

Some of the tasks involved in macro-level practice include supervising professional staff, working with communities to conduct **needs assessments**, participating in budgeting, writing **grants** and **proposals**, developing and implementing programs, and conducting program **evaluations**. Tasks often also include **community organizing** activities such as negotiating and bargaining with diverse groups, encouraging consumer participation in decision making, establishing and carrying out interagency agreements, and engaging in **advocacy** efforts for client needs. Societal or **policy**-related tasks are also often key; this involves group activities such as **coalition** building, **social action**, **lobbying**, testifying, tracking legislative developments that directly

> ### Anti-Bullying Programs for Elementary, Middle and High Schools
>
> Sadly, youth violence is becoming an increasing concern. Currently, it is the second leading cause of death for young people between the ages of 10 and 24. Due to this and the fact that youth violence is preventable, macro-level prevention efforts and strategies have been put into place to stop youth violence before it begins. For example, the website vetoviolence.cdc.org, developed for the Centers of Disease Control (CDC) health partners, practitioners, community leaders, school administrators, and every day citizens, provides invaluable resources, tools, training approaches, and success stories related to youth violence. Among its offerings is accredited training and resources for preventing bullying, gang violence, and peer violence. This organization is a perfect example of a macro-level response to a critical societal need.

affect clients, and carrying out efforts designed to effect legal and regulatory frameworks.

All of these activities are the foundation for the creation and development of new social programs, modification of existing programs, and elimination of obsolete or ineffective programs. In the field of human services, there is a never-ending need to meet the changing necessities of client populations. For example, in 1975, there was no need to create agencies that serviced clients suffering from AIDS-related problems because HIV/AIDS had not yet become a social problem. However, by the mid-1990s, many programs and legislation had been created to deal with this issue. Today, with significant demographic shifts (e.g., the increase of the older adult population and immigration) and other social issues (many of which are discussed in Chapter 7), new and innovative programs are becoming increasingly necessary. Read the Anti-Bullying Programs for Elementary, Middle, and High Schools box as an example.

Interestingly, with current technological innovations, many human services workers are using the Internet as a tool for engaging in macro-level work, such as promoting social change, raising awareness, and increasing communication between colleagues and partners (Hick & McNutt, 2002).

DEVELOPING PROGRAMS AND POLICIES

The following section describes actions related to creating, implementing, and evaluating programs. (Note: While macro-level practice also includes providing direct community intervention, such as during community disaster responses, this will be discussed in Chapter 6).

For the macro-level practitioner, the community is the client just as an individual is a client to the micro-level practitioner. A community has its own resources and limitations and coping mechanisms to deal with problems, and it must take responsibility for its actions just as an individual or family does (Homan, 1994). Macro-level practitioners engage in the process of examining these aspects of the community to assess its needs just as the micro-level practitioner examines an individual or family regarding these aspects when assessing their needs.

The first step in macro-level practice is conducting a needs assessment, which is the process of assessing and defining needs, opportunities, and resources involved in developing and implementing programs and interventions in the community. This "analysis is not done *on* the community but *with* the community" (Haglund, Weisbrod, & Bracht, 1990, p. 91). Community members and leaders are involved in the process to increase awareness, accountability, and ownership of the program. The assessment or analysis varies by community but often includes several of the following components: (1) general community profile, including collecting data on demographic factors (e.g., age, gender, and ethnicity of population), social factors (e.g., family structure, housing conditions, and education levels), and economic factors (e.g., employment rates and welfare benefits); (2) behavioral, social, and environmental risks or problems (such as social support systems and air quality); (3) a health or wellness profile; (4) current programs and their effectiveness; and (5) special studies of target groups (e.g., adolescents), and their awareness levels and perceived needs; and (6) community capacity (e.g., available resources). The macro-level practitioner will obtain this information by conducting interviews, developing and collecting data from surveys, collecting statistics from prior research, and engaging in data analysis, as well as thoroughly researching the background and history of the problem.

The data collected in the needs assessment are compiled and shared with the community leaders, professionals, board members, and the target population of the project. The second author participated in a community needs assessment years ago for a small town in Arizona. The community was struggling with a growing prevalence of teen pregnancies. After several months of conducting a needs assessment, interviewing residents of the community, including parents, teachers, community leaders, and the teenagers themselves, it was determined that the teens needed more after-school programming, mentorship, and leadership. The community responded by building a community center staffed with adult volunteers and peer mentors that offered after-school tutoring, weekend recreational programs, teen pregnancy prevention education, and support groups. A year later, the community was reassessed and significant positive changes were occurring, including reduced unwanted pregnancies.

If the project is going to be legislative change, coalition building is necessary. A coalition may be described as a "loosely developed association of constituent groups and organizations, each of whose primary identification is outside the coalition" (Netting, Kettner, & McMurtry, 1993, p. 113). Coalitions are vital when there is a need for action and cooperation. The coalition is able to present a strong voice in the pursuit of funding and legislative change. An example of a coalition to help pass an **initiative** for increased funding for schools might be made up of a national teachers' association, the national PTA association, and the police association. Overall, based on the research conducted and the feedback of the community, the macro-level workers decide whether their project will be part of an existing program, be a modification of an existing program, be a new agency, or need a new legislative policy. Often, lobbying is also necessary. Lobbying is a specialized form of persuasion that is central to most levels of government. Lobbyists seek access to lawmakers to influence policy making and decision making (Alle-Corliss & Alle-Corliss, 1999). For some social policy changes, lawmakers assume full responsibility in enacting legislative change. Other social policy changes are placed in the hands of voters. Certain social policy changes may be enacted if enough voters sign a petition to have the policy placed on an official ballot where voters have an opportunity to decide whether the policy should be passed. Election time is usually preceded by a media blitz in which backers (coalitions) of the initiative try to persuade voters to pass the proposal.

If the project is the creation of a new nonprofit agency or a new program at an existing agency, acquiring funding for the new program is the next process. This involves deciding on and building a budget and obtaining financial resources, such as through **fundraising** efforts through private donors, as well as through writing grants and proposals to appropriate governmental and/or foundation agencies. When these entities have funding, they issue **funding announcements**, often referred to as a request for application (RFA) or request for proposals (RFP). (See the box titled Program Brief for Grants to Encourage Arrest Policies and Enforcement of Protection Orders Program From the Office on Violence Against Women for an example of the qualifications and guidelines needed to apply for a grant from the Office on Violence Against Women).

Program Brief for Grants to Encourage Arrest Policies and Enforcement of Protection Orders Program from the Office on Violence against Women

The Grants to Encourage Arrest Policies and Enforcement of Protection Orders Program (Arrest Program) encourages jurisdictions to treat domestic violence as a serious violation of criminal law. The Arrest Program also promotes mandatory or pro-arrest policies as an effective domestic violence intervention that is part of a coordinated community response. Arrest should be one element in a comprehensive criminal justice system response to hold offenders accountable and enhance victim safety.

Arrest, accompanied by a thorough investigation and meaningful sanctions, demonstrates to offenders that they have committed a serious crime and communicates to victims of domestic violence that they do not have to endure an offender's abuse. Arrest should be followed by immediate arraignment and a thorough investigation. Orders of protection should be enforced, and cases should be vigorously prosecuted. Designated dockets can enhance the management of domestic violence cases and expedite the scheduling of trials. Frequent judicial oversight and the use of graduated sanctions can help courts monitor the behavior of domestic violence offenders. Probation and parole agencies should closely monitor offenders and strictly enforce the terms and conditions of probation or parole.

At each juncture in the criminal justice process, actions should be guided by concerns for victim safety. Mechanisms should be put in place to allow the voices and experiences of victims of domestic violence, particularly those who have sought assistance from the criminal justice system, to inform the development of policies. These mechanisms should ensure that the diverse experiences of victims

(Continued)

are considered—particularly the experiences of women of color, immigrant victims, the elderly, victims with disabilities, and victims from other traditionally underserved segments of the community.

Criminal justice agencies must collaborate among themselves and in respectful partnership with victim advocates from nonprofit, nongovernmental victim service agencies, including local shelters, victim advocacy organizations, and domestic violence coalitions, to ensure that victim safety is a paramount consideration in the development of any strategy to address domestic violence. Nonprofit, non-governmental agencies may include faith-based or community-based organizations. The Arrest Program challenges victim advocates, police officers, pretrial services personnel, prosecutors, judges and other court personnel, probation and parole officers, and community leaders to work together to craft solutions to respond to domestic violence.

Scope of Program

Ensuring victim safety and offender accountability are the guiding principles underlying the Arrest Program. The scope of this program includes the statutory program purposes and the special interest categories outlined below. Proposed projects need not address multiple program purposes or special interest categories to receive support.

The Violence Against Women Act of 2000 directs that Program funds be used to:

- Implement mandatory arrest or pro-arrest programs and policies in police departments, including mandatory or pro-arrest programs and policies for protection order violations.
- Develop policies, educational programs, and training in police departments to improve tracking of cases involving domestic violence and dating violence.
- Centralize and coordinate police enforcement, prosecution, or judicial responsibility for domestic violence cases in groups or units of police officers, prosecutors, probation and parole officers, or judges.
- Coordinate computer tracking systems to ensure communication between police, prosecutors, parole and probation officers, and both criminal and family courts.
- Strengthen legal advocacy service programs for victims of domestic violence and dating violence, including strengthening assistance to such victims in immigration matters.
- Educate judges in criminal and other courts about domestic violence and improve judicial handling of such cases.
- Provide technical assistance and computer and other equipment to police departments, prosecutors, courts, and tribal jurisdictions to facilitate the widespread enforcement of protection orders, including interstate enforcement, enforcement between States and tribal jurisdictions, and enforcement between tribal jurisdictions.
- Develop or strengthen policies and training for police, prosecutors, and the judiciary in recognizing, investigating, and prosecuting instances of domestic violence and sexual assault against older individuals (as defined in section 102 of the Older American Act of 1965) and individuals with disabilities (as defined in section 3(2) of the Americans with Disabilities Act of 1990).

Program Priority Areas

By statute, 42 U.S.C. Section § 3796(hh-1)(b) priority will be given to applicants that:

- Illustrate that the jurisdiction does not currently provide for centralized handling of cases involving domestic violence by police, prosecutors, and courts;

(Continued)

- Demonstrate a commitment to strong enforcement of laws, and prosecution of cases involving domestic violence, including the enforcement of protection orders from other States and jurisdictions (including tribal jurisdictions);
- Have established cooperative agreements or can demonstrate effective ongoing collaborative arrangements with neighboring jurisdictions to facilitate the enforcement of protection orders from other States and jurisdictions; and Intend to utilize grant funds to develop and install data collection and communication systems, including computerized systems, and training on how to use these systems effectively to link police, prosecutors, courts, and tribal jurisdictions for the purpose of identifying and tracking protection orders and violations of protection orders in those jurisdictions where such systems do not exist or are not fully effective.

Special Interest Categories

The Office on Violence Against Women (OVW) is interested in funding States, Indian tribal governments, State and local courts, or units of local government that have implemented—or plan to implement—promising approaches that respond to domestic violence as a serious violation of criminal law. Although applications that address any of the statutory program purposes outlined above are eligible for funding, OVW is especially interested in supporting projects that address the following special interest categories. All applicants are required to collaborate with nonprofit, nongovernmental victim service agencies. The following list does not imply any order of priority.

- Involve faith-based and/or community-driven initiatives to address violence against women among diverse and traditionally underserved populations. Include dedicated parole and probation officers within existing or newly created domestic violence units to actively participate in holding perpetrators accountable.
- Develop innovative programs to improve judicial handling of domestic violence cases. For example, specialized courts or dockets for domestic violence cases, enhanced judicial monitoring of domestic violence offenders, or the creation or enhancement of technology to provide prosecutors and judges access to case information on prior arrests.
- Develop and implement coordinated initiatives to address incidents of sexual assault and/or stalking occurring in the context of domestic violence
- Address system accountability by conducting a safety audit of the jurisdiction's criminal justice system.

Program Eligibility

Eligible grantees for this program are States, Indian tribal governments, State and local courts, and units of local government. For purposes of this program, a unit of local government is any city, county, township, town, borough, parish, village, or other general-purpose political subdivision of a State; an Indian tribe that performs law enforcement functions as determined by the Secretary of Interior; or, for the purpose of assistance eligibility, any agency of the District of Columbia government or the U.S. Government performing law enforcement functions in and for the District of Columbia and the Trust Territory of the Pacific Islands. Police departments, pretrial service agencies, district or city attorneys' offices, sheriffs' departments, probation and parole departments, shelters, nonprofit, nongovernmental victim service agencies, and universities are not units of local government for the purposes of this grant program. These agencies or organizations may assume responsibility for the development

(Continued)

and implementation of the project, but they must apply through a State, State or local court, Indian tribal government, or unit of local government.

By statute, to be eligible to receive funding through this program, applicants must:

- Certify that their laws or official policies encourage or mandate arrests of domestic violence offenders based on probable cause that an offense has been committed and encourage or mandate arrest of domestic violence offenders who violate the terms of a valid and outstanding protection order.
- Demonstrate that their laws, policies, or practices and their training programs discourage dual arrests of offender and victim.
- Certify that their laws, policies, or practices prohibit issuance of mutual restraining orders of protection except in cases where both spouses file a claim and the court makes detailed findings of fact indicating that both spouses acted primarily as aggressors and that neither spouse acted primarily in self-defense.
- Certify that their laws, policies, and practices do not require, in connection with the prosecution of any misdemeanor or felony domestic violence offense, or in connection with the filing, issuance, registration, or service of a protection order, or a petition for a protection order, to protect a victim of domestic violence, stalking, or sexual assault, that the victim bear the costs associated with the filing of criminal charges against the offender, or the costs associated with the filing, issuance, registration, or service of a warrant, protection order, petition for a protection order, or witness subpoena, whether issued inside or outside the State, tribal, or local jurisdiction.

"Grants to Encourage Arrest Policies and Enforcement of Protection Orders Program," from the Office on Violence Against Women, within the U.S. Department of Justice, found at www.usdoj.gov/ovw.

These are the packets that contain full instructions and all required forms for submitting a proposal for financial support to develop the intended project. The program proposal must describe the nature of the program, the target population, the social problem to be addressed, as well as how monies will be used. This typically includes monies for people/staff, equipment and supplies, space/location, transportation, communication and marketing, and special needs like child-care services. In the case shared earlier about developing a community center in Arizona, funding was actually provided by the local Native American Tribal Reservation of which many of the community residents were members.

Grant writing can be detailed and technical. Therefore, any agency lucky enough to employ a competent grant writer would be willing to pay that person fairly well; they are the ones who bring funding to an agency after all. However, many agencies cannot pay to hire an outside grant writer and often rely on their current employees to do it. It is thus in the best interest of any human services professional to have their own grant writing skills and experience.

> **Writing Grants Is a Key Skill to Have in the Field of Human Services**
>
> The second author teaches an undergraduate grant writing and program planning course. She regularly tells her students that while grant writing is a very tedious, labor-intensive, and time-consuming endeavor, it is necessary for the work we do in our field. Without grant opportunities, many of the programs and services we rely on to help and support our clients and to improve the well-being of individuals, families, and communities would not be available. Particularly today, when the United States has been experiencing major economic challenges, resulting for example in dramatic cuts to an already inadequate public mental health system, the ability to secure grant monies through private donors and corporations, as well as available government grant sources, is critical. Having grant writing skills is not only marketable for students but is an essential role for staff at nonprofit agencies and educational and health care organizations across the country.

EVALUATING PROGRAMS AND POLICIES

Writing grants can be quite competitive. Therefore, it is typically required that grant proposals include a mechanism by which the program or service will be evaluated. Many write into their budget the hiring of a program evaluator. Program evaluation is essentially the process of determining whether or not the types of services offered are worthwhile, effective, and cost efficient for clients. In other words, program evaluation allows you to know if your program is a "good" program (more on this is discussed later in this chapter). For example, Lynam and colleagues (1999) evaluated the DARE program, a widely used and expensive drug prevention program, by following up on the program 10 years after it ensued. They compared children who participated in the DARE program with children who participated in a less-structured and less-expensive education program. Their results indicate that there were no differences between the two groups, as determined by usage of marijuana and other illicit drugs and measures of self-esteem. In addition, other evaluation efforts indicated that DARE is not effective in eliminating substance use. If you were the principal of an elementary school, would you pay for the DARE program? Thanks to evaluation research such as this, you would likely look for a more effective and affordable drug prevention program.

Program evaluation has gained popularity as human services professionals, practitioners, and researchers are increasingly required to base their decisions and program-related efforts on the best available evidence. This seems like it should be common sense, but often programs and practices become popular based on good marketing, word of mouth, tradition, and politics. Thankfully, the movement toward evidence-based reform and utilization of high-quality evidence increases the likelihood that clients will experience useful, successful, and healthy outcomes.

There are several different approaches to evaluation. Three are presented here. **Formative evaluation** is typically used to assist in the forming of new programs or during the early stages of a new program in order to adjust and enhance interventions and outcomes. They are used to provide feedback on what services were provided, to whom, when, how often, and in what settings (Moskowitz, 1989) and whether or not the program had been implemented as originally planned. The person(s) conducting the formative evaluation might assess for dropout rates, management/administrative issues, problems that have occurred, and actual costs of the working program. If the program did not achieve its expected outcomes, formative evaluation can lend some insight into weakness in the process of its planning and implementation. Formative evaluation–related findings can also point to ways in which projects should be changed if they are expanded or continued.

Another form of evaluation is **process evaluation**, which describes the services and activities that were used to implement the program. Findings from process evaluations are used to help determine the quality and accuracy of the intervention delivered to program participants (often referred to as assurances). They can also help researchers to understand which specific components of the intervention or program were most effective. This is especially critical if the program offers several interventions, such as group counseling, one-on-one counseling, and self-help program. Determining the effects of all of the offered components not only informs future studies of how to save costs but sheds light on the nature of each component in making an impact (or lack thereof) on the participants. Questions a process evaluator might ask include: What need did the program fill? What people or organizations were involved? What is the culture of the program? What are the components of the program offered? What is the socioeconomic makeup of the program? How effective are staff members? What are the costs? And what changes have been made? (Royse, Thyer, & Padgett, 2010). Answers to these questions help to understand key indicators of program process, including frequency of service, intensity of service, size of group receiving service, and responsiveness of participants. Unlike formative evaluation, which occurs early in the program, process evaluation can occur at any point. Information from process evaluations is important in that it can inform other communities who may want to replicate the program.

Finally, **outcome evaluation** is used to measure a program's results or outcomes in a way that determines whether or not the program produced the changes or outcomes that were intended. Did changes occur to participants' knowledge, attitudes, skills, belief systems, and/or behaviors? Were conditions *increased, improved,* or *greater* than prior to the intervention, such as increased coping skills or parenting knowledge? Likewise, were conditions *decreased, fewer,* or *removed,* such as decreased incidence of bullying behaviors or fewer behavioral outbursts among children? The goal of outcome evaluation is thus to assess if positive outcomes resulted from the program or policy change. Additionally, outcomes are often indicated by short-term, intermediate, and long-term results as measured by pre-post designs, comparison groups, and experimental designs.

Overall, whatever form of evaluation is being conducted, program evaluators typically analyze their collected data and write reports to present to the relevant community members or stakeholders. As mentioned earlier, program evaluation is a critical component of working in the human services field. Developing skills to review literature, collaborate with others, collect and analyze data, and write reports (or at the very least, be able to interpret such reports) are essential for all current and future human service professionals.

> **Critical Thinking/Self-Reflection Corner**
> - Would you enjoy conducting a community-based needs assessment?
> - How would you build trust with community members in order to conduct an effective needs assessment?
> - Who do you consider as part of your community? How would you feel if someone came in to your community and wanted to assist you in conducting a needs assessment?
> - How do you know if a program is good? That is, what characteristics and qualities constitute a good program?
> - If you were conducting a program evaluation, who would you want to collaborate with and why?
> - Discuss with your classmates any nonprofit you are familiar with. What programs does it offer? If you were asked to evaluate one of its programs, where would you begin? What questions would you start with? What would you want to measure in terms of outcomes sand effectiveness?

ADVOCACY AND POLICY

Advocacy and policy go hand in hand within the field of human services. At the macro level, these actions shape, either directly or indirectly, how we serve clients, secure funding sources, and solve problems facing children, youth, and families. Hepworth and Larsen (1986) describe advocacy as "the process of working with and/or on behalf of clients (1) to obtain services or resources for clients that would not otherwise be provided, (2) to modify extant policies, procedures, or practice that adversely impact clients, or (3) to promote new legislation or policies that will result in the provision of needed resources or services." From a human services perspective, advocacy can be seen as a way to remove barriers that hinder prevention activities. Several activities are involved in advocacy, including influencing policy and legislation (discussed in more detail later in this chapter), engaging in outreach, fostering coalitions, providing education, promoting community education, and strengthening individual and community knowledge and skills. Grassroots movements, nonprofit organizations, and lobbying (also discussed in more detail later) are three ways in which individual and humans services professionals are able to effectively advocate for themselves or others on a larger scale.

There are several types of advocacy, three of which are presented here. Self-advocacy is when clients or consumers learn their rights and how to protect them. Thankfully, the consumer movement has been well served over the years by a variety of leaders—outspoken consumer champions who refused to let the people be taken advantage of by big business, big government, or big brother. Due to efforts of key historical and contemporary political activists, such as Dorothea Dix (Chapter 1), Ralph Nader, and Erin Brokovich, and many visionary presidential leaders who passed key legislation, major battles were fought and won for consumers. Another type of advocacy is community advocacy, which involves educating the community about problems and organizing them to take action. As discussed earlier in this chapter, this often begins with a community needs assessment and coalition building. Finally, legislative advocacy is promoting and influencing legislation that benefits populations in need.

Advocacy often leads directly to policy, defined as the guidelines, principles, legislation, and activities that affect human welfare and that are set to improve, or meet, human needs related to housing, health, education, safety, justice, and more. In Chapter 2, several modern policies were discussed. Without such policies, and without policy makers, many more individuals and families would struggle to connect to necessary resources, services, and opportunities related to their well-being and often their survival.

Similar to community practice (discussed earlier in this chapter), policy practice is also about bringing about change; in this context though, it is done through the political system by influencing government policy and legislation at the local, state, federal, or global level. Policy activities typically include reforming current policies or developing new ones. Engaging in policy practice requires extensive knowledge of an issue, the population it affects, consideration of social conditions that contribute to the related problem, and of course, knowledge of governmental processes, laws, regulations, and rules. Engaging in effective policy practice also requires a belief that social problems can be fixed if their underlying structures are changed. For example, to decrease poverty, individuals should not be blamed, but rather, the focus should be on improving the existing structural barriers that limit successful access to employment opportunities. Other types of structural barriers can include institutionalized racism, laws that oppress specific groups, and lack of cultural knowledge.

Many human services workers who engage in policy practice take a **person-in-environment perspective**, whereby a person is understood within the context or environment (cultural, familial, environmental, geographic, etc.) that he or she interacts and is socialized, nurtured, and educated within. Understanding how individuals are shaped by their environments, which can hinder or facilitate one's development, becomes the motivation to engage in policy practice and essentially improve one's environment. Indeed policy practice is a core component of the National Organization for Human Services' Code of Ethics: "The Human Service Professionals' Responsibility to the Community and Society," which includes "advocating for change in regulations and statutes when such legislation conflicts with ethical guidelines and/or client rights. Where laws are harmful to individuals, groups, or communities, human service professionals consider the conflict between the values of obeying the law and the values of serving people and may decide to initiate social action."

Several steps are involved in the policy-making process. These typically include identifying problems, formulating proposals, legitimizing policy, implementation, and evaluation. While this is quite simplistic, this does provide a comprehensive overview of the many facets involved in policy practice. Identification of problems involves publicized demands for government action; that is, getting policy makers to make your proposed issue an agenda item. Many human services workers will work with special interest groups, nonprofits, media sources, and lobbyists (or become a lobbyist themselves) to influence government officials and pertinent committees or agencies responsible for writing and enforcing laws. Next, policy-planning organizations, interest groups, government bureaucracies, state legislatures, as well as the president and Congress may all engage in formulating policy proposals. This is the process of creating, adopting, and implementing a policy, as well as developing alternatives of options for dealing with a problem. Due to limited time and resources, policy makers have to be selective about which problems to act on. Many lobbyists will attempt to influence government decisions by writing letters, making phone calls, donating money, urging legislators to prose certain legislation, and voting during elections. They often also write and submit a **white paper**, a policy or position paper documenting justification for change of a problem. If legitimized, executive orders, budgets, laws, and more will be instituted. Once the policy has been adopted, it is in the process of being implemented. Unfortunately, sometimes nothing happens, and the policy process continues. The hope, of course, is that once a law is passed, significant change will follow.

Lastly, as discussed earlier, evaluation is a key final step to ensuring that programs, or in this case laws and policies, are effective. Indeed, evaluation is a growing priority in government settings to ensure that the policies that have been initiated are having the desired effects for the intended population, as well as vested **stakeholders**.

The Sin by Silence Bill

In 2002, Penal Code 1473.5 became law after extensive lobbying efforts in California to make government officials aware of the issues surrounding women who are convicted of killing their abusive husbands, including data indicating that 93 percent of the women who had killed their significant others had been battered; 67 percent of these women attempted to protect themselves or their children; and that of the 7,000 plus women imprisoned in California's state prisons the majority have survived domestic violence (AB 593/AB 1593). Through persistent phone calls, social media, and letters, as well as support from Assemblywoman Fiona Ma, California became the first state in the nation to permit women convicted of killing their batterers (prior to 1992) to file a writ of habeas corpus (legal action that ensures that an arrested person be allowed to come before a judge and not be held illegally) and challenge their original conviction in order to have more time to voice their story and to have their cases tried under new laws that were not in place during their original trials.

U.S. Department of Education, Accountability Report of the No Child Left Behind Act

In 2010, the U.S. Department of Education published an accountability report of the No Child Left Behind Act (2001), among which the goals were to ensure that all children would become proficient in reading and math. The report is based on data collected from two independent research firms who examined the effectiveness and quality of the act on several measures, including teacher quality and level of access to fair, equal, and high-quality educational services. Among the extensive findings and positive outcomes, it was also found that one-third of teachers in targeted schools reported that "inadequate numbers of textbooks and instructional materials presented a major challenge to their improvement efforts" and that "more than one-half of districts in corrective action reported that they did not receive any of the mandated interventions" (U.S. Department of Education, 2010). Such findings are critical to the evaluation process and to increasing the chance that procedure and plans related to the act will be adapted to achieve more successful outcomes in the future.

Critical Thinking/Self-Reflection Corner

- Consider an organization you are part of. What boundaries exist? How do these boundaries help or challenge efforts to engage in advocacy?
- Think about a group or population that is in need. What sort of policies do you think should be in place to improve its well-being?
- What group or population do you feel deserves to be advocated for?
- If you were a lobbyist, what challenges do you think you would face?
- Some bills are controversial, such as the Sin by Silence Bill discussed earlier. What are the pros and cons of the passing of this bill?

CHAPTER SUMMARY

Macro-level practice focuses on ensuring that the social problems and needs of the community are met by the development of community resources. Macro-level practitioners work to create social changes by changing laws and by developing programs in the community. Macro-level intervention also includes programs such as trauma response to community disasters (discussed in Chapter 6).

Human services is a dynamic field; it is constantly changing, as culture, social and political conditions, and demographics evolve. As such, macro-level practices will also evolve, resulting in a regular ebb and flow of adapting and creating programs and policies. The key to success in the field is a commitment to provide resources to clients and consumers by utilizing their strengths and listening to their voices. In doing so, organizations, communities, and societies will thrive.

Suggested Applied Activities

1. Think of an agency that you would like to create in your community. Outline a proposal using the following questions to guide you: What populations will your agency serve? Why is there a need for this agency? What services currently exist for this population, and why are they not enough to meet the needs of the population? Which community leaders support your program? How will it be staffed? Who will be on your board of directors? Describe the services that will be delivered? How will you evaluate the agency and its effectiveness?

2. Think of three propositions that you would like to see pass on a ballot. Do you think they would have a chance? How could you lobby for them to pass?

3. Make a list of the pros and cons of being a macro-level worker in the human services field.

Chapter Review Questions

1. What is the general goal of macro-level practice?

2. What is a community needs assessment? How might you conduct a needs assessment?

3. What is advocacy? What techniques or strategies are used to engage in advocacy work?

   _____

   _____

4. What is a grant? What role do grants play in the field of human services?

   _____

   _____

5. What types of evaluation exist? Why is each one important?

   _____

   _____

6. What is the person-in-environment perspective, and why should macro-level workers take this into account when developing programs and policies?

   _____

   _____

Glossary of Terms

Advocacy is any action that promotes or defends a cause.

Coalition is a group of associations and organizations that work together to create social change or develop programs.

Community organizing is the process by which people come together to work toward a shared cause related to social change.

Evaluation is conducted by a funding source in which an evaluator examines the effectiveness and problems of a program that is receiving the funding.

Formative evaluation includes efforts to assist in the formation of new programs or to evaluate during the early stages of a new program in order to adjust and enhance interventions and outcomes.

Funding announcements are notices of available funding opportunities.

Fundraising is the process of gathering voluntary contributions of monies and resources to support a cause, program, or social action.

Grants are funding offers from either government agencies or private foundations to agencies that have submitted an application for funding.

Initiative is a balloted proposal for legislative change that citizens vote on during general elections.

Lobbying is communicating with members of Congress and the executive branch by testifying and providing information related to a proposed policy, as well as assisting in the writing and proposing of legislation.

Macro-level practices are interventions at the community, county, or state level that focus on working with and creating organizational and social policy.

Needs assessments use neighborhood interviews and surveys to determine what a community believes are its problems.

Outcome evaluation is used to measure a program's results or outcomes in a way that determines whether or not the program produced the changes or outcomes that were intended.

Person-in-environment perspective is a framework for understanding human behavior by taking into account the various aspects of an individual's environment, including social, political, familial, economic, and physical conditions and influences.

Policy is a course of action, guiding principle, or procedure intended to influence and determine decisions and action.

Process evaluation describes the services and activities used to implement a program and to help determine the quality and accuracy of the intervention delivered to program participants.

Proposal is a document in which the details of a new program are described.

Social action is the ability of social workers and consumers of services to confront and change power relationships and the structure and function of important social institutions in communities.

Stakeholders are all of those groups and individuals who have an interest in the outcomes of a policy practice initiative.

White paper is a document that states a position and a call to action regarding a social problem that needs change.

Case Presentation and Exit Quiz

General Description

Helen is working on behalf of a nonprofit that serves homeless families. She has noticed that are several potential problems with the shelter run by the nonprofit. For example, she notices that children sleep separately from their parents; that despite support from the nonprofit, too many families are "regulars" of the shelter; and that the food provided is not as nutritious as it should be. Unfortunately, the nonprofit has limited funding for the shelter and wants to ensure that any monies spent are used effectively. She talks with the families and learns that they would like more training and support to find employment and child care.

Exit Quiz

1. Helen wants to make changes at the shelter. However, to be ethical and to ensure she is meeting the needs of the families, Helen should do what first?
    a. Write a grant
    b. Engage in advocacy
    c. Conduct a community needs assessment
    d. Write her local legislator about the shelter's problems

2. In order for Helen to secure more monies for employment training and child-care support, Helen should do what?
    a. Write a white paper
    b. Look for an RFP or RFA (funding announcements) and submit a grant
    c. Fundraise
    d. Both b and c

3. Helen receives funding to hire an employment specialist/educator to work with the families at the shelter and develop educational seminars related to

finding and securing employment. After 6 months, the program is evaluated, and it is found that the employment outcomes were not met. It is determined that the original plan of offering these educational seminars once a month was too little and that the program should offer its educational seminars at least twice week. This recommendation most likely resulting from which form of evaluation?

  a. Formative
  b. Process
  c. Outcome

4. Later, Helen works with her local legislators to get community business owners to mentor and train interested parents who utilize the shelter. Helen understands that removing any structural barriers that may exist to accessing employment opportunities is essential to the families' well-being. Helen believes in the person–in–environment perspective.

  a. True
  b. False

Exit Quiz Answers

1. c
2. d
3. b
4. a

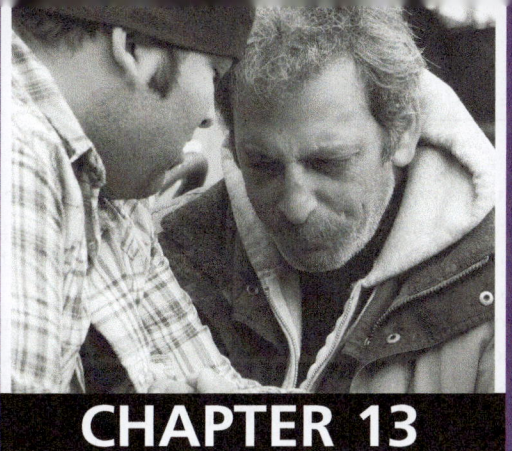

CHAPTER 13

Leadership and Organizational Structure

INTRODUCTION

Previous chapters focused on human services workers and people who use human services–related services and activities. This chapter, however, takes a close look at public and nonprofit agencies, which contribute the largest number of human services agencies. Aspects relating to agency and organizational structure and leadership styles are explored. The advantages and disadvantages of working and receiving services from each type of agency are also discussed.

While many of the characteristics of human services agencies can be seen in other types of agencies, the focus here is on agencies whose primary function is to meet the emotional, social, family, educational, psychological, and basic welfare needs of individuals, families, and groups. The terms "**organization**" and "**agency**" are often used interchangeably but may be used to indicate distinct entities as well.

An organization can be thought of as a purposeful social unit constructed to achieve certain goals or to perform tasks. Organizations are generally "composed of many different individuals who perform specified roles in an effort to provide needed services to certain populations in the community" (Alle-Corliss & Alle-Corliss, 1999, p. 213). Some organizations work directly with people while others are indirectly involved with clients and perform advocacy and **lobbying** functions.

An agency can be defined as an organization that exists to achieve various goals and usually provides services directly or indirectly to the community. The functioning of an agency is usually organized through the establishment of positions that work together to provide services. Most people think of an agency as an actual physical establishment where services are provided and consumers visit. While this same definition is also true for an organization, some organizations don't necessarily provide direct services but are focused instead on fundraising efforts and policy discussions.

Some examples of common agencies are community centers, counseling clinics, adoption agencies, community service programs, diversion programs, halfway houses, and group homes. Organizations that are not necessarily considered agencies might include the National Organization for Women (NOW), the **American Red Cross**, and the United Way. While all of the organizations focus on serving people in need, these larger organizations usually farm out the direct services to smaller agencies that are physically located in various communities. The organization may have a national headquarters where decisions and policies are made.

Throughout this chapter, *agency* and *organization* may be used synonymously because the distinction between the two terms is small, and in reality, most people use the two terms interchangeably.

GENERAL CHARACTERISTICS OF HUMAN SERVICES AGENCIES

Before beginning a career in the human services, it is wise to understand the general structure of these types of agencies. The characteristics discussed in this section are not necessarily unique to human services agencies, and so this information will be relevant to any type of organization. Human services workers in particular will benefit from knowing about these aspects because they may be a source of work stress some time in the future. Understanding typical issues involved in working at human services agencies allows for more objective reactions when these factors cause problems and conflicts. The structural characteristics presented in this section include agency norms, the **shadow organization**, leadership styles, and **number numbness**.

Norms

As with any group of people, agencies operate within the scope of both written and unwritten norms. Norms are the rules and guidelines that are understood and followed by members of a group, and a worker can become familiar with an organization by becoming familiar with these norms (Russo, 1980). At times workers may find themselves in conflict with agency norms. Conflicts are not resolved quickly or easily most of the time. When a human services worker's own values are in conflict with an organization's norms, it may be helpful to communicate respectfully and assertively with a supervisor. While this may be scary, it may also be an opportunity to grow. It may also be an opportunity for an organization to modify its norms. An easy-to-understand example has to do with sexual harassment in the workplace. At one time, it was the norm of many agencies to condone or ignore sexual harassment. Eventually, enough workers complained about this behavior to make it illegal at any place of employment. This process took many years, but because employees spoke up, change did occur, which was helpful for employees and organizations. In this case, change was a good thing, but as with all change it was risky. Many changes create work for staff members and require that the public be educated about the changes (Russo, 1980). Keeping things the same (status quo) is sometimes preferred because although the status quo may be miserable, the unknown may be worse.

Shadow Organization

In addition to the formal norms of an organization, human services workers should be aware of the informal organizational norms, sometimes referred to as the shadow organization. This is how the agency really operates (Russo, 1980). Although workers should follow the formal guidelines, many times groups of people who work with each other over time develop their own way of doing things. At times, these ways may differ from those written in organizational manuals. Much of the shadow organizational norms are related to social interaction patterns among various staff at the agency. Some agencies do spell out in a manual how to treat others, but often this type of behavior is not written out in formal language and must be learned on the job. New employees should take notice of this shadow organization and make decisions about how to interact based on their own values and interpersonal style. For example, a new employee sees the majority of staff gossiping about their boss but feels uncomfortable about this type of behavior. The new employee can decide not to participate in the gossip rather than report those who are doing it. While it may still feel uncomfortable knowing that others are engaging in the behavior of gossiping, if the new employee were to tell, there could be serious consequences such as getting picked on by others, being given a heavier workload, and even being framed for an illegal activity. **Whistle-blowing** is not always appreciated and should be done when the consequences of the shadow organization are seriously affecting the lives and well-being of others. Another example is the air-traffic controller who recently blew the whistle on fellow workers who were playing chicken with the airplanes (letting the planes almost collide just for the thrill). She reported them and suffered major consequences as a result. But by whistle-blowing, she probably saved the lives of innocent travelers.

Leadership Styles

Every agency has administrative positions. As discussed in Chapter 4, these people are in charge of ensuring that the agency runs smoothly and effectively. They must keep track of budgetary concerns, employee performance, and serve as liaison between the agency and the community. Leadership styles vary among administrators. Many have categorized management style into two types: **instrumental** (theory X) and **expressive** (theory Y) (Blake & Mouton, 1968; Etzioni, 1965; Guba & Bridwell, 1957; McGregor, 1960; Parsons, Bales, & Shills, 1955). The instrumental leader needs respect from employees, manages hostility among employees with authority, focuses on production, and worries about the budget and how it is distributed. The expressive leader is less able to handle hostility, has a need to maintain close relationships with employees, and shows great concern for people (Etzioni, 1965).

Number Numbness

Regardless of management's leadership style, most agency administrators spend a great deal of time discussing budgets either with board members (if it is a nonprofit agency) or with upper management (if it is a public agency). These human services workers don't deal directly with clients but focus on managing the numbers that keep an agency operating. These numbers include daily averages, daily attendance at programs, rates of pledge payments, credit hours, and, of course, any donations or payments. They also focus on operating costs, wages, and many other numbers. Maxwell (1973) has labeled this phenomenon "number numbness." Human services workers who are motivated by human growth and development and human contact often find these activities boring and stressful. However, an agency can only function at its total capacity after all of the numbers are examined and managed. Of course, program efficiency and client services are important to management, but at times these matters take a backseat to funding activities and operating costs. The bottom line is that an agency cannot provide any human services to clients without an organized financial system. Every agency is accountable to funding sources, and numbers crunching is a large aspect of being accountable.

Human services workers who deal directly with clients (often referred to as **line staff**) must understand their individual role in keeping this financial system operating efficiently. This means that line staff may have to maintain accurate records of their own productivity rates, time spent in various activities, and other data relevant to the operation of the agency. These data can then be used by the data managers to conduct analyses. These analyses are then turned over to management and board members for **evaluation** and recommendations. Line staff workers often experience this number numbness as demoralizing because they usually enter the field of human services to provide service and care to clients not to conduct data analyses. Line staff should guard against developing number numbness themselves. Social workers, counselors, advocates, and other human services workers must leave the numbers crunching to management for the most part and keep their focus on the clients, while at the same time maintain vital data for those coworkers who must focus on numbers.

TYPES OF HUMAN SERVICES AGENCIES

The specific structure and operations of both publicly funded and nonprofit agencies, including mental health, social welfare, correctional, and educational agencies are presented in this section.

Public Agencies

Public agencies receive government funding from municipal, state, and federal taxes. The benefit of working in a public setting is its stability, good wages, and benefits, such as health insurance, sick pay, and vacation pay. Some of the disadvantages of working for public agencies might be their focus on accountability, red tape (paperwork), and routine work hours. Sometimes the focus can be shifted away from client needs and put on policy, procedures, and numbers.

Most government-run human services agencies operate under a classic bureaucratic model. Because most federal, state, county, and city agencies employee hundreds and thousands of workers, there is a need for a highly structured approach in organizing these agencies. The classical bureaucratic approach, which can be traced back to the Industrial Revolution during the mid-1800s (Brueggemann, 1996), introduced the idea that when a large number of individuals work together in an orderly fashion they can accomplish more than the same number of individuals working independently (Netting, Kettner, & McMurtry, 1993). This model allows for efficiency and achievement of organizational goals. This structured approach emphasizes task specialization and matching individual workers to appropriate positions. Management must ensure that workers understand their roles and must maintain worker morale for the good of the organization.

Some people view bureaucracies negatively because of their inflexible rules, mandatory paperwork, accountability, hierarchy, and reluctance to modify programs. Each human services worker must decide whether the benefits outweigh some of the annoying aspects of a public agency before beginning a career at one.

Most public agencies operate under a well-organized hierarchy. A hierarchy is a way of organizing workers by power and authority. Most public agencies develop elaborate and efficient flow charts that visually illustrate the **chain of command**. Typically, more workers are at the bottom of a hierarchy than at the top. The workers at the bottom are generally line staff workers who deal directly with clients and support staff such as administrative assistants. These workers are supervised by the first level of management, who are accountable to middle management, who in turn are accountable to upper management. Upper management is accountable to funding sources and other government officials (the mayor, the governor, or the county board of supervisors). The higher up on the chain of command a worker is, the more responsibility he or she has for the operation of the agency.

Most organizations frown on jumping chain of command. The preferred mode of communication is from one level of the hierarchy to the next. For example, if a line staff worker complains to upper management without first talking to his or her immediate supervisor, upper management might question why the supervisor wasn't contacted first and may even tell the line staff worker that he or she must talk to the supervisor before upper management will listen to the complaint. Breaking the chain of command is often considered a slap in the face to those at the level that was skipped. Most policy documents inform workers of the proper way to communicate in the chain of command.

Nonprofit Agencies

Some nonprofit agencies deal with clients who receive direct services from the agency itself. Other agencies provide an arena for fundraising and community outreach and education. They tend to be more flexible in hiring community college and bachelor level human services workers. The advantage for the

True Stories from Human Service Workers

Bureaucracy in a Public Mental Health Agency

County facilities have a reputation for being mired in red tape—that is, they require a lot of paperwork. The following example illustrates the type of paperwork a mental health worker might encounter while working for county-operated mental health services.

Example: One of the authors worked for four years at the County of Orange Mental Health Services in southern California, where she first experienced red tape. "I was hired as a mental health worker II while I was working on a master's degree in counseling. While much of my time was spent providing individual counseling (about 50 percent), a good portion of my time was spent in meetings, reviewing cases, and filling out forms. As a mental health worker, I had to complete a psychosocial assessment, a mental-status exam, a multiaxial diagnosis form, a treatment plan, and a progress report for each client I treated. The information on each form had to be linked in content to information on the other forms. This paperwork was burdensome and took several years to learn how to complete efficiently. The worst part for me was that my immediate supervisor's job was to check all of the paperwork to ensure it as completed accurately, and if there were any mistakes, if anything was missing, or if I forgot to sign my name, I would find the chart in my box ordering me to fix my errors. This is an example of red tape. However, I do see the point to it all. The agency was funded primarily by a state program called Medi-Cal, which required paperwork to be completed uniformly so that counselors would be accountable for their services. Once this accountability was satisfactorily provided, the agency would continue to receive funding. Without this funding, clients could not continue to be served."

This example illustrates the link between a line staff worker, management, paperwork, accountability, and funding typical of bureaucratic organizations. While the author's focus was always on client service, she also realized that completing the paperwork was vital to being able to continue to provide services to clients.

worker is a more informal atmosphere where program development and client needs are emphasized and there is autonomy and flexibility in work hours. Workers at nonprofit agencies also have the opportunity to give back to the community, increased job satisfaction for helping people, opportunity for increased responsibilities and training in a new field, opportunity to use professionals skills to make a difference, work with caring and motivated people, and gain rewards beyond a paycheck (McAdam, 1986). The disadvantage is often instability in funding and lower salaries. The focus of these agencies is to provide high-quality service to people to meet their needs.

According to Weinstein (1994), more than 983,000 nonprofit organizations operate in the United States. In the 1990s, the average annual salary for people who work in these agencies was about $17,500 compared to $24,000 in the for-profit sector. Nonprofit agencies depend on volunteers but the number of paid employees has increased from 8.8 million in 1977 to 14.4 million in the 1990s. An estimated 98 million Americans volunteer at nonprofit agencies, and the estimated value of this volunteer time is over $170 billion. Weinstein found that nonprofit employers with the largest number of employees were in the following disciplines: health services; educational/research services; religious organizations; social and legal services; civic, social, and fraternal organizations; arts and culture; and foundations. Human services are obviously well represented in the nonprofit sector.

Although nonprofits may have some characteristics of the bureaucratic structure found in public agencies, nonprofits tend to follow the **human relations** model of organizational structure. This model can be traced back to the 1929 stock market crash that preceded the Great Depression. The federal government responded to this economic disaster by implementing New Deal agencies, which were established to restore hope in the government as well as to assist people in finding employment. These new agencies were structured differently from the organizational bureaucracies that were receiving so much criticism at the time. The New Deal agencies instead focused on employee rights and social concerns. The workplace was considered a secondary social system, and concern about employees' needs, interests, and issues had a powerful effect on workplace efficiency and output (Brueggemann, 1996). Organizations with large numbers of workers, such as public and government agencies, found that merging a more structured approach with a focus on employee well-being worked best. Without structure, chaos might ensue. Although the bureaucratic model wouldn't suggest that workers' needs should be ignored, meeting every worker's needs all the time simply isn't practical. Large numbers of employees necessitate some rigidity in policy.

The human relations model became the foundation for many nonprofit agencies. It was a nice fit with the growing sense of humanism and civil rights that was seen in the 1960s and 1970s. Nonprofit agencies became an alternative method of providing service to people who were often resistant to governmental policy and philosophies. This anti-establishment era was ripe for services provided within a human relations organizational structure. Not only were employees more happy under this structure, but many clients were as well. Under this type of management, nonprofit agencies operated in more casual ways than public agencies. The focus was more on client needs and program development rather than on numbers and accountability. This was possible because many of the nonprofit agencies from the 1960s through the 1980s got much of their funding from private donations and fundraising events, and they were staffed primarily by volunteers who provided much of the professional services.

During the 1990s and 2000s, nonprofit funding began relying more heavily on special **grants** and funding available through government programs. As a result, these previously autonomous agencies had to become accountable to their government funding sources. The increased availability of funding gave agencies an opportunity to hire paid staff, which may have also increased the need for more structure and policy. Despite the growing complexity of these agencies' infrastructures, they were able to maintain their human relations orientation.

The foundation of most nonprofit agencies is the **board of directors**, which is typically made up of people from the community who have an interest in the agency's purpose and goals. They may be professionals such as lawyers, judges, doctors, teachers, or just average citizens who may have volunteered for similar agencies in the past or have used similar agencies in their own lives. This board usually meets about once a month and receives no pay for their services. Their job is to collaborate with the executive director to oversee all the services provided by the agency. They communicate directly with the executive director of the agency and may speak on behalf of the agency at fundraising events. They may advise the executive director of the agency about how to seek funding, how to evaluate the agency programs, and when an employee may need to be terminated. They play a large role in the hiring and firing of the agency executive director.

Executive directors usually work directly with agency boards as well as its employees. Directors often have advanced degrees and oversee all services at an agency. They also work directly with the various program coordinators at the agency and the assistant director and spend a great deal of time on fundraising activities and grant writing. They represent their agencies at fundraisers and often participate in public meetings and social activities that might benefit the agency. Directors are often in charge of hiring, training, monitoring, and terminating staff and also monitor client activities and ensure that regulations are followed.

Most nonprofit agencies also employ an assistant to the director and program coordinators. These employees meet with the director, and together they organize, plan, or modify the day-to-day operation of the agency. This includes the management of volunteers, budget, fundraising activities, and direct services.

True Stories from Human Service Workers

Working at a Nonprofit Agency

Working at nonprofit agencies has its advantages and disadvantages. The climate is probably best for people who enjoy autonomy at work and can cope with occasional uncertainties and minimal pay.

Example 1: Jan Tyler, program director at Heritage House, a drug and alcohol rehabilitation program in Costa Mesa, California, says, "I manage the agency by consensus as much as possible. Some of the benefits in working at the agency is seeing lives change and improve dramatically and having a part in it. Some disadvantages in working for this nonprofit agency is that finding and hiring qualified personnel is very difficult. Also, low pay, burnout, and intense emotional involvement of the staff with each other and with clients are disadvantages."

Example 2: According to Brenda Titus, of Sexual Assault Victim Services, "A major advantage in working for a nonprofit agency is that the type of work performed by each individual is necessary and results in observable positive outcomes. A major disadvantage is that funding for the agency is often unreliable."

Nonprofit agencies focus on service to clients and a truly caring environment is evident. Along with these positive aspects, unfortunately, is the reality that funding is precarious.

Some agencies are fortunate to have enough in their budget to employ line staff workers who provide direct services to the clients. Other agencies depend on volunteers to provide all direct services. Most agencies have paid employees as well as volunteers and interns. Nonprofit agencies simply cannot operate without volunteers. They truly are the foundation of the nonprofit agency.

Some nonprofit agencies have grown in size (i.e., the American Red Cross and the United Way) and must operate under a more classical bureaucratic structure to efficiently organize the thousands of people working at the agency. Other nonprofit agencies are relatively small in terms of the number of workers and can efficiently operate with more flexibility, and workers often experience a sense of autonomy and personal support in these smaller agencies.

Critical Thinking/Self-Reflection Corner

- What motivates you in a job? Pay? Autonomy? Helping others? Power?
- Would you see yourself fitting in better at a nonprofit agency or a public agency? Why?
- Can you see yourself serving in an administrative position? In what way? If not, why not?

CHAPTER SUMMARY

Both public and nonprofit human services agencies serve similar functions in the community. Both provide services to similar populations with the aim of preventing and eliminating a variety of social problems, deviant behaviors, and emotional disorders. While both types of agencies may use the bureaucratic or the human relations approach to management, human services workers will probably see a combination of both types of structure. Traditionally, public agencies have operated within a bureaucratic structure because of the large numbers of employees working for city, county, state, and federal agencies. Bureaucracy may be useful for these agencies to aid in maintaining accountability and preventing chaos.

Nonprofit agencies have traditionally been able to function under the human relations model because of the smaller number of staff usually employed at the agency. Because nonprofits use volunteers to keep the agency operating, they often encourage a more supportive, family-like organization to ensure that volunteers feel welcome and appreciated. Also, because nonprofit agencies tend to pay lower than public agencies, workers may benefit from the human relations model because workers are rewarded by the support and caring attitude of supervisors and increased job challenges.

Funding for public agencies is typically obtained through taxes paid to various levels of government while funding for nonprofit agencies is through grants, fundraisers, and charitable donations. Volunteers make up the largest number of workers at nonprofit agencies while most workers at public agencies are paid employees.

Human services agencies are designed to meet the needs of the community in which it exists. They may be structured in classical bureaucratic style if the number of workers is high such as in government-operated agencies. Nonprofit agencies usually employ a smaller number of workers and may be managed under a human relations style of administration. Government-operated agencies tend to be more rigid and operate under chain of command. There is much focus on accountability and standardized paperwork. Nonprofit agencies focus on providing support to employees and volunteers and emphasize program effectiveness. Funding for nonprofit agencies is more tenuous than for public agencies.

Now that most of the practices and theories related to the field of human services have been presented, the reader is encouraged to review the Appendix. By answering some of the questions, the reader may begin to have an idea about the specific human services career path for which she or he may be best suited. Of course, this path may change throughout one's life, but it may serve as a beginning guide.

Suggested Applied Activities

1. Think of an agency that you would like to create in your community. Outline a proposal using the following questions to guide you: What populations will your agency serve? Why is there a need for this agency? What services currently exist for this population, and why are they not enough to meet the needs of the population? Which community leaders support your program? How will it be staffed? Who will be on your board of directors? Describe the services that will be delivered. How will you evaluate the agency and its effectiveness?

2. Think of three propositions that you would like to see pass on a ballot. Do you think they would have a chance? How could you lobby for them to pass?

Chapter Review Questions

1. How is a public agency usually funded?

2. How are nonprofit agencies funded?

3. What are two aspects of a bureaucratic-run agency?

4. What is the difference between theory X and theory Y in terms of organizational practice?

5. What is a board of directors?

6. What is red tape?

7. What is chain of command?

Glossary of Terms

Agency is an organization that works to achieve various goals and usually provides services directly or indirectly to a community.

American Red Cross is an organization established to assist people who have been devastated by a disaster.

Board of directors is a group of people who serve as an advisory council for a nonprofit agency.

Chain of command is the hierarchal structure found in bureaucracies in which lower level employees must communicate only with the person directly above them in the hierarchy.

Expressive leadership style is a management style that focuses on minimizing interpersonal hostility and on fostering close, supportive relationships among employees.

Grants are funding offers from either government agencies or private foundations to agencies that have submitted an application for funding.

Human relations model is an approach to management that focuses on the needs of its employees and social forces in the workplace.

Instrumental leadership style is a rigid style of management whose main concern is with production and profit margins and respect for the organization's hierarchical structure.

Line staff are human services workers who deal directly with clients.

Number numbness occurs when human services workers focus on budget, accountability, policy, and procedures rather than on program development and human needs.

Organization is a purposeful social unit constructed to achieve certain goals or to carry out a task.

Shadow organization refers to the informal norms and behaviors found at most agencies that often dictate acceptable ways to interact and communicate with colleagues, staff, and supervisors.

Whistle-blowing occurs when a worker speaks up about questionable practices that may be detrimental to the operation of an organization.

Case Presentation and Exit Quiz

General Description

Janice Nash just accepted a position as an elementary school teacher at a public school. For the past five years, Janice had been working for a government-funded program for low-income preschoolers called Head Start while she was working on her teaching credentials. That had been her only work experience. She started volunteering during high school at the Head Start Preschool, and after two years she was hired as a teacher/outreach coordinator. She earned some of her internship credit at Head Start when they increased her responsibilities to include training and supervising new volunteers.

Janice will be teaching second grade at her new job. When Janice arrives for orientation, she is overwhelmed. Her classroom is huge compared to the classrooms at Head Start. More than 50 other teachers from the school are at the first staff meeting. The principal is a 58-year-old woman with a doctoral degree in education. She is dressed in a pantsuit and speaks in a very formal manner. At Head Start, the head teacher had been a 35-year-old woman with a bachelor's degree in child development, and staff members were all on a first-name basis with each other and interactions were informal. At this new school, the principal addressed teachers more formally, using their last names, and even referred to herself as Dr. Blain.

At the meeting, Janice receives many forms, schedules, attendance rosters, and other paperwork that she must complete daily. Janice is told that by the following week, she must turn in daily lesson plans for the next six months. Each lesson plan must meet state standards and use the required texts and contain material that prepares students for the state-mandated testing in April.

Teachers did not mingle or speak with each other or with the principal. Janice had been accustomed to being involved in the planning of the programs at Head Start. When she was supervising volunteers, she'd take time to introduce each new volunteer to the other volunteers and staff members at each meeting. All the other teachers seemed to know what they were doing. They had all been teaching at the school for at least three years. Janice is the only new teacher.

One teacher, Mrs. Baker, introduces herself to Janice after the meeting. They are both teaching second grade. Mrs. Baker had been teaching 14 years and last year was named teacher of the year. She tells Janice that things will all work out, but that it takes time to get used to Dr. Blain. Mrs. Baker informs Janice that principals stay at the school for about five years, so they might have better luck next time. Mrs. Baker tells Janice that as long as she does the required paperwork and has her lesson plans documented appropriately, Dr. Blain will stay off her back. Mrs. Baker tells Janice that some of the teachers are sometimes uncooperative and may even try to sabotage the work of a new teacher. Mrs. Baker suggests that Janice lay low and discover with whom she feels comfortable before she gets too close to anyone.

After her talk with Mrs. Baker, Janice was approached by Dr. Blain. Dr. Blain explains that when Janice has any questions or problems, she should first go to one of the vice principals for help. If they couldn't help her, then she'll be referred to Dr. Blain directly.

Exit Quiz

1. Dr. Blain operates under which management style?
   a. Expressive
   b. Theory Y
   c. Instrumental
   d. Theory Z

2. The head teacher at Head Start operates under which management style?
   a. Expressive
   b. Theory X
   c. Instrumental
   d. Theory Z

3. The focus on attendance, policy, and daily reports may lead some teachers to experience
   a. a heightened sense of job enrichment
   b. a feeling of meaning in their lives
   c. number numbness
   d. all of the above

4. Mrs. Baker was telling Janice about
   a. the shadow organization
   b. how to win teacher of the year award
   c. how to make Dr. Blain like her
   d. all of the above

5. If some of the teachers behave in negative ways with Janice, she should
   a. go straight to Dr. Blain
   b. try to get back at them
   c. talk about them to other teachers behind their backs
   d. none of the above

6. Janice should go to the vice principal with problems to
   a. avoid Dr. Blain
   b. adhere to chain of command
   c. learn about the shadow organization
   d. none of the above

7. Head Start most likely follows the
   a. bureaucratic model
   b. theory X model
   c. human relations model
   d. none of the above

Exit Quiz Answers

1. c
2. a
3. c
4. a
5. d
6. b
7. c

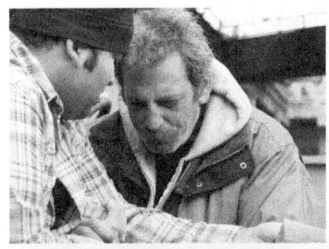
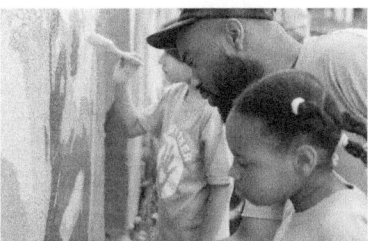
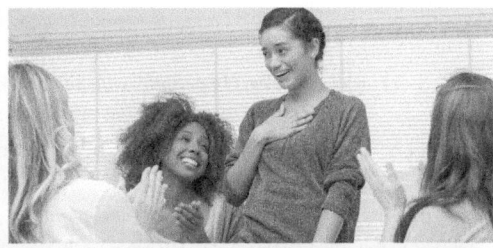

References

Chapter 1 Human Services: Foundational Concepts and Historical Background

Alle-Corliss, L., & Alle-Corliss, R. (1998). *Human service agencies: An orientation to fieldwork*. Pacific Grove, CA: Brooks/Cole.

Clodd, E. (1997). *Animism: The seed of religion*. Whitefish, MT: Kessinger Publishing.

Columbia electronic encyclopedia (6th ed.). (2006). New York: Columbia University Press. Retrieved from http://www.infoplease.com/encyclopedia/people/kr

Compayri, G. (2002). *Horace Mann and the public school in the United States* (M. D. Frost, Trans.). Portland, OR: University Press of the Pacific.

Corey, G., & Corey, M. S. (1993). *Becoming a helper* (2nd ed.). Pacific Grove, CA: Brooks/Cole.

Cutler, D., Bevilacqua, J., & McFarland, B. (2003). Four decades of community mental health: A symphony in four movements. *Community Mental Health Journal, 39*(5), 381–398.

Davis, K. G. (1990). *Don't know much about history*. New York: Perennial.

Dean, D. (1996). *Law-making and society in late Elizabethan England: The parliament of England, 1584–1601*. In A. Fletcher, J. Guy, & J. Morrill (Series Eds.), *Cambridge studies in early modern British history*. Cambridge, UK: Cambridge University Press.

El-Hai, J. (2004). *The lobotomist: A maverick medical genius and his tragic quest to rid the world of mental illness*. New York: Wiley.

The Free Online Dictionary, Thesaurus and Encyclopedia. (2013). *Ablism*. Retrieved February 14, 2013, from http://www.thefreedictionary.com/ablism

Grob, G. (1994). *The mad among us: A history of the care of America's mentally ill*. New York: Free Press.

Harper, R. F. (2002). *The code of Hammurabi, king of Babylon*. Portland, OR: University Press of the Pacific.

Hollingshead, G. (2004). *Bedlam*. New York: HarperCollins.

The Holy Bible (1611, Revised Standard Version, W. Tyndale, Trans.). New York: Thomas Nelson & Sons.

Howard, A. (1972). *Legislative history of S 1305 and S 1769: Bills to amend the economic opportunity act of 1964 to authorize a legal services program by establishing a national legal services corporation*. Chicago: University of Chicago Law School.

Kramer, R. M. (1981). *Voluntary agencies in the welfare state*. Berkeley, CA: University of California Press.

Library of Congress. (1989–1990). *Community Mental Health Centers Construction Act of 1989*. Author.

Lindemann, E. (1944). Symptomatology and management of acute grief. *American Journal of Psychiatry, 101*, 141–148.

Lombroso, C., & Ferrero, G. (2004). *Criminal woman, the prostitute and the normal woman* (N. H. Rafter & M. Gibson, Eds. and Trans.). Durham, NC: Duke University Press. (Original work published in Italian in 1893.)

Maslow, A. (1968). *Toward a psychology of being* (2nd ed.). New York: Harper & Row.

Miles, S. H. (2003). *The Hippocratic oath and the ethics of medicine.* New York: Oxford University Press.

Mommsen, T. E. (1942). Petrarch's conception of the Dark Ages. *Speculum, 17*(2), 226–242.

Neukrug, E. (1994). *Theory, practice and trends in human services.* Pacific Grove, CA: Brooks/Cole.

Rosenthal, H. (2003). *Human services dictionary.* London: Psychology Press.

Schaefer, R. T. (1988). *Racial and ethnic groups.* Glenview, IL: Scott Foresman.

Sears, D. O., Peplau, L. A., & Taylor, S. E. (1991). *Social psychology.* Englewood Cliffs, NJ: Prentice Hall.

Slaikeu, K. A. (1990). *Crisis intervention: A handbook for practice and research* (2nd ed.). Boston: Allyn & Bacon.

Summers, M. (1969). *Malleus maleficarum.* New York: Beaufort Books.

Weiner, D. B. (1979). The apprenticeship of Philippe Pinel: A new document, observations of citizen Pussin on the insane. *American Journal of Psychiatry, 136,* 1128–1134.

Zastrow, C. (1995). *The practice of social work* (3rd ed.). Pacific Grove, CA: Brooks/Cole.

Chapter 2 Modern-Day Human Services: Policies and Programs, Interventions, and Demographic Considerations

Allard, S. W. (2008). *Helping hand for the working poor: The role of nonprofits in today's safety net.* Paper presented at the 2008 West Coast Poverty Center conference, "Old Assumptions, New Realities: Economic Security for Working Families in the 21st Century," University of Washington, September 10–12, 2008. p. 1

Alle-Corliss, L., & Alle-Corliss, R. (1998). *Human service agencies: An orientation to fieldwork.* Pacific Grove, CA: Brooks/Cole.

Caplan, G. (1964). *Principles of preventive psychiatry.* New York: Basic Books.

Center for Health Workforce Studies. (2006). *The impact of the aging population on the health workforce in the United States.* Washington, DC: National Center for Health Workforce Analysis, Bureau of Health Professions, Health Resources and Services Administration, U.S. Department of Health and Human Services.

Chin, J. L. (2000). Culturally competent health care. *Public Health Reports, 115,* 25–33.

Department of Health and Human Services. (2011). *Immigrant access to health and human services.* Retrieved from http://aspe.hhs.gov/hsp/11/ImmigrantAccess/index.shtml

Himes, C. L. (2002). Elderly Americans. *Population Bulletin, 56*(4), 1–44.

Hogan-Garcia, M. (1999). *The four skills of cultural diversity competence.* Pacific Grove, CA: Brooks/Cole.

Hsu, J., Tseng, W., Ashton, G., McDermott, J., & Char, W., (1985). Family interaction patterns among Japanese American and Caucasian families in Hawaii. *American Journal of Psychiatry, 142,* 577–581.

Jones, M. L. (1993). *The color of culture.* Impact Communications.

Kanel, K. (2005). *Ataque de nervios: Is it time to designate it as a clinical syndrome on its own?* Unpublished manuscript. (Kar, Kramer, Skinner, & Zambrana, 1995)

Kar, S., Kramer, J., Skinner, J., & Zambrana, R. E. (1995). Panel V1: Ethnic minorities, health care systems, and behavior. *Health Psychology, 14,* 641–646.

Kim, B. S. K., Liang, C. T. H., & Li, L. C. (2003). Counselor ethnicity, counselor nonverbal behavior, and session outcome with Asian American Clients: Initial findings. *Journal of Counseling & Development, 81*(2), 202–207.

Koss-Chioino, J. D. (1999). Depression among Puerto Rican women: Culture, etiology and diagnosis. *Hispanic Journal of Behavioral Sciences, 21*(3), 330–350.

Levin, J., & Rabrenovic, G. (2007). The sociology of violence. In C. D. Bryant & D. L. Peck (Eds.), *21st century sociology: A reference handbook.* Thousand Oaks, CA: Sage Publications.

Liebowitz, M. R., Salman, E., Jusion, C. M., Garfinkel, R., Street, L., Cardenas, D. L., Silvestre, J., Fryer, A. J., Carrasco, J. L., Davies, S., Guarnaccia, J. P., & Klein, D. (1994). Ataque de nervios and panic disorder. *American Journal of Psychiatry 151*(6), 871–875.

Newton, J. (1988). *Preventing mental illness.* London: Routledge & Kegan Paul.

Oquendo, M. A. (1995). Differential diagnosis of ataque de nervios. *American Journal Orthopsychiatry, 65*(1), 60–64.

Passel, J. S., & Cohn, D. (2011). *Unauthorized immigrant population: National and state trends, 2010.* Pew Research Hispanic Trends Report. Retrieved from http://www.pewhispanic.org/2011/02/01/unauthorized-immigrant-population-brnational-and-state-trends-2010/

Price, R. H., Cowen, E. L., Lorion, R. P., & Ramos-McKay, J. (1988). *Fourteen ounces of prevention: A casebook for practitioners.* Washington, DC: American Psychological Association.

Schechter, D. S., Marshall, R., Salman, E., Goetz, D., Davies, S., & Liebowitz, M. R. (2000). Ataque de nervios and history of childhood trauma. *Journal of Traumatic Stress, 13*(3), 529–534.

Smith, S. R. (2002). Social services. In L. M. Salamon (Ed.), *The State of Nonprofit America.* Washington, DC: The Brookings Institution Press.

Chapter 3 Ethical and Multicultural Issues in the Human Services

Abudabbeh, N., & Aseel, H. A. (1999). Transcultural counseling and Arab Americans. In J. McFadden (Ed.), *Transcultural counseling* (2nd ed., pp. 283–296). Alexandria, VA: American Counseling Association.

Al-Abdul-Jabbar, J., & Al-Issa, I. (2000). Psychotherapy in Islamic society. In I. Al-Issa (Ed.), *Al-Junun: Mental illness in the Islamic world* (pp. 277–293). Madison, CT: International Universities Press.

Al-Krenawai, A., & Graham, J. R. (2000). Culturally sensitive social work practice with Arab clients in mental health settings. *Health & Social Work, 25*(1), 9–22.

Allison, S. R., & Vining, C. B. (1999). Native American culture and language. *Bilingual Review, 24*(1/2), 193–207.

American Association for Marriage and Family Therapy. (2001). *AAMFT code of ethics.* Washington, DC: Author.

American Counseling Association. (2005). *Code of ethics.* Alexandria, VA: Author.

American Psychiatric Association. (2001). *Principles of medical ethics with annotations especially applicable to psychiatry.* Washington, DC: Author.

American Psychological Association. (2002). Ethical principles of psychologists and code of conduct. *American Psychologist, 57*(12), 1060–1073.

American School Counselor Association. (2004). *Ethical standards for school counselors.* Alexandria, VA: Author.

Association for Counselor Education and Supervision. (1995). Ethical guidelines for counseling supervisors. *Counselor Education and Supervision, 34*(3), 270–276.

Benitez, B. R. (2004). Confidentiality and its exceptions (including the U.S. Patriot Act). *The Therapist, 16*(4), 32–36.

Brohl, K., & Ledford, R. (2012). *Continuing education for California social workers and marriage and family therapists.* California: Elite CME Publishers.

Canadian Counselling Association. (1999). *CCA code of ethics.* Ottawa: Author.

Canda, E. R. (2009, Fall Semester). *Spiritual aspects of social work practice: Course description and syllabus* [Online]. Lawrence, KS: University of Kansas.

Council for Standards in Human Service Education. (2005). *CSHSE legacy: Past, present & future.* Retrieved January 29, 2013, from www.cshse.org

Feminist Therapy Institute. (2000). *Feminist therapy code of ethics* (rev. 1999). San Francisco: Author.

Hare-Mustin, R. T. (1983). An appraisal of the relationship between women and psychotherapy: 80 years after the case of Dora. *American Psychologist, 32*, 889–890.

Herr, E. L., & Cramer, S. H. (1987). *Controversies in the mental health professions.* Muncie, IN: Accelerated Development.

Hogan-Garcia, M. (1999). *The four skills of cultural diversity competence.* Pacific Grove, CA: Brooks/Cole.

Hsu, J., Tseng, W., Ashton, G., McDermott, J., & Char, W., (1985). Family interaction patterns among Japanese American and Caucasian families in Hawaii. *American Journal of Psychiatry, 142*, 577–581.

Jensen, D. G. (2003). HIPAA overview. *The Therapist, 15*(3), 26–27.

Kim, B. S. K., Atkinson, D. R., & Umemoto, D. (2001). Asian cultural values and counseling process: Current knowledge and directions for future research. *The Counseling Psychologist, 29*, 570–603.

Kim, B. S. K., Liang, C. T. H., & Li, L. C. (2003). Counselor ethnicity, counselor nonverbal behavior, and session outcome with Asian American clients: Initial findings. *Journal of Counseling & Development, 81*(2), 202–207.

Loza, N. (2001, May). *Insanity on the Nile: The history of psychiatry in pharaonic Egypt.* Paper presented at the Second Biannual National Conference on Arab American Health Issues, Dearborn, MI.

Mattes, L. J., & Omark, D. R. (1994). *Speech and language assessment for the bilingual handicapped.* San Diego, CA: College-Hill Press.

Nassar-McMillan, S. C. (1999, May). *Mental health considerations in the Arab community*. Paper presented at the Conference on Arab American Health Issues, Dearborn, MI.

Nassar-McMillan, S. C., & Hakim-Larson, J. (2003). Counseling considerations among Arab Americans. *Journal of Counseling & Development, 81*(2), 150–159.

National Association of Social Workers. (1999). *Code of ethics*. Washington, DC: Author.

National Organization for Human Services. (2000). Ethical standards of human service professionals. *Human Service Education, 20*(1), 61–68.

National Organization for Human Services. (2013). *Ethical standards for human service professionals*. Retrieved January 29, 2013, from http://www.nationalhumanservices.org/ethical-standards-for-hs-professionals

Native American Research and Training Center. (1995). *Some alarming facts*. Tucson, AZ: University of Arizona.

Nydell, M. (1987). *Understanding Arabs: A guide for westerners*. Yarmouth, ME: Intercultural Press.

Shields, S. A. (1995). The role of emotion, beliefs, and values on gender development. In N. Eisenberg (Ed.), *Review of personality and social psychology* (Vol. 15, pp. 212–232). Thousand Oaks, CA: Sage.

Siegel, M. (1979). Privacy, ethics, and confidentiality. *Professional Psychology, 10*, 249–258.

Swoboda, J. S., Elwork, A., Sales, B. D., & Levine, D. (1978). Knowledge of a compliance with privileged communication and child-abuse reporting laws. *Professional Psychology, 9*, 448–457.

Uba, L. (1994). *Asian Americans: Personality patterns, identity, and mental health*. New York: Guilford Press.

United States Department of Health and Human Services. (2003). OCR Privacy Brief: Summary of the HIPAA Privacy Rule and other consumer information materials.

Zylstra, S. (2006). Untitled [Letter to the editor]. *The Therapist, 18*(1), 6.

Chapter 4   Human Services Workers

Bureau of Labor Statistics. (2012). *Current population survey: Education pays*. Handout from the California Association of Alcohol and Drug Educators 2013 Conference.

Day, S. (2010). *My experiences working in human services after obtaining a 2-year degree*. Retrieved June 19, 2013, http://voices.yahoo.com

Kazdin, A. E. (2001). *Behavior modification in applied settings* (6th ed.). Pacific Grove, CA: Brooks/Cole.

Locsin, A. (2013). List of careers in human services. *The Houston Chronicle*. Retrieved June 19, 2013, http://work.chron.com/list-careers-human-services-6907.html

National Organization for Human Services. (2013). *New information on the student application: Human Services-Board Certified practitioner*. Retrieved June 19, 2013, http://www.nationalhumanservices.org/certification

Occupational Outlook Handbook. (2013). *Social and human service assistants*. Retrieved June 19, 2013, http://www.bls.gov/ooh/community-and-social-service/social-and-human-service-assistant

Recruiter.com. (2013). *Human services careers*. Retrieved June 19, 2013, http://www.recruiter.com/careers/human-services.html

Salary Wizard. (2013). *Job description for human services worker*. Retrieved June 19, 2013, http://www1.salary.com/Human-Services-Worker-Salary.html

Chapter 5   Basic Counseling Skills, Personal Characteristics of Human Services Workers, and Theoretical Approaches in Counseling

Adler, A. (1959). *Understanding human nature*. New York: Premier Books.

Bateson, G., Jackson, D. D., Haley, J., & Weakland, J. (1956). Toward a theory of schizophrenia. *Behavioral Science, 1*, 251–264.

Beck, A. T., Rush, A., Shaw, B., & Emery, G. (1979). *Cognitive therapy of depression*. New York: Guilford Press.

Borntrager, C., Chorpita, B. F., Higa-McMillan, C. K., Daleiden, E. L., & Starace, N. (2013). Usual care for trauma-exposed youth: Are clinician-reported therapy techniques evidence-based? *Children and Youth Services Review, 35*, 1, 133–141.

Bowen, M. (1992). *Family therapy in clinical practice*. New York: Jason Aronson.

Brenner, C. (1974). *An elementary textbook of psychoanalysis*. Garden City, NY: Anchor Books.

Bugental, J. F. T. (1978). *Psychotherapy and process: the fundamentals of an existential-humanistic approach*. New York: Random House.

Burroughts, T., & Somerville, J. (2012). Utilization of evidenced based dialectical behavioral therapy in assertive community treatment: Examining feasibility and challenges. *Community Mental Health Journal*. Springer Science+Business Media, LLC2012 10.1007/s10597-120-9485-2. Retrieved June 18, 2013, http://link.springer.com/article/10.1007/s10597-012-9485-2/fulltext.html

Caplan, G. (1964). *Principles of preventive psychiatry*. New York: Basic Books.

Carkhuff, R., & Berenson, B. (1967). *Beyond counseling and therapy*. New York: Holt, Rinehart & Winston.

Corey, G. (2005). *Theory and practice of counseling and psychotherapy* (7th ed.). Pacific Grove, CA: Brooks/Cole.

Department of Mental Health. (2013). *Evidence-based practices*. Retrieved June 20, 2013, http://mental health.vermont.gov/ebp

Drake, R. E, Goldman, H. H., Leff, H. S., Lehman, A. F., Dixon, L., Mueser, K. T., Torrey, W. C., et al. (2001). Implementing evidence-based practices in routine mental health service settings. *Psychiatric Services, 52*(2), 52–58.

Ellis, A. (1962). *Reason and emotion in psychotherapy*. Secaucus, NJ: Citadel Press.

Feigenbaum, J. (2007). Dialectical behavior therapy: An increasing evidence base. *Journal of Mental Health, 16*(1), 51–68.

Freud, S. (1966). *The complete introductory lectures on psychoanalysis* (J. Strachey, Trans.). New York: W.W. Norton. (Original work published in 1933.)

Gabbard, G. O. (2000). *Psychodynamic psychiatry in clinical practice* (3rd ed.). Washington, DC: American Psychiatric Press.

Geller, J. L. (1986). In again, out again: Preliminary evaluation of a state hospital's worst recidivists. *Hospital & Community Psychiatry, 37*, 386–390.

Gibb, J. R. (1970). The effects of human relations training. In A. E. Bergin, & S. L. Garfield (Eds.), *Handbook of psychotherapy and behavior change* (Chapter 22, pp. 2114–1276). New York: John Wiley & Sons.

Glasser, W. (1975). *Reality therapy: A new approach to psychiatry*. New York: Harper & Row.

Guntrip, H. (1973). *Psychoanalytic theory, therapy, and the self*. New York: Basic Books.

Haley, J. (1976). *Problem-solving therapy: New strategies for effective family therapy*. San Francisco: Jossey-Bass.

Hutchins, D. E., & Cole, C. (1992). *Helping relationships and strategies* (2nd ed.). Pacific Grove, CA: Brooks/Cole.

Ivey, A. E., Gluckstern, N. B., & Ivey, M. G. (1997). *Basic attending skills* (3rd ed.). North Amherst, MA: Microtraining Associates.

Kanel, K. (2002). Mental health needs of Spanish-speaking Latinos in southern California. *Hispanic Journal of Behavioral Sciences, 24*(1), 74–91.

Kanel, K. (2014). *A guide to crisis intervention* (5th ed.). Pacific Grove, CA: Brooks/Cole.

Laing, R. D., & Esterson, A. (1977). *Sanity, madness, and the family*. New York: Penguin Books.

Linehan, M. M. (1993). *Cognitive-behavioral treatment of borderline personality*. New York: Guilford Press.

Madanes, C. (1981). *Strategic family therapy*. San Francisco: Jossey-Bass.

Mahler, M. S., Pine, F., & Bergman, A. (1975). *The psychological birth of the human infant: Symbiosis and individuation*. New York: Basic Books.

Meichenbaum, D. (1985). *Stress inoculation training*. New York: Pergamon.

Meichenbaum, D. (1986). Cognitive behavior modification. In F. H. Kanfer & A. P. Goldstein (Eds.), *Helping people change: A textbook of methods* (pp. 346–380). New York: Pergamon.

Minuchin, S. (1974). *Families and family therapy*. Cambridge, MA: Harvard University Press.

Okun, B. (1992). *Effective helping* (4th ed.). Pacific Grove, CA: Brooks/Cole.

Pavlov, I. P. (1927). *Conditioned reflexes* (G. V. Anrep, Trans.). New York: Liveright.

Rogers, C. (1958). The characteristics of a helping relationship. *Personnel and Guidance Journal, 37*, 6–16.

Rogers, C. (1961). *On becoming a person*. Boston: Houghton Mifflin.

Rogers, C. (1970). *Carl Rogers on encounter groups*. New York: Harper & Row.

Rogers, C. (1987). Steps toward world peace, 1948–1986: Tension reduction in theory and practice. *Counseling and Values, 32*(1), 12–16.

Satir, V. (1983). *Conjoint family therapy* (3rd ed.). Palo Alto, CA: Science and Behavior Books.

Skinner, B. F. (1948). *Walden II*. New York: Macmillan.

Skinner, B. F. (1953). *Science and human behavior*. New York: Macmillan.

Swigar, M. E., Astrachan, B., Levine, M. A., Mayfield, V., & Radovich, C. (1991). Single and repeated admissions to a mental health center: Demographic, clinical and use of service characteristics. *International Journal of Social Psychiatry, 37*, 4, 259–266.

Whitaker, C. A. (1976). The hindrance of theory in clinical work. In P. J. Guerin, Jr. (Ed.), *Family therapy: Theory and practice* (pp. 182–192). New York: Gardner Press.

Wolpe, J. (1990). *The practice of behavior therapy* (4th ed.). Elmsford, NY: Pergamon.

Wynne, L., Tyckoff, I., Day, J., & Hirsch, S. H. (1958). Pseudomutuality in schizophrenia. *Psychiatry, 21*, 205–220.

Yalom, I. D. (1980). *Existential psychotherapy*. New York: Basic Books.

Yalom, I. D. (1985). *The theory and practice of group psychotherapy*. New York: Basic.

Chapter 6 Crisis Intervention, Suicide Prevention, PTSD, Community Disasters and Trauma Response, and Military Trauma

American Psychiatric Association. (2000). *Diagnostic and statistical manual of mental disorders, fourth edition, text revision (DSM-IV-TR)*. Washington, DC: Author.

Boyd, C., & Asmussen, S. (2013). Traumatic brain injury (TBI) and the military. In A. Rubin, E. L. Weiss, & J. E. Coll (Eds.), *Handbook of military social work* (pp. 163–178). Hoboken, NJ: John Wiley & Sons, Inc.

Claver, M., Dobalian, A., Fickel, J. J., Ricci, K., & Horn-Mallers, M. (2013). Comprehensive care for vulnerable elderly veterans during disasters. *Archives of Gerontology and Geriatrics, 56*(1), 205–213. DOI:10.1016/j.archger.2012.07.010

Claver, M., Friedman, D., Dobalian, A., Ricci, K., & Horn-Mallers, M. (2012). The role of Veterans Affairs in emergency management: A systematic literature review. *PLoS Currents, 12*(4), e198d344bc40a75f927c9bc5024279815. DOI:10.1371/198d344bc40a75f927c9bc5024279815

Department of Defense. (2009). *Numbers for traumatic brain injury*. Silverspring, MD: DVBIC.org

Gabbard, G. O. (2000). *Psychodynamic psychiatry in clinical practice* (3rd ed.). Washington, DC: American Psychiatric Press Inc.

Hoge, C. W., Castro, C. A., Messer, S. C., McGurk, D., Cotting, D. I., & Koffman, R. L. (2004). Combat duty in Iraq and Afghanistan, mental health problems, and barriers to care. *New England Journal of Medicine, 351*, 13–22.

Kanel, K. L. (2013). Veterans' mental health: Challenges and issues of college enrolled OIF and OEF veterans. *Social Work in Mental Health*. DOI:10.1080/15332985.2013.812541

Kanel, K. L. (2015). *A guide to crisis intervention* (5th ed.). Pacific Grove, CA: Brooks/Cole.

Lindy, J. D., Grace, M. C., & Green, B. L. (1984). Building a conceptual bridge between civilian trauma and war trauma: Preliminary psychological findings from a clinical sample of Vietnam veterans. In B. A. van der Kolk (Ed.), *Post-traumatic stress disorder: Psychological and biological sequelae* (pp. 43–57). Washington, DC: American Psychiatric Press

Mental Health Center of North Iowa. *Background phases of disaster* [Online]. Mason City, IA: Author. Retrieved May 23, 2014, from www.mhconi.org/Topic DisasterBkgrd.htm

National Center for Posttraumatic Stress Disorder. (2005). *Treatment of PTSD* [Online Fact Sheet]. White River Junction, VT: Author. Available at www.ncptsd.org/facts/treatment/fs_treatment.html

Shapiro, F., (2002). EMDR twelve years after its introduction: Past and future research. *Journal of Clinical Psychology, 58*, 1–22.

Wyman, S. (1982). *Suicide evaluation and treatment*. Paper presented at a seminar of the California Association of Marriage and Family Therapists, Orange County Chapter.

Yarvis, J. S. (2013). Posttraumatic stress disorder (PTSD) in veterans. In A. Rubin, E. L. Weiss, & J. E. Coll (Eds.), *The handbook of military social work* (pp. 81–97). Hoboken, NJ: John Wiley & Sons, Inc.

Yarvis, J. S., & Schiess, L. (2008). Subthreshold PTSD as a predictor of depression, alcohol use, and health problems in soldiers. *Journal of Workplace Behavioral Health, 23*, 4.

Chapter 7   Human Services Populations

Alzheimer's Association. (2013). *What is Alzheimer's?* Retrieved from http://www.alz.org/alzheimers_disease_what_is_alzheimers.asp

Bial, M. (2005). Looming workforce shortages in aging services: Getting ready on college campuses. *The Journal of Pastoral Counseling, 40*, 49–60.

Bonnie, R., & Wallace, R. (2003). *Elder mistreatment: Abuse, neglect and exploitation in an aging America.* Washington, DC: National Academies Press.

CDC. (2011). Youth risk behavior surveillance—United States, *Morbidity and Mortality Weekly Report, 61*, SS-4.

CDC. (2013). *Adolescent and school health. Sexual risk behavior: HIV, STD, & teen pregnancy.* Retrieved from http://www.cdc.gov/HealthyYouth/sexualbehaviors/

Center for American Progress. (2013). *Elderly poverty: The challenge before us.* Retrieved from http://www.americanprogress.org/issues/poverty/report/2008/07/30/4690/elderly-poverty-the-challenge-before-us/

CSUN. (2007). *Television and health.* Retrieved from http://www.csun.edu/science/health/docs/tv&health.html

Deal, R. L. (2013). *Marriage, family, stepfamily statistics.* Retrieved from http://www.smartstepfamilies.com/view/statistics

DiClemente, R. J., Ponton, L. E., & Hartley, D. (1991). Prevalence and correlates of cutting behavior: Risk for HIV transmission. *Journal of the American Academy of Child and Adolescent Psychiatry, 30*, 735–739.

Domenico, D. M., & Jones, K. H. (2007). Adolescent pregnancy in America: Causes and responses. *The Journal for Vocational Special Needs Education, 30*(1), 4–12.

Hooyman, N. R., & Kiyak, H. A. (2011). *Social gerontology: A multidisciplinary perspective* (9th ed.). Boston: Allyn and Bacon.

Jason Foundation. (2013). *Youth suicide statistics.* Retrieved from http://jasonfoundation.com/prp/facts/youth-suicide-statistics/

Menacker, F., Martin, J. A., MacDorman, M. F., & Ventura, S. J. (2004). Births to 10–14 year-old mothers, 1990–2002: Trends and health outcomes. *National Vital Statistics Reports, 53*(7), 1–18.

National Alliance on Mental Health (NAMI). (2010). *Mental illnesses.* Retrieved from http://www.nami.org/Template.cfm?Section=By_Illness&template=/ContentManagement/ContentDisplay.cfm&ContentID=88551

National Children's Alliance. (2013). *National statistics on child abuse.* Retrieved from http://www.nationalchildrensalliance.org/NCANationalStatistics

National Conference of State Legislature (NCSL). (2013). Homeless and runaway youth. Retrieved from http://www.ncsl.org/research/human-services/homeless-and-runaway-youth.aspx

National Gang Center. (n.d.). Office of Juvenile Justice and Delinquency Prevention. Bureau of Justice Assistance. U.S. Department of Justice. *Frequently asked questions about gangs.* Retrieved May 23, 2014, from http://www.nationalgangcenter.gov/About/FAQ

National Institute of Drug Abuse. (2012). *Drug facts: High school and youth trends.* Retrieved from http://www.drugabuse.gov/publications/drugfacts/high-school-youth-trends

Repetti, R. L., Taylor, S. E., & Seeman, T. E. (2002). Risky families: family social environments and the mental and physical health of offspring. *Psychological Bulletin, 128*(2), 330–366.

Simpson, C., Pruitt, R., Blackwell, D., & Sweringen, G. S. (1997, April). Preventing teen pregnancy: Early adolescence. *Advance for Nurse Practitioners,* 24–29.

Spear L. P. (2000). The adolescent brain and age-related behavioral manifestations. *Neuroscience and Biobehavioral Reviews, 24*, 417–463.

TeenHelp.com. (2013). *Teen violence statistics.* Retrieved from http://www.teenhelp.com/teen-violence/teen-violence-statistics.html

Teen Violence Statistics. (2009). *School shootings.* Retrieved from http://www.teenviolencestatistics.com/content/school-shootings.html

Twentman, C. T., & Plotkin, R. C. (1982). Unrealistic expectations of parents who maltreat their children: An educational deficit that pertains to child development. *Journal of Clinical Psychology, 38*, 407–503.

U.S. Department of Justice. (2002). *National incidence studies of missing, abducted, runaway or thrownaway children (NISMART).* Retrieved from http://www.missingkids.com/en_US/documents/nismart2_runaway.pdf

U.S. Department of Justice. (2012). *Comprehensive anti-gang initiative.* Retrieved from http://www.ojjdp.gov/programs/antigang/index.html

Whitlock, J. (2010). Self-injurious behavior in adolescents. *PLOS Med, 7*(5), e1000240. doi:10.1371/journal.pmed.1000240

Williamson, J. M., Bordin, C. M., & Howe, B. A. (1991). The ecology of adolescent maltreatment: A multilevel examination of adolescent physical abuse, sexual abuse, and neglect. *Journal of Consulting and Clinical Psychology, 59*(3), 449–457.

Chapter 8   Mental Illness, Poverty, Disabilities, Crime/Violence, and Substance Abuse

American Psychiatric Association. (2013a). *Addictions*. Retrieved from http://www.apa.org/topics/addiction/

American Psychiatric Association. (2013b). *Diagnostic and statistical manual of mental disorders* (5th ed.). Arlington, VA: American Psychiatric Publishing.

ASPE. (2012). *Information on poverty and income statistics: A summary of 2012 current population survey data*. Retrieved from http://aspe.hhs.gov/hsp/12/Poverty AndIncomeEst/ib.shtml

Bureau of Justice Statistics. (2013). *Prevalence of imprisonment in the U.S. population, 1974–2001*. Retrieved from http://www.bjs.gov/index.cfm?ty=pbdetail&iid=836

CDC. (2012). *Health United States, 2011*. Retrieved from http://www.cdc.gov/nchs/data/hus/hus11.pdf

Cornell University. (2012). *2011 Disability Status Report United States*. Retrieved from http://www.disability statistics.org/StatusReports/2011-PDF/2011-Status Report_US.pdf?CFID=5729736&CFTOKEN=4e4 b5785ee3fb320-772B731D-5056-B400-0D232789 0ED11DE8&jsessionid=8430179b460fc482cf3c720 71782f7e5b381

Families USA. (2013). *2013 federal poverty guidelines*. Retrieved from http://www.familiesusa.org/resources/tools-for-advocates/guides/federal-poverty-guidelines.html

Federal Bureau of Investigation. (2012). *Crime in the United States, 2012*. Retrieved from http://www.fbi.gov/about-us/cjis/ucr/crime-in-the-u.s/2012/crime-in-the-u.s.-2012/persons-arrested/persons-arrested

Froh, J. J., & Bono, G. (forthcoming, 2013). *Making grateful kids: A scientific approach to helping youth thrive*. West Conshohocken, PA: Templeton Press.

Group Health. (n.d.). *The epidemiology of use of analgesics for chronic pain*. Retrieved May 23, 2014, from http://www.fda.gov/downloads/Drugs/NewsEvents/UCM308128.pdf

Hasin, D. S., Stinson, F. S., Ogburn, E., & Grant, B. F. (2007). Prevalence, correlates, disability, and comorbidity of DSM-IV alcohol abuse and dependence in the United States. *Journal of the American Medical Association, 64*(7), 830–842.

HHS. (1999). *A report to Congress on substance abuse and child protection. Understanding addiction, substance abuse treatment, and recovery. Chapter 2*. Retrieved from http://aspe.hhs.gov/hsp/subabuse99/chap2.htm

Mayerson, A. (1992). *The history of the ADA: A movement perspective*. Disability Rights Education and Defense Fund. Retrieved from http://dredf.org/publications/ada_history.shtml

National Institute of Mental Health (NIMH). (n.d.). *The number count: Mental disorders in the America*. Retrieved May 23, 2014, from http://www.nimh.nih.gov/health/publications/the-numbers-count-mental-disorders-in-america/index.shtml

National Institute on Drug Abuse. (2011). *Substance abuse among older adults*. Retrieved from http://www.drugabuse.gov/news-events/nida-notes/2011/12/substance-abuse-among-older-adults

National Institute on Drug Abuse. (2012a). *National survey of drug use and health*. Retrieved from http://www.drugabuse.gov/national-survey-drug-use-health

National Institute on Drug Abuse. (2012b). *Principles of drug addiction treatment: A research-based guide* (3rd ed.). Retrieved from http://www.drugabuse.gov/publications/principles-drug-addiction-treatment-research-based-guide-third-edition/principles-effective-treatment

National Institute on Drug Abuse. (n.d.a). *DrugFacts: Nationwide trends*. Retrieved May 23, 2014, from http://www.drugabuse.gov/publications/drugfacts/nationwide-trends

National Institute on Drug Abuse. (n.d.b). *Addiction science: From molecules to managed care*. Retrieved May 23, 2014, from http://www.drugabuse.gov/publications/addiction-science-molecules-to-managed-care/introduction/drug-abuse-costs-united-states-economy-hundreds-billions-dollars-in-increased-health

Oswald, W. T. (2005). *The poverty trap: A critical look at how we define the causes of poverty*. Retrieved from http://www.caringcouncilsd.org/Documents/The PovertyTrap.PDF

SAMHSA. (n.d.). *Adults with both mental illness and substance use disorder in 2011*. Retrieved May 23, 2014, from http://www.samhsa.gov/data/

Chapter 9 Interpersonal Partner Abuse, Sexual Assault, HIV/AIDS, and LGBT Issues

Black, M. C., Basile, K. C., Breiding, M. J., Smith, S. G., Walters, M. L., Merrick, M. T., …, Stevens, M. R. (2011). *The national intimate partner and sexual violence survey: 2010 summary report*. Retrieved from http://www.cdc.gov/violenceprevention/pdf/nisvs_report2010-a.pdf

California State University, Northridge. (2013). *Queer studies*. Retrieved October 25, 2013, http://www.csun.edu/qs

Centers for Disease Control and Prevention. (2002). Guidelines for preventing opportunistic infections among HIV-infected persons: Recommendations of the U.S. Public Health Service and the Infectious Diseases Society of American. *Morbidity and Mortality Weekly Report, 51*, RR-8.

Committee on the Judiciary, U.S. Senate, 102nd Congress. (1992). *Violence against women: A majority staff report* (p. 3). Washington, DC: Author.

Department of Defense 6495.01. (2005). *Sexual assault prevention and response program*. Washington, DC: Author.

Ferguson, C. J. (2012). Positive female role-models eliminate negative effects of sexually violent media. *Journal of Communication, 62*(5), 888–899. doi:10.1111/j.1460-2466.2012.01666.x

Good Therapy.org. (2013). *Therapy for LGBT issues*. Retrieved October 25, 2013, http://www.goodtherapy.org/therapy-for -LGBT-issues.html

Heise, L., Ellsberg, M., & Gottemoeller, M. (1999, December). Ending violence against women. *Population Reports* (Series L, No. 11, Volume XXVII, Number 4). Baltimore, MD: Population Information Program of the Johns Hopkins University School of Public Health.

Kanel, K. (2007). *A guide to crisis intervention* (3rd ed.). Pacific Grove, CA: Brooks/Cole.

Katz, L. S., Bloor, L. E., Cojucar, G., & Draper, T. (2007). Women who served in Iraq seeking mental health services: Relationships between military sexual trauma, symptoms and readjustment. *Psychological Services, 4*(4), 239–249.

Kitfield, J. (2012, September 18). The enemy within. *National Journal*. Retrieved from http://www.nationaljournal.com/magazine/the-military-s-rape-problem-20120913

Knickerbocker, B. (2013). American Catholics like what they're hearing from Pope Francis. Boston, MA: The Christian Science Monitor.

Magallon, T. (1987, June). Counseling patients with HIV infections. *Medical Aspects of Human Sexuality*, 129–147.

Merriam-Webster Dictionary. (2013). *Queer Theory*. Retrieved October 25, 2013, http://www.merriam-webster.com/dictionary/queer%20theory

Moore, B. A., & Kennedy, D. H. (2011). *Wheels down: Adjusting to life after deployment*. Washington, DC: APA Lifetools.

National Gay and Lesbian Task Force. (2013). *Marriage equality is just the beginning*. Retrieved October 25, 2013, http://www.ngltf.org/issues/aging/challenges

Pierce, P. E. (2006). The role of women in the military. In T. W. Britt, A. B. Adler & C. A. Castro (Eds.), *Military life: The psychology of serving in peace and combat* (pp. 97–118). Westport, CT: Greenwood.

Price, R. E., Omizo, M. M., & Hammitt, V. L. (October 1986). Counseling clients with AIDS. *Journal of Counseling and Development, 65*, 96–97.

Rennison, C. M. (2003, February). Intimate partner violence, 1993–2001 (NCJ 197838). *Bureau of Justice Statistics crime data brief*. Washington, DC: U.S. Department of Justice.

Rothman, E. F., Exner, D., & Baughman, A. (2011). The prevalence of sexual assault against people who identify as gay, lesbian or bisexual in the United States: A systematic review. *Trauma Violence Abuse, 12*(2), 55–66.

Safe Horizon. (2013). *Domestic violence: Statistics and facts*. Retrieved June 19, 2013, http://www.safehorizon.org

Safe House Center. (2013). *LGBT Crisis Prevention Centers*. Retrieved October 25, 2013, http://www.safehousecenter.org/additional-information/lgbt-crisis-prevention-centers/

Schading, B. (2007). *A civilian's guide to the U.S. military: A comprehensive reference to the customs, language and structure of the armed forces*. Cincinnati, OH: Writer's Digest Books.

Slader, S. (1992). *HIV/IV drug users*. Paper presented at a meeting held at California State University, Fullerton.

Third World Solidarity. (2013). *The unique challenges facing queer people of color*. Retrieved from http://462 thridworldsolidarity.wordpress.com/the-unique-challenges-facing-queer-people-of-color/

USAID. (2013). *Gender-based violence*. Retrieved from http://www.usaid.gov/what-we-do/gender-equality-and-womens-empowerment/gender-based-violence

U.S. Bureau of Justice. (2013a). Female Victims of Sexual Violence, 1994-2010. Retrieved October 23, 2010, http://www.bjs.gov/index.cfm?ty=pbdetail&iid-4594

U.S. Bureau of Justice. (2013b). *Rape statistics*. Retrieved October 23, 2013, http://www.statisticbrain.com/rape-statistics

U.S. Department of Justice. (2005). *2005 National Crime Victimization Study*. Retrieved from http://www.bjs.gov/index.cfm?ty=pbdetail&iid=766

U.S. Department of Justice. (n.d.). *Facts about children and violence*. Retrieved May 23, 2014, from http://www.justice.gov/defendingchildhood/facts.html

U.S. Statistics. (2013). *HIV in the United States*. Retrieved February 19, 2013, http://aids.gov/hiv-aids-basics/hiv-aids-101/statistics/

Walker, L. E. A. (1984). *Battered woman syndrome*. New York: Springer Publishing.

Chapter 10   Stress Management

Almeida, D. M. (2005). Resilience and vulnerability to daily stressors assessed via diary methods. *Current Directions in Psychological Science, 14*(2), 62–68.

Almeida, D. M., & Horn, M. C. (2004). Is daily life more stressful during middle adulthood? In O. G. Brim, C. D. Ryff, & R. C. Kessler (Eds.), *How healthy are we? A national study of well-being at midlife* (pp. 425–451). Chicago: University of Chicago Press.

Anonymous. (2005). The change agenda. *Management Today*, p. 45.

Caplan, J. (2005). Training: What's hot in 2005. *China Staff, 11*(2), 20–24.

Chang, J. (2005). Pressure points. *Sales and Marketing Management, 157*(4), 18.

Ellis, A. (1962). *Reason and emotion in psychotherapy*. Secaucus, NJ: Citadel Press.

Ellis, A. (2001). *How to control your anxiety before it controls you*. New York: Citadel Press.

Freudenberger, H. J. (1975). The staff burnout syndrome in alternative institutions. *Psychotherapy: Theory, Research and Practice, 12*, 73–82.

Fry, W. F., & Salameh, W. A. (Eds.). (1993). *Advances in humor and psychotherapy*. Sarasota, FL: Professional Resources Press.

Goldman, L., & Lewis, J. (2005). The emphasis on stress. *Occupational Health, 57*(3), 12–14.

Gomez, J. S., & Michaelis, R. C. (1995). An assessment of burnout in human service providers. *Journal of Rehabilitation, 61*, 23.

Haley, J. (1976). *Problem solving therapy*. San Francisco: Jossey-Bass.

Horn Mallers, M., Charles, S. T., Neupert, S. D., & Almeida, D. M. (2010). Perceptions of childhood relationships with mother and father: Daily emotional and stressor experiences in adulthood. *Developmental Psychology, 46*(6), 1651–1661.

Kanel, K. (2007). *A guide to crisis intervention* (3rd ed.). Pacific Grove, CA: Brooks/Cole.

Lazarus, R. S. (1999). *Stress and emotion: A new synthesis*. New York: Springer.

Lee, C., Dolezalek, H., & Johnson, G. (2005). Top 10. *Training, 42*(3), 26–41.

Maslach, E., & Jackson, S. E. (1986). *Maslach burnout inventory: Manual* (2nd ed.). Palo Alto, CA: Consulting Psychologists Press.

McEwen, B. S. (1998). Protective and damaging effects of stress mediators. *New England Journal of Medicine, 338*, 171–179.

McGuire, P. A. (1999). More psychologists are finding that discrete uses of humor promote healing in their patients [Online]. *APA Monitor Online, 30*(3). Available at www.apa.org/monitor/mar99/humor.html

Mendoza, M. (2005, April). Breaking point. *Human Resources*, pp. 24–27.

Palazzoli, M. S., Cecchin, G., Prata, G., & Boscolo, L. (1978). *Paradox and counter paradox*. New York: Aronson.

Pines, A., & Maslach, C. (1978). Characteristics of staff burnout in mental health settings. *Hospital and Community Psychiatry, 29*, 223–233.

Russo, J. R. (1980). *Serving and surviving as a human-service worker.* Prospect Heights, IL: Waveland Press.

Selye H. (1976). *The stress of life* (rev. ed.). New York: McGraw-Hill.

Sparks, P. J., Simon, G. E., Katon, W. J., Altman, L., C., Ayars, G. H., & Johnson, R. L. (1990). An outbreak of illness among aerospace workers. *Western Journal of Medicine, 153,* 28.

Vettor, S. M., & Kosinski, F. A., Jr. (2000). Work-stress burnout in emergency medical technicians and the use of early recollections. *Journal of Employment Counseling, 37,* 216.

Chapter 11 Case Management

DeLeon, P. H., Uyeda, M. K., & Welch, B. L. (1985). Psychology and HMDS: New partner-ships or new adversary? *American Psychologist, 40*(10), 1122–1124.

The Global Community of Information Professionals. (2013). *What is case management.* Retrieved June 19, 2013, http://www.aiim.org/whaat-is-Case-Management

Herr, E. L., & Cramer, S. H. (1987). *Controversies in the mental health professions.* Muncie, IN: Accelerated Development.

Hollis, J. W., & Donn, P. A. (1980). *Psychological report writing theory and practice.* Muncie, IN: Accelerated Development.

Renata, R. (2013). *Human services case management definition.* Retrieved June 19, 2013, http://www.ehow.com/about_6726091_human-services-case-management-definition.html

State of New Jersey Department of Human Services Division of Developmental Disabilities. (2013). *Case management.* Retrieved June 19, 2013, http://www.state.nj.us/humanservices/ddd/services/case/

Tulkin, S. R., & Frank, G. W. (1985). The changing role of psychologists in health maintenance organizations. *American Psychologist, 40*(10), 1125–1136.

University of Davis Extension Center for Human Services. (2013). *Certificate program in human services case management.* Retrieved June 19, 2013, http://humanservices.ucdavis.edu/Custom/CAse/CAseMgmt/index.aspx

Chapter 12 Macro-level Practice

AB 593/AB 1593. *The Sin by Silence Bills.* Retrieved from http://legislation.sinbysilence.com/about-ab-593/facts

Alle-Corliss, L., & Alle-Corliss, R. (1999). *Advanced practice in human service agencies.* Pacific Grove, CA: Brooks/Cole.

Brueggemann, W. G. (1996). *The practice of macro social work.* Chicago: Nelson-Hall.

Haglund, B., Weisbrod, R. R., & Bracht, N. (1990). Assessing the community: Its services, needs, leadership and readiness. In N. Bracht (Ed.), *Health promotion at the community level* (pp. 91–108). Newbury Park, CA: Sage.

Hepworth, D. H., & Larsen, J. A. (1986). *Direct social work practice: Theory and skills.* Chicago, Illinois: Dorsey Press.

Hick, S. F., & McNutt, J. G. (2002). *Advocacy, activism, and the Internet.* Chicago: Lyceum Books.

Homan, M. S. (1994). *Promoting community change: Making it happen in the real world.* Pacific Grove, CA: Brooks/Cole.

Kirst-Ashman, K. K., & Hull, G. H., Jr. (1993). *Understanding generalist practice.* Chicago: Nelson Hall.

Lynam, D. R., Milich, R., Zimmerman, R., Novak, R., Logan, T. K., Martin, C., et al. (1999). Project DARE: No effects at 10-year follow-up. *Journal of Consulting and Clinical Psychology, 67,* 590–593.

Meenaghan, T. M., & Gibbons, W. E. (2000). *Generalist practice in larger settings.* Chicago: Lyceum Books, Inc.

Moskowitz, J. M. (1989). Preliminary guidelines for reporting outcome evaluation studies of health promotion and disease prevention programs. *New Directions for Program Evaluation, 43,* 101–112.

Netting, E. F., Kettner, P. M., & McMurtry, S. (1993). *Social work macro practice.* New York: Longman.

Richmond, M. E. (1917). *Social diagnosis.* New York: Russell Sage Foundation.

Royse, D., Thyer, B. A., & Padgett, D. K. (2010). *Program evaluation: An introduction.* Belmont, CA: Wadsworth.

U.S. Department of Education. (2010). *State and Local Implementation of the No Child Left Behind Act. Volume IX—accountability under NCLB: final report.* Retrieved from http://www2.ed.gov/rschstat/eval/disadv/nclb-accountability/nclb-accountability-final.pdf

Chapter 13 Leadership and Organizational Structure

Alle-Corliss, L., & Alle-Corliss, R. (1999). *Advanced practice in human service agencies.* Pacific Grove, CA: Brooks/Cole.

Blake, R. R., & Mouton, J. S. (1968). *Corporate excellence through grid organization development.* Houston, TX: Gulf Publishing.

Brueggemann, W. G. (1996). *The practice of macro social work.* Chicago: Nelson-Hall.

Etzioni, A. (1965). Dual leadership in complex organizations. *American Sociological Review, 30,* 5.

Guba, E. G., & Bridwell, C. E. (1957). *Administrative relationships.* Chicago: Midwest Administration Center, University of Chicago.

Homan, M. S. (1994). *Promoting community change: Making it happen in the real world.* Pacific Grove, CA: Brooks/Cole.

Kanel, K. (2007). *A guide to crisis intervention* (3rd ed.). Pacific Grove, CA: Brooks/Cole.

Kirst-Ashman, K. K., & Hull, G. H., Jr. (1993). *Understanding generalist practice.* Chicago: Nelson Hall.

Maxwell, A. D. (1973). Number numbness. *Liberal Education, 59*(3), 405–416.

McAdam, T. W. (1986). *Careers in the nonprofit sector: Doing well by doing good.* Farmington Hill, MI: Taft Group.

McGregor, D. (1960). *The human side of enterprise.* New York: McGraw-Hill.

Netting, E. F., Kettner, P. M., & McMurtry, S. (1993). *Social work macro practice.* New York: Longman.

Parson, T., Bales, R., & Shills, E. (1955). *Family socialization and interaction process.* Glencoe, IL: Free Press.

Russo, J. R. (1980). *Serving and surviving as a human service worker.* Prospect Heights, IL: Waveland Press.

Weinstein, B. (1994). *I'll work for free: A short-term strategy with a long-term payoff* [audio-cassette]. New York: Henry Holt.

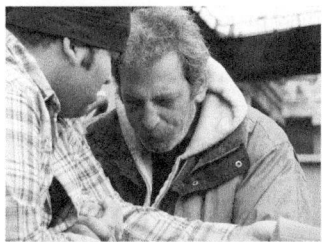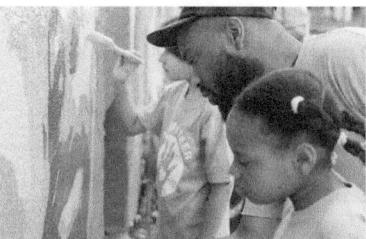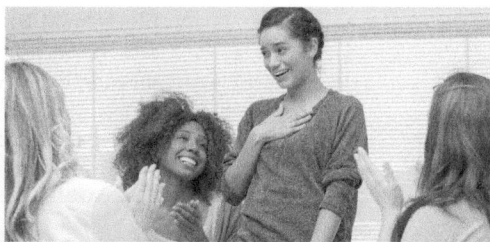

Appendix

HUMAN SERVICES CAREER INVENTORY

1. Do I want to deal directly with clients?

   _____

   _____

2. What types of clients do I want to work with?

   _____

   _____

3. If I don't want to work with clients directly, for what client population am I interested in providing indirect services?

   _____

   _____

4. What specific duties do I want to engage in at work? (Reread Chapter 4. You may select more than one, of course.)

   _____

   _____

5. Do I need to engage in some type of self-awareness process to do my job effectively? What areas do I need to develop or eliminate in order to provide service appropriately?

6. Do I want to work for a public or a nonprofit agency? Why?

7. Do I want to work at a residential or an outpatient facility?

8. Do I want to participate in lobbying and coalition building?

9. Do I want to write program proposals?

10. How much money do I need to make to live satisfactorily?

11. Are my career plans realistic for these financial desires?

12. How much education am I willing to obtain?

13. What are the realistic options for me at my educational attainment goal?

   _____

   _____

14. What am I going to do to ensure that I don't become burnt out as a human services worker?

   _____

   _____

15. Do I still want to go into the field of human services?

   _____

   _____

Good luck! Kristi Kanel

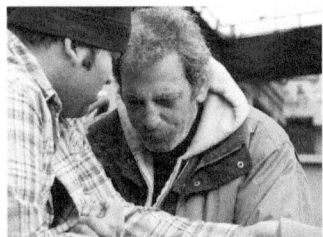
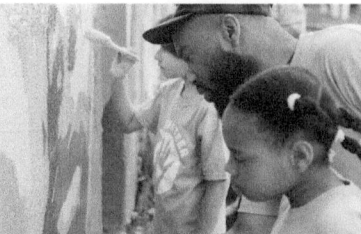
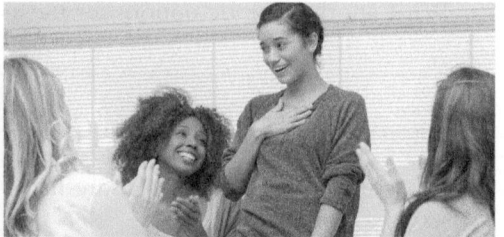

Name Index

A
Abudabbeh, N., 73
Addams, J., 17–18
Adler, A., 127–128, 130, 132
Al-Abdul-Jabbar, J., 73
Al-Issa, I., 73
Al-Krenawai, A., 73
Allard, S. W., 35
Alle-Corliss, L., 2, 39, 297, 311
Alle-Corliss, R., 2, 39, 297, 311
Allison, S. R., 74
Almeida, D. M., 247, 252
Altman, L., C., 250
Aristotle, 10, 11
Aseel, H. A., 73
Ashton, G., 43, 72
Asmussen, S., 157
Atkinson, D. R., 72
Ayars, G. H., 250

B
Bales, R., 313
Bateson, G., 133
Baughman, A., 229
Beck, A. T., 132
Benitez, B. R., 60, 62
Berenson, B., 117
Bergman, A., 126
Bevilacqua, J., 19
Bial, M., 182
Black, M. C., 224
Blake, R. R., 313

Bonnie, R, 177
Bono, C., 239
Bono, G., 195
Bordin, C. M., 164
Borntrager, C., 122
Boscolo, L., 257
Bowen, M., 133–134
Boyd, C., 157
Brenner, C., 123, 124, 126
Bridwell, C. E., 313
Brohl, K., 60
Brokovich, E., 304
Brueggemann, W. G., 294, 315, 317
Bugental, J. F. T., 117
Burroughts, T., 122
Bush, G., 32, 37

C
Canda, E., 74–75
Caplan, G., 19, 39, 114
Caplan, J., 258
Carkhuff, R., 117
Cecchin, G., 257
Chang, J., 248, 251
Char, W., 43, 72
Charles, S. T., 247
Chin, J. L., 44
Claver, Dobalian, Fickel, Ricci, & Mallers (2013), 153
Claver, Friedman, Dobalian, Ricci, & Horn Mallers (2012), 153
Clinton, B., 32, 34

Clodd, E., 10
Cole, C., 109, 115
Compayri, G., 15
Corey, G., 2, 116, 124, 126
Corey, M. S., 2
Cramer, S. H., 54, 274
Crow, J., 240
Cutler, D., 19

D
Darche (1990), 170
Davis, K. G., 17, 20
Day, J., 133
Day, S., 89
Deal, R. L., 167
Dean, D., 14
Degeneres, E., 239
DeLeon, P. H., 273
Diclemente, Ponton, & Hartley (1991), 170
Dix, D., 16–17, 304
Dolezalek, H., 258
Domenico, D. M., 172
Donn, P. A., 286
Drake, R. E., 121–122

E
El-Hai, J., 11
Ellis, A., 132, 254–255
Ellsberg, M., 229
Elwork, A., 60
Emery, G., 132

Epictetus, 254
Esterson, A., 133
Etzioni, A., 313
Exner, D., 229

F
Feigenbaum, J., 122
Ferguson, C. J., 230
Ferrero, G., 16
Finkelhor, Turner, Ormrod, Hamby, & Kracke, 2009, 226
Frank, G. W., 274
Freud, S., 16, 18, 123, 125–128
Freudenberger, H. J., 250
Froh, J. J., 195
Fromm, E., 127
Fry, W. F., 263

G
Gabbard, G. O., 126, 127, 151–152
Geller, J. L., 122
Gibb (1970), 116
Gibbons, W. E., 294
Glasser, W., 129–130
Gluckstern, N. B., 109
Goldman, L., 250, 259, 260
Gomez, J. S., 248
Gottemoeller, M., 229
Grant, B. F., 213
Grob, G., 16
Guba, E. G., 313
Guntrip, H., 123, 126

H
Haglund, Weisbrod, & Bracht (1990), 296
Hakim-Larson, J., 73
Haley, J., 133–134, 257
Hammitt, V. L., 238
Hare-Mustin, R. T., 70
Harper, R. F., 13
Hasin, D. S., 213
Heise, L., 229
Hepworth, D. H., 303
Herr, E. L., 54, 274
Hick, S. F., 295
Himes, C. L., 41
Hippocrates, 11, 12
Hirsch, S. H., 133

Hogan-Garcia, M., 41, 69–70
Hoge, C. W., 155
Hollingshead, G., 14
Hollis, J. W., 286
Homan, M. S., 295
Hooyman, N. R., 177
Horn, M. C., 252
Horney, K., 127
Horn Mallers, M., 247
Howard, A., 20
Howe, B. A., 164
Hsu, J., 43, 72
Hull, G. H., Jr., 294
Hutchins, D. E., 109, 115

I
Ivey, A. E., 109, 112

J
Jackson, D. D., 133
Jackson, S. E., 248, 250
Jefferson, T., 15
Johnson, G., 258
Johnson, L., 20
Johnson, R. L., 250
Jones, K. H., 172
Jones, M. L., 44

K
Kanel, K., 43, 113–115, 120, 145, 149, 151, 155, 156, 235, 237, 241, 251, 253
Kar, Kramer, Skinner, & Zambrana (1995), 43
Katon, W. J., 250
Katz, L. S., 232
Kazdin (2001), 83
Kennedy, D. H., 231–232
Kennedy, J. F., 19–20
Kettner, P. M., 296, 315
Kim, B. S. K., 43, 72
King, M. L., Jr., 22
Kirst-Ashman, K. K., 294
Kitfield, J., 231
Kiyak, H. A., 177
Knickerbocker, B., 239
Kosinski, F. A., Jr., 248, 249
Koss-Chioino, J. D., 43
Kraepelin, E., 16
Kramer, R. M., 4

L
Laing, R. D., 133
Larsen, J. A., 303
Lazarus, R. S., 247
Ledford, R., 60
Lee, C., 258
Levin, J., 44
Levine, D., 60
Lewis, J., 250, 259, 260
Li, L. C., 43, 72
Liang, C. T. H., 43, 72
Liebowitz et al., 1994, 43
Lindemann, E., 19
Lindy, J. D., 152
Linehan, M. M., 122
Locsin, A., 90, 92
Lombroso, C., 16
Loza, N., 73
Lynam, D. R., 301

M
MacDorman, M. F., 170
Madanes, C., 134
Magallon, T., 238
Mahler, M. S., 126
Mann, H., 15
Martin, J. A., 170
Maslach, C., 248
Maslach, E., 248, 250
Maslow, A., 2
Mattes, L. J., 74
Maxwell, A. D., 314
Mayerson, A., 201
McAdam, T. W., 316
McDermott, J., 43, 72
McEwen, B. S., 247
McFarland, B., 19
McGregor, D., 313
McGuire, P. A., 263–264
McMurtry, S., 296, 315
McNutt, J. G., 295
Meenaghan, T. M., 294
Meichenbaum, D., 132
Menacker, F., 170
Mendoza, M., 253
Michaelis, R. C., 248
Miles, S. H., 12
Minuchin, S., 134
Mommsen, T. E., 13
Moore, B. A., 231–232

Moskowitz, J. M., 302
Mouton, J. S., 313

N
Nader, R., 304
Nassar-McMillan, S. C., 73
Netting, E. F., 296, 315
Neukrug, E., 2
Neupert, S. D., 247
Newton (1988), 40
Nydell, M., 73

O
Obama, B., 34, 37, 240
Ogburn, E., 213
Okun, B., 109, 118
Omark, D. R., 74
Oquendo (1995), 43
Oswald, W. T., 197, 198

P
Padgett, D. K., 302
Palazzoli, M. S., 257
Parson, T., 313
Passel & Cohn (2011), 42
Pavlov, I. P., 131
Pierce, P. E., 231–232
Pine, F., 126
Pinel, P., 15
Pines, A., 248
Plato, 11
Plotkin, R. C., 164
Prata, G., 257
Price, Cowen, Lorion, & Ramos-McKay (1988), 39
Price, R. E., 238

Q
Queen Elizabeth of England, 10, 14

R
Rabrenovic, G., 44
Reagan, N., 217
Renata, R., 271

Rennison, C. M., 226
Repetti, R. L., 171
Richmond, M. E., 294
Rogers, C., 18, 112–113, 116
Roosevelt, F., 1, 20
Rosenthal, H., 8
Rothman, E. F., 229
Royse, D., 302
Rush, A., 132
Russo, J. R., 248, 249, 258, 312–313

S
Sales, B. D., 60
Satir, V., 134
Schading, B., 231
Schaefer (1988), 7, 8
Schechter et al. (2000), 43
Schiess, L., 155
Sears, Peplau, & Taylor (1991), 7
Seeman, T. E., 171
Selye, H., 247
Shapiro, F., 151
Shaw, B., 132
Shields, S. A., 70
Shills, E., 313
Siegel, M., 60
Simon, G. E., 250
Simpson, Pruitt, Blackwell, & Sweringen (1997), 169
Skinner, B. F., 130–131
Slader, S., 238
Slaikeu, K. A., 19
Smith (2002), 35
Snelling, C., 199
Socrates, 11
Somerville, J., 122
Sparks, P. J., 250
Spear, L. P., 169
Stinson, F. S., 213
Strachey, J., 123, 126
Sullivan, H. S., 127
Summers, M., 14

Swigar, M. E., 122
Swoboda, J. S., 60

T
Taylor, S. E., 171
Thyer, B. A., 302
Tseng, W., 43, 72
Tulkin, S. R., 274
Twentyman, C. T., 164
Tyckoff, I., 133
Tyndale, W., 13

U
Uba, L., 43, 72
Umemoto, D., 72
Uyeda, M. K., 273

V
Ventura, S. J., 170
Vettor, S. M., 248, 249
Vining, C. B., 74

W
Walker (1984), 225
Wallace, R., 177
Weakland, J., 133
Weiner, D. B., 15
Weinstein, B., 316–317
Welch, B. L., 273
Whitaker, C. A., 134
Whitlock, J., 170
Williamson, J. M., 164
Winfrey, Oprah, 36
Wolpe, J., 131
Wyman, S., 149
Wynne, L., 133

Y
Yalom, I. D., 127–130
Yarvis, J. S., 151, 155

Z
Zastrow, C., 8
Zylstra, S., 74

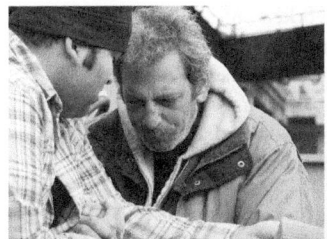
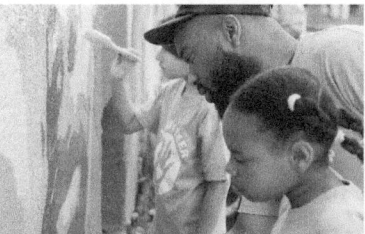
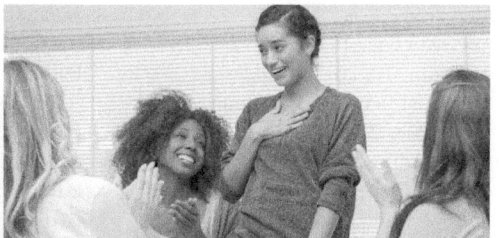

Subject Index

A

ABC model of crisis intervention, 145–146, 159
  basic attending skills, 145
  coping, 145–146
  identifying the problem, 145
Ableism, 8
Absenteeism, burnout and, 251
Abstinence, 213, 215, 216
ACBSW (Accredited Bachelor of Social Work), 91
Acceptance, 116
Accredited Bachelor of Social Work (ACBSW), 91
Acquired immunodeficiency syndrome (AIDS), 44, 85, 87, 234–239, 295
  causality models, 236
  definition of, 235, 244
  emergency situations and, 237–238
  facts and statistics, 235
  historical background, 234–235
  human services for, 237–239
  needs and issues, 236–237
  prevalence, 235
  primary prevention, 239
  secondary intervention and, 238
  tertiary intervention and, 238–239
Active listening, 111–112, 138
Activities of daily living (ADLs), 177
Acute conditions, 177, 186
Addams, Jane, 25, 1718

Addiction Equity Act, 32
ADHD (attention-deficit hyperactivity disorder), 207
Administration on Aging (AoA), 178
Administrators, 82
Adolescence, 169–176
  causality models, 171–172
  drug usage, 171
  gangs and delinquency, 169, 186
  pregnancy, 169–170
  prevalence, 169–171
  runaways, 170, 186
  self-mutilation, 170, 186
Adult Children of Alcoholics (ACA), 166
Adult protective services (APS), 32, 51, 180, 186
Advocacy
  community, 304
  defined, 294, 308
  legislative, 304
  and policy, 303–306
  self, 304
Advocates, responsibilities, 82, 84
African Americans, 73–74
  poverty rates for, 196
Ageism, 7–8
Agencies, defined, 311, 321
Age of reason, 14–16
Aggressive, 260, 266
Aggressive, *versus* assertive, 260–263

Aging adults, 176–182
  alcohol abuse, 178
  Alzheimer's disease, 179
  causality models, 179–180
  dementia, 180, 186
  elder mistreatment, 177–178, 186
  emergency situations, 180–181
  frail elderly, 179, 186
  human services, 180–182
  oldest-old, 177, 186
  old-old, 177, 186
  poverty, 178–179
  prevalence, 177
  primary prevention, 181–182
  secondary intervention, 181
  tertiary intervention, 181
  young-old, 177, 186
AIDS. *See* Acquired immunodeficiency syndrome (AIDS)
AIDS-related complex (ARC), 238, 243
Alcohol abuse, 178
  aging adults, 178
Alcoholics Anonymous (AA), 216
Allostatic load, 247, 266
America, graying of, 41–42
American Red Cross, 312, 319, 321
Americans with Disabilities Act (1990), 203, 220
America's Law Enforcement and Mental Health Project, 35
Anaheim Free Clinic, 21

Anal stage, 125
Ancient civilizations, 11–12
Animism, 10, 25
Antisocial personality disorder, 207, 208, 220
Anxiety disorders, 191, 220
APALC (Asian Pacific American League Center), 45
APS (Adult Protective Services), 32, 51
Arab Americans, 73
ARC (AIDS-related complex), 238, 243
Asian American counselors, 72
Asian Pacific American League Center (APALC), 45
ASPE (Assistant Secretary for Planning and Evaluation), 42
Assertive, 260, 266
Assertive community treatment (ACT), 121
Assertive, *versus* aggressive, 260–263
Assessment, defined, 275, 289
Assistants, 82
Assistant Secretary for Planning and Evaluation (ASPE), 42
Associate's degree of arts (an A.A.), 89
Associate's degree of science (an A.S.), 89
Associate's degrees, human services workers and, 89–90
Ataque de nervios, 43
At-risk adolescents
 emergency situations and, 172–173
 primary prevention and, 175
 secondary intervention and, 173–174
 tertiary intervention and, 174–175
Attention-deficit hyperactivity disorder (ADHD), 204, 207, 220
Autistic stage, 126
Autonomy, 171, 186

B
Baby boomers, 41, 51
Bachelor of arts (BA), 90
Bachelor of science (BS), 90
Bachelor of social work degree (BSW), 91
Bachelor's degrees, human services workers and, 90–91

Basic Attending Skills (Ivey, Gluckstern, and Ivey), 109
Battered woman's shelters, 226–227, 243, 281
Battered woman's syndrome, 225–226, 243
Battering cycle, 228, 243
Bedlam, 14, 25
Behavioral approaches, 130–132
Behavioral deterioration
 burnout and, 250
Behavioral theories, 130–132, 138
Behavior changer, 83–84
Behavior change specialists, 83, 103
Being in the closet, 71, 76
Benefit theory, 45
Bethlem Royal Hospital, 14
Bias, 6
Biopsychosocial model, 8, 25
Bipolar disorder, 191, 194, 207, 216, 220
Birth-control, 21, 66, 88, 98
Bisexual, defined, 240
Blaming, 255, 261–263
Board-and-care homes, 277, 289
Board of directors, 317, 321
Body mass index (BMI), 168
Borderline personality disorders (BPD), 121
Brokers, 85
BSW (Bachelor of social work degree), 91
Burnout
 cognitive symptoms, 250
 defined, 246, 248–249, 266
 emotional symptoms, 250
 impact of, 249–252
 managing, 252–264
 physical symptoms of, 250

C
Caplan, Gerald, 19, 25
Caregivers, 85
Caring professionalism, 120, 138
Carl Rogers on Encounter Groups (Rogers), 129
Carl Rogers's approach, 129
Case management, 270–288
 defined, 270–271
Case plans, 282, 289

Caseworkers, 85
Causality models
 criminal behavior and, 207
 disabilities, 202
 mental disorders and, 191–193
 mental illness and, 191–193
 poverty and, 197–199
 substance abuse, 213–214
Causality, psychological models of, 135–136
Centenarian, 177, 186
Chain of command, 315, 321
Changing behaviors, focus on, 84
Child abuse, 164–167
 emergency situations and interventions, 164–165
 and neglect, 162, 163, 186
 play therapy, 165
 primary prevention, 166–167
 secondary intervention, 165
 tertiary intervention, 165–166
Child Abuse Prevention and Treatment Act (CAPTA), 33, 61, 162
Childhood obesity, 168, 186
Child maltreatment, 162–163
 causality models, 163–164
 prevalence, 163
Child protective services (CPS), 32, 51, 164, 174, 186, 279–280
Child protective workers, 85
Children, 162–168
 causality models, 163–164
 childhood obesity, 168, 186
 child maltreatment, 162–163
 counseling for, 165
 familial divorce, 167
 remarriage, 167
Chronically poor, 200, 220
Chronic condition, 177, 186
Chronic problems, 40, 51
Civil rights movement, 22, 25
Classical conditioning, 130, 131, 138
Classism, 8
Clients, human services, 2, 25
 as key term, 5–8
 with multiple needs, 5
Clinical depression, 170, 186
Closet, being in, 71

SUBJECT INDEX

Closet gay, defined, 240
Coalitions, 294, 296–297, 303, 304, 308
Cocaine Anonymous (CA), 216
Code of Hammurabi, 13, 25
Codes of Ethics, human services and, 55–56
Cognitive behavioral therapy (CBT), 171, 254
Cognitive restructuring, 257, 266
Cognitive symptoms, burnout and, 250
Cognitive theory, 132–133, 138
  distortions, 132
Cognitive therapy, 19
Communication
  effective skills and, 111–115
  goals of, 109–110
  improving, 259–263
Community advocacy, 304
Community Mental Health Centers Act (1963), 19–20, 25, 32, 51
Community organizing, 294, 308
Comorbidity, 191, 220
Compassionate communication, 116, 138
Competence, ethics and, 68–69
Concreteness, 117
Conditioned response, 124, 131, 138
Conditioned stimulus, 131, 138
Confidentiality, 55, 60–62, 76
  exceptions to, 61–62
Congruence, 116, 138
Conservators, 95, 103
Consultants, 85–86
Continuing education, ethical competence and, 60, 68–69
Correctional facilities
  bachelor's degrees, 100
  doctoral degrees, 100
  master's degrees, 100
  modern, 83, 100
  two-year degrees, 100
Correctional system, modern, 35–36
Council of Standards in Human Service Education (CSHSE), 56
  standards of, 57
Counseling, theoretical approaches to, 121–134

County behavioral health services, 32
County of Orange Mental Health Services, 316
CPS (Child Protective Services), 32, 51
Crime, 35
Crime perpetrator, 206–210
  causality models of, 207
  emergency situations and, 208
  historical background, 206
  human services delivery for, 208–210
  needs and issues, 207–208
  primary prevention and, 210
  secondary intervention and, 208–209
  tertiary intervention and, 209–210
Crisis intervention, 19, 25, 40, 51, 144–146
  ABC model of, 145–146
  defined, 144, 159
Crisis workers, 86
Critical and irrational thoughts, 257–258
Critical incident debriefing, 152, 159
CSHSE (Council of Standards in Human Service Education), 56
Cultural bias, 69, 76
Culture, defined, 41, 51, 69–70
Cycle of poverty, 198–199, 220
Cyclically poor, 200, 220

D

Daily living activities (ADLs), 177, 186
Dancing with the Stars, 239
D.A.R.E. (Drug Awareness Resistance Education), 40, 217–218, 301
Data managers, 82, 103
Deinstitutionalization of the mentally ill, 19, 25
Delirium, 191, 220
Delusional disorders, 191, 220
Dementia, 180, 186, 191, 220
Demographic shifts, 41–45
Denial, 124, 138
Department of Health and Human Services (DHHS), 33
Department of Human Services establishment of, 1

Department of Justice (DOJ), 35
Department of Probation, 35
Depression, 145, 146, 151, 155–157
Deserving poor, 198, 220
Determination, 148, 159
Developed sense of well-being, 117–118, 138
DHHS (Department of Health and Human Services), 33
Diagnostic and Statistical Manual of Mental Disorders (DSM-V), 191, 211, 220
Diagnostic and Statistical Manuel of Mental Disorders (DSM-IV), 150
Differentiate, 171, 186
Disabilities, 201–205
  causality models, 202
  definition of, 201
  historical background, 201
  human services to, 202–205
  prevalence, 202
Disabled persons
  emergency situations and, 202–203
  human services to, 202–205
  primary prevention and, 205
  secondary intervention and, 203–204
  tertiary intervention and, 204–205
Disasters, 152–154
Discrimination, 7, 69, 71
Disengaged, 193, 221
Disillusionment, or Recoil and Rescue, phase, 154
Disparity, 6–7, 25
Disparity, notion of, 20
Displacement, 124, 138
Disputation, 256, 266
Distress, 247, 266
Diversion program, 84, 209, 221
Dix, Dorothea, 16, 25
Dizziness, burnout and, 250
Doctoral degrees, human services workers and, 93
Doctor of philosophy (PhD), 93
Doctor of psychology (PsyD), 93
Doctor of social work (DSW), 93
DOJ (Department of Justice), 35

Domestic violence
    emergency situations and, 226–227
    feminist view of, 226
    primary prevention and, 229
    secondary intervention and, 227–228
    statistics and facts, 225
    tertiary intervention and, 228–229
    women, 224–225
Don't Ask Don't Tell policy, 240
Drug Awareness Resistance Education (D.A.R.E.), 40, 217–218, 301
Drug prevention programs, 175
DSM-IV (Diagnostic and Statistical Manual of Mental Disorders), 150
Dual relationships
    defined, 62, 77
    examples of, 63–64
    reasons to avoid, 63
Duty to warn, 61, 77
Dyslexia, 204

E
EADACPA (Elder Abuse and Dependent Adult Civil Protection Act), 61
Early christianity, 12–14
Eating disorders, 193, 221
Eclectic approach, 1, 25
Economic Opportunity Act (1964), 20
Educational groups, 275
Educational reform, 22
Educational system, modern, 36–37
Educators, 87
Effective Helping (Okun), 109
Ego, 123, 138
Ego defense mechanisms, 123, 138
Elder Abuse and Dependent Adult Civil Protection Act (EADACPA), 61
Elder Justice Act, 61, 178
Elder mistreatment, 177–178, 186
Electric shock therapy, 93
Electroconvulsive therapy, 93
Elizabethan Poor Laws, 10, 14, 25
Elmira Reformatory, 18, 25
EMDR (Eye movement desensitization and reprocessing), 151, 159, 232, 243

Emergency situations
    aging adults, 180–181
    AIDS clients and, 237–238
    at-risk adolescents and, 172–173
    child abuse, 164–165
    crime perpetrator and, 208
    disabled persons and, 202–203
    domestic violence and, 226–227
    mental illness and, 193–194
    poverty and, 199
    sexual assault and, 232–233
    substance abuse and, 214
    violence perpetrator and, 208
Emotional abuse, 163, 178
Emotional symptoms, burnout and, 250
Emotions, reflecting, 113–114
Empathy, 111, 117, 138
Enmeshed, 193, 221
Ethics
    defined, 54, 77
    necessity of, 55–60
Ethnic disparity, 182, 186
Ethnicity, 71–74
Ethnic/racial considerations, 42–43
Ethnocentrism, 8
Ethnoracial, 42, 51
European American counselors, 72
Eustress, 247, 266
Evaluation, 294, 308, 314
Evaluation, program and policies, 301–303
Evaluators, 86
Evidence-based practice, 121–123
Existential humanistic counseling approach, 117
Existential-humanistic theory, 128–130
Existential Psychotherapy (Yalom), 129
Expressive leadership style, 313, 322
Eye movement desensitization and reprocessing (EMDR), 151, 159, 232, 243

F
Family therapy, 133–134, 274
Fatigue, burnout and, 250
Federal Short-Doyle Act, 32
Feedback, 114–115, 138
Feminists, 226, 244

Fight-or-flight, 250
Fixated stage, 125, 138
Flexibility, 118–119, 138
Formative evaluation, 301–302, 308
Frail elderly, 179, 186
Freud, Sigmund, 16, 25
Funding announcements, 297, 308
Fundraisers, 87
Fundraising, 297, 308

G
Gallows, 13
Gangs, 169, 186
Gay community, 71
Gay, defined, 240
Gay, lesbian, bisexual, transgender (GLBT), 71
Gender, 70
Generalist human services model, 2, 26
Generalist model, 8
Genital stage, 126
Genuineness, 116, 138
Gestalt therapy, 19
Givens, 129, 138
GLBT (Gay, lesbian, bisexual, transgender), 71
Grants, 294, 308, 317–320, 322
Grant writers, 87
Grassroots movements, 20, 26
Great Depression, 317
Group therapy, 129, 138

H
Harm reduction models, 40–41, 52
Headaches, burnout and, 250
Health and Safety Executive in the United Kingdom, The (Goldman and Lewis), 259
Health Insurance Portability and Accountability Act (HIPAA), 60, 77
Health Maintenance Organization Act (1973), 273
Health maintenance organizations (HMOs), 4, 33, 52, 273–275, 289
Heart palpitations, burnout and, 250
Helping Relationships and Strategies (Hutchins and Cole), 109

Heritage House, 318
Heroic or impact, phase, 153–154
Heteronormativity, 239, 244
Heterosexism, 8, 71, 240
Hierarchy, 315
High blood pressure, burnout and, 250
High school diplomas, human services workers and, 88–89
HIPAA (Health Insurance Portability and Accountability Act), 60, 77
Hippocrates, 11, 26
Hispanics, poverty rates for, 196
HIV. *See* Human immunodeficiency virus (HIV)
HMOs (health maintenance organizations), 4, 33, 52, 273–275, 289
Holistic approach, 1, 26
Homeless youth. *See* Runaways
Homeostasis, 247, 266
Homophobia, 71, 240
Homosexuality, 71
Honeymoon, or immediate post-disaster, phase, 154
Houston Chronicle, 90
Hull House, 17, 18, 26
Human immunodeficiency virus (HIV), 44, 85, 87, 234–239, 295
  casuality models, 236
  definition of, 235, 244
  emergency situations and, 237–238
  facts and statistics, 235
  historical background, 234–235
  HIV clients, 239
  human services for, 237–239
  needs and issues, 236–237
  prevalence, 235
  secondary intervention and, 238
Human relations model, 317, 322
Human service agencies, types of, 314–319
Human services
  to aging adults, 180–182
  careers in, 9
  defined, 2, 26
  delivery in child abuse situations, 164–167
  historical background, 1–22
  interaction with aging adults, 182
  key terms in, 5–8
  master-level careers in, 92–93
  modern, 16–18
  populations, 162–183
  20th century, 18–22
Human services agencies
  administration in, 83
  characteristics of, 312–314
Human services professionals
  ethical standards for, 58
  responsibility towards colleagues, 59
  responsibility towards community, 56, 58–59
  responsibility towards profession, 59
Human service workers
  defined, 2, 26
  educational requirements of, 88–94
  job functions of, 82–88
  personal characteristics of, 116
  as professionals, 2
  true stories, 83, 84, 89, 91, 98, 99, 152
Humours, 12, 26
  maintaining sense of, 263–264
Hurricane Katrina, 40, 152
Hurricane Sandy, 152
Hypersomnia, 156

I
Iceberg effect of elder abuse, 178, 186
Id, 123, 138
Immigration, 42
Incest Survivors Anonymous (ISA), 166
Indigent, 199, 221
Individual counseling, 271–272
Individual psychology, 128, 138
Individual therapy, 275
Initiative, 296, 308
Inpatient treatment, 277, 289
Insight, 128, 138
Insomnia, 156
Instrumental activities of daily living (IADLs), 177, 186
Instrumental leadership style, 313, 322
Intake, defined, 278, 289
Intake process, 278–282, 289
Intake workers, 278, 281
Intellectualization, 124, 139
Interns, 3–4, 26
Interpersonal communication, 259–263
Interpersonal partner abuse, 224–229
  prevalence, 225
Interpersonal therapy (IPT), 171
Invisible wounds, 155, 159
Involuntary hospitalization, 149–150, 159
Irrational and self-defeating thoughts, 254, 255, 266
Irvin Yalom's model, 129

J
John 8:7, 13
Joint custody, 167
Juvenile delinquents, 169, 186

K
Keeping Children and Families Safe Act, 61
Key terms, 5–8
King, Martin Luther Jr., 22, 26
Knowledgeable, 119–120
Kraepelin, Emil, 16, 26

L
Latent stage, 126
Latino Legal Voice for Civil Rights, 45
Laziness, poverty and, 197–198
Leadership styles, 313
Learned helplessness, 197, 207, 221
Leeching, 12
Legislative advocacy, 304
Lesbian community, 71
Lesbian, defined, 240
Lesbian, gay, bisexual, transgender (LGBT), 170, 239–242
Lesbian, gay, bisexual, transgender, queer, and intersexed (LGBTQI), 43

Letting, 12
LGBT (Lesbian, Gay, Bisexual, transgender), 170, 239–242
  elders, 241
  general issues by, 241
  intervention with, 242
  issues faced by, 241
  older people, 241
  people of color, 241
LGBTQI (Lesbian, gay, bisexual, transgender, queer, and intersexed), 43
Libido, 123, 139
Licensed professional counselor (LPC), 92
Lifestyle, maintaining healthy, 258–259
Lindemann, Eric, 19, 26
Line staff, 314–315, 322
Lobbying, 294, 296–297, 303, 308, 311
Lobotomy, 11, 26. *See also* Electric shock therapy
Lombroso, Cesare, 16, 26
Low birth-weight babies, 170, 186

M

Macro level, 275–278, 278–282, 289
Macro-level interventions, 39, 52
Macro-level practice
  advocacy and policy, 303–306
  defined, 294, 308
  developing program and policies, 295–301
  evaluating program and policies, 301–303
Macro-level practitioner, 294–296
Major depressive disorder, 191, 221
Malleus Maleficarum (book), 14
Managed care, 19, 26
Mandatory reporting standards, 61, 77
Manmade disasters, 152, 153–154, 159
Mann, Horace, 15, 26
Marianisma, 43
Master-level therapists, 81
Master of arts (MA), 92
Master of science (MS), 92
Master of social work (MSW), 92
Master's degrees, human services workers and, 92–93

Means, of suicide, 146, 148, 159
Medicaid, 34, 52
Medi-Cal, 316
Medical degrees, human services workers and, 93–94
Medical detoxification, 216, 221
Medicare, 34, 52
Medication, 272, 289
Mental disorders
  categories of, 192
  definition of, 191
  prevalence of, 191
Mental health agencies, 96–99, 103
  bachelor's degrees, 97
  doctoral degrees, 99
  master's degrees, 97–99
  two-year degrees, 96–97
Mental health agencies, modern-day, 32–34
Mental health, development in, 18–19
Mental Health Parity Act (1996), 32
Mental illness, 190–195
  emergency situations and, 193–194
  historical background, 190
  human services delivery for, 193–195
  needs and issues, 193
  primary prevention and, 194
  secondary intervention and, 194
  tertiary intervention and, 194
Mental retardation, 201, 204
Mezzo level, 272–275, 289
Mezzo-level interventions, 39, 52
Micro level, 271–272, 289
Micro-level interventions, 39, 52
Middle ages, 12–14
Military sexual trauma (MST), 232, 244
  intervention for, 232
Military trauma, 154–158
Minimal encouragers, 112, 139
Minimization, 124, 139
Model, human services
  defined, 2, 26
  as key term, 5
Modern Family, 239
Morale, 249, 253
MSW (Master of social work), 92
Multicultural competence, 69–75

Multicultural programs and policies, 43–44
Multicultural violence prevention program, 45
Multidisciplinary team approach, 6, 26
Multineeds clients, 5, 26

N

NAMI (National Alliance for the Mentally Ill), 32
Narcissistic personality disorders, 207, 221
Narcotics Anonymous (NA), 216
National Alliance for the Mentally Ill (NAMI), 32
National Association of Human Services, 56–60
National Association of Social Work (NASW), 91
National Institutes on Aging, 41
National Organization for Women (NOW), 312
National Organization of Human Services (NOHS), 56
Native Americans, 74
Natural disasters, 152, 159
Nausea, burnout and, 250
Needs assessments, 294, 296, 308
Negative reinforcement, 131, 139
Neo-Freudians, 127–128, 139
Neutral stimulus, 131, 139
New Deal, 20, 26, 317
New Freedom Commission on Mental Health, 32
New Freedom Initiative, 32
No Child Left Behind Act, 306
NOHS (National Organization of Human Services), 56
Nonprofit agencies, 4, 26, 315–319
Nonprofit agencies that deal with correctional issues, 38
Nonprofit educational programs, 38
Nonprofit mental health agencies, 38
Nonprofits, 37–38
Nonprofit social welfare agencies, 38
Normal (infantile) autism, 126, 139
Norms, 312–313
No-suicide contract, 148, 159
Number numbness, 312, 314, 322

O

Object, 126, 139
Object-relations theory, 126–127, 139
Obsessive compulsive disorder, 191, 194, 221
Occupational Outlook Handbook (2013), 90
Occupational therapist, 88
Office of Juvenile Justice and Delinquency Prevention (OJJDP), 35
Office on Violence Against Women (OVW), 299
OJJDP (Office of Juvenile Justice and Delinquency Prevention (OJJDP), 35
Older Americans Act, 178
Oldest-old, 177, 186
Old-old, 177, 186
Ombudsman, 95, 104
On Becoming a Person (Rogers), 129
Open-ended questions, 114, 139
Openness, 114, 119, 139
Operant conditioning, 130–131, 139
Operation Enduring Freedom (OEF), 155, 231, 244
Operation Iraqi Freedom (OIF), 154, 155, 231, 244
Oral stage, 125
Organization, 311, 322
Organizational culture, 69, 77
Outcome evaluation, 302, 308
Outpatient treatment, 281–282, 289
Outreach workers, 87–88

P

Panic disorder, 191, 221
Paraphrasing, 113, 139
Paraprofessionals, 2–3, 26
Parasuicide, 170, 186
Parents, counseling for, 165
Partial hospitalization, daycare, or day-treatment, 276, 290
Passive, 260–263, 266
Patient Protection and Affordable Care Act, 34, 52, 61
Patriot Act (2001), 62, 77
Pedophiles, 164, 207, 221
Peer pressure, 171, 172
Persian Gulf syndrome, 156
Personality disorders, 126, 139, 191, 221
Personal Responsibility and Work Opportunity Reconciliation Act (PRWORA), 34, 200, 221
Person-centered model, 129, 139
Person-in-environment perspective, 304, 309
Pervasive developmental disorder, 191, 221
PET (psychiatric emergency team), 150
Pete Domenici Mental Health Parity, 32
Phenomenological, 128, 139
Phobias, 193, 221
Physical abuse, 162, 163, 178
Pinel, Philippe, 15, 26
Planning, treatment, 282–283
Plan, suicide, 146, 147, 159
Play therapy, children, 165
Policy
  and advocacy, 303–306
  defined, 294, 309
  developing, 295–297
  evaluating, 301–303
Policy-making process., 305
Policy practice, 304, 305
Politics, 44, 52
Positive regard, 117
Positive reinforcement, 131, 139
Post-traumatic stress disorder (PTSD), 150–152, 159, 191, 232, 234
  group therapy, 151
  interventions for, 151–152
  military service, 155–156
  research study of, 156–157
  symptoms of, 151
  veterans, 155–157
Poverty
  aging adults, 178–179
  defined, 195–196, 221
  emergency situations and, 199
  prevalence of, 196–197
  primary prevenion and, 200–201
  secondary intervention and, 199–200
  tertiary interventions and, 200
Precipitating event, 256, 266
Pregnancy, 169–170
Prehistoric humans, 10–11
Prejudice, 7
Prevention and Elder Abuse, Neglect, and Exploitation Program, 178
Primary intervention, defined, 39–40, 52
Primary prevention
  aging adults, 181–182
  AIDS clients and, 239
  at-risk adolescents and, 175
  child abuse and, 166–167
  crime perpetrator and, 210
  disabled persons and, 205
  domestic violence and, 229
  mental illness and, 194
  poverty and, 200–201
  substance abuse and, 217–218
  violence perpetrator and, 210
Prison pet partnership, 210
Prison reform, 20–22
Privacy, 60
Private agencies, 4–5, 26
Privilege, 60, 77. *See also* Confidentiality
Process evaluation, 302, 309
Professional, human service worker, 2, 26
Prognosis, 40, 287, 290
Progress notes, 283–286, 290
  SOAP method, 285–286, 290
Project Head Start, 40
Projection, 124, 139
Proposals, writing, 294, 309
Protestant-based culture
  psychoanalytic approach, 18
  psychoanalytic surgery, 16
PRWORA (Personal Responsibility and Work Opportunity Reconciliation Act), 34, 200, 221
Psychiatric emergency team (PET), 194, 221
Psychoanalysis, 123–126
Psychoanalytic theories, 16, 26, 123, 139
Psychosexual stages, 125, 139
Psychosurgery, 11, 26
Psychotherapists, 88
PTSD (Post-traumatic stress disorder), 150–152, 159, 191, 232, 234
Public agencies, 4, 27, 314–315

Q
Queer, defined, 240
Questions, open-ended, 114

R
Racism, 7
Rationalization, 124, 139
Reaction formation, 124, 139
Reality therapy, 19, 129–130, 139
Reason and Emotion in Psychotherapy (Ellis), 132
Reciprocal inhibition, 131, 139
Reconstruction and Recovery phase, 154
Recreational therapist, 88
Recruiter.com, 91
Red Ribbon Week, 175, 217–218
Reflecting emotions, 113–114
Reflection, 113, 140
Reform, educational, 22
Regional centers, 202, 221
Regression, 124, 140
Religion, issues surrounding, 74–75
Renaissance, 14
Reports, defined, 286, 290
Report writing, 286–288
Repression, 123, 140
Request for application (RFA), 297
Request for proposals (RFP), 297
Residential facilities, 40, 277, 290
Resourceful, 119–120, 140
Respect, 117
Response cost, 131, 140
Roe *vs.* Wade, 21
Runaways, 170, 186

S
Salary, nonprofit agencies and, 316–317
Salary Wizard (2013), 90
Salem witch trials, 15
SAMHSA (Substance Abuse and Mental Health Services Administration), 33
Sandy Hook Elementary School, shooting, 153
Saving Private Ryan, 155
Scared Straight program, 40, 210
Schizophrenia, 32, 191, 221
School violence, 176
Science and Human Behavior (Skinner), 130
Secondary interventions, 275, 290
 aging adults, 181
 AIDS clients and, 238
 at-risk adolescents and, 173–174
 child abuse and, 165
 crime perpetrator and, 208–209
 defined, 40, 52
 disabled persons and, 203–204
 domestic violence and, 227–228
 mental illness and, 194
 poverty and, 199–200
 sexual assault and, 233
 substance abuse and, 214–216
 violence perpetrator and, 208–209
Self advocacy, 304
Self-awareness, 65, 77, 118, 140
 benefits of, 67
Self-critical thoughts, 254–255, 266
Self-criticism, 255
Self-defeating thoughts, 255, 266
Self-examination, 59, 64, 65, 67, 77
Self-mutilation, 170, 186
Self-preservation, 120–121, 140
Self-regulating mechanism, 133, 140
Senescence, 177, 186
Sense of humor, maintaining, 263–264
Separation/individuation, 127, 140
September 11, 2001, 40, 153, 154
Sexism, 7
Sexual abuse, 163, 164, 165, 171, 178, 179
Sexual assault, 229–234
 emergency situations and, 232–233
 military, 231–232
 prevalence, 229–231
 secondary intervention and, 233
 tertiary intervention and, 234
Sexual Assault Victim Services, 318
Sexually transmitted diseases (STDs), 239
Sexually transmitted infections (STIs), 169, 186
Sexual orientation, 71
Shadow organization, 312, 313, 322
Sin by Silence Bill, 305
Single women, poverty rates for, 196
SOAP method, progress reports and, 285–286, 290
Social action, 294, 309
Social deterioration, burnout and, 250
Social disorganization theory, 45
Social values, 44, 52
Social welfare agencies, 94–96
 bachelor's degrees, 95–96
 doctoral degrees, 96
 master's degrees, 96
 two-year degrees, 94–95
Social welfare development, 20
Social welfare programs, modern, 34–35
Socioeconomic classes, 20
Sociological theories, 44, 52
Southern Regional Education Board (SREB), 82
Specialized education programs, 100–101
 bachelor's degrees, 101
 doctoral degrees, 101
 master's degrees, 101
 two-year degrees, 100–101
Spiritual Aspects of Social Work Practice (Study), 74
Split custody, 167
SREB (Southern Regional Education Board), 82
Stakeholders, 305, 309
Status quo, 313
Stereotypes, 7
Stigma, 69, 77
Stocks, 13
Stoning, 13
Strain theory, 45
Stress
 blaming, 255
 cognitive symptoms, 250
 defined, 246–248, 266
 emotional symptoms, 250
 four-pronged aproach to managing, 253–254
 impact of, 249–252
 managing, 252–264
 physical symptoms of, 250
 work environment and, 253

Stress management, 246–264
  defined, 247, 266
Sublimation, 124, 140
Substance abuse
  causality models, 213–214
  defined, 211–213, 221
  emergency situations and, 214
  historical background, 211
  human service delivery for, 214–218
  needs and issues, 214
  primary prevention and, 217–218
  secondary intervention and, 214–216
  tertiary intervention and, 216–217
Substance Abuse and Mental Health Services Administration (SAMHSA), 33
Substance dependence, 211, 221
Suicidal ideation, 148, 159, 170, 186
Suicide
  assessment, 146
  determination, 148
  involuntary hospitalization, 149–150
  means of, 146, 148, 159
  no-suicide contract, 148
  plan, 146, 147
  prevention, 146–150
  risk, 146, 159
  suicidal ideation, 148
  voluntary hospitalization, 149–150
Suicide assessment
  defined, 146, 159
  stages used in, 146–149
Suicide hotlines, 278–279
Suicide prevention, 146–150
Suicide risk, 146, 159
Superego, 123, 140
Supervisors, work environment and, 253
Supplemental Nutrition Assistance Program (SNAP), 200
Supplemental Security Income (SSI) program, 200
Support groups, 145, 159, 273, 275, 290
Symbiosis, 126–127, 140

T
Tardiness, burnout and, 251
TBI (Traumatic brain injury), 155, 157, 159
Temporary restraining orders, 227, 244
Tertiary intervention
  aging adults, 181
  AIDS clients and, 238–239
  at-risk adolescents and, 174–175
  child abuse and, 165–166
  crime perpetrator and, 209–210
  defined, 40, 52
  disabled persons and, 204–205
  domestic violence and, 228–229
  mental illness and, 194
  poverty and, 200
  sexual assault and, 234
  substance abuse and, 216–217
  violence perpetrator and, 209–210
Tertiary interventions, 275, 290
Thanatos, 123, 140
Theory and Practice of Group Psychotherapy, The (Yalom), 129
Therapeutic community (TC), 216, 222
Therapists, 88
Therapists, master's level, 81
Thorazine, 19
Transference, 64, 77
Transgender, 71, 240
Transphobia, 239, 244
Trauma response, 152
Traumatic brain injury (TBI), 155, 159
  intervention for, 157
  symptoms of, 157
Traumatic community disorder, 152–154
Trepanning, 10, 11, 27
Trephining, 11, 27
Tribal communities, 74
Twelve-step facilitation (TSF), 215, 222
Twelve-step programs, 272–273, 290

U
Ulcers, burnout and, 250
Unconditional positive regard, 116–117, 140
Unconditioned response, 131, 140
Unconditioned stimulus, 131, 140
Unconscious, 123, 140
UNICEF (United Nations Children's Fund), 34
Unintended pregnancy, 169, 186
United Nations Children's Fund (UNICEF), 34
United Way, 312, 319

V
Values, 65–67
  clarification, 65
  examples of self-monitoring, 66
Verbal following, 112–113, 140
Veterans, 153, 155
  interventions for, 157–158
  PTSD and, 155–157
  research study of, 156–157
Veterans Administration (VA), 153
Vietnam War, 155
Violence, 44–45
Violence, against women, 45
Violence Against Women Act (2000), 298
Violence perpetrator, 206–210
  causality models of, 207
  emergency situations and, 208
  historical background, 206
  human services delivery for, 208–210
  needs and issues, 207–208
  primary prevention and, 210
  secondary intervention and, 208–209
  tertiary intervention and, 209–210
Virginia Tech University, shooting, 153
Voluntary hospitalization, 149–150, 159
Volunteers, 3–4, 27

W
Walden Two (Skinner), 130
War on Poverty, 20, 27
Welfare Reform Act (1996), 200
Well-being, 117–118
Wellesley Project, 19
Whistle-blowing, 313, 322

White paper, 305, 309
WHO (World Health Organization), 33
Witch trials, 15
Women
    and domestic violence, 224–225
    violence against, 45
Women, Infant, and Children (WIC) program, 200
Work environment
    coworkers and, 253
    stress and, 253
    supervisors and, 253
Work performance, burnout and, 251–252

World Health Organization (WHO), 33
World Trade Center attacks, 153
World War II, veterans of, 155
Writing Grants, 294, 297, 301

Y
Young-old, 177, 186